Handhelds in Medicine

Handhelds in Medicine
A Practical Guide for Clinicians

Scott M. Strayer, MD, MPH

Assistant Professor, Department of Family Medicine,
UVA Health System, University of Virginia School of Medicine,
Charlottesville, Virginia

Peter L. Reynolds, MD

Major, United States Air Force, Staff Family Physician, United States
Medical Clinic, Geilenkirchen, Germany

Mark H. Ebell, MD, MS

Associate Professor, Department of Family Medicine, Michigan State
University, East Lansing, Michigan

Editors

With 633 Illustrations and a CD-Rom

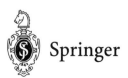

Springer

Scott M. Strayer, MD, MPH
Assistant Professor
Department of Family Medicine
UVA Health System
University of Virginia School
  of Medicine
Charlottesville, VA 22908
USA

Peter L. Reynolds, MD
Major
United States Air Force
Staff Family Physician
United States Medical Clinic
52511 Geilenkirchen
Germany

Mark H. Ebell, MD, MS
Associate Professor
Department of Family Medicine
Michigan State University
East Lansing, MI 48824
USA

Cover illustration: The cover illustration is by Roy Wiemann, New York, 2003.

Library of Congress Cataloging-in-Publication Data
Strayer, Scott M.
    Handhelds in medicine : a practical guide for clinicians / Scott M. Strayer, Peter L.
Reynolds, Mark H. Ebell.
      p. cm.
    Includes index.
    ISBN 0-387-40329-9 (alk. paper)
    1. Diagnosis. 2. Clinical medicine. 3. Portable computers. 4. Pocket
    computers. I. Reynolds, Peter, 1947– II. Ebell, Mark H. III. Title.
  RC71.3.S77 2003
  004.16′02461—dc21   2003052967

ISBN 0-387-40329-9   Printed on acid-free paper.

We dedicate this book to our spouses:
Karen Strayer, Katie Reynolds, and Laura Bierema

To our children:
Denton, Riley, Madeline, Sophie, Samuel, and especially, Lukas,
who spent too little time with us, but taught us so much

To our medical colleagues everywhere who seek out
self-improvement through technical innovation

Preface

Have you ever wanted to calculate the predicted peak flow for one of your asthmatic patients without spending valuable minutes searching for that confounded little slide rule gizmo? How about being able to enter your patient's risk factors and cholesterol number, and have the goal LDL cholesterol level spit out for you without having to read the latest version of the National Cholesterol Education Program's guidelines in their entirety—let alone remembering how to use them in your busy daily practice? Wouldn't it be great if you could somehow remember all Mrs. Jones' medications when the nursing home calls to see if it's OK to treat her acutely elevated blood pressure with some atenolol? What would you give to be able to look up the dosing instructions for that newly released medication in seconds, without lugging out the 10-pound PDR (would it even be in there if the medication was just released)?

All these medical tasks and many, many more can be easily accomplished using the current models of handheld computers. While earlier generations of handheld computers suffered from clumsy interfaces, short battery lives, and poor software, the latest models available from Palm®, Handspring, TRG, Sony, Hewlett-Packard, Toshiba, Casio, and others come very close to being the ideal information tool for clinicians at the point of care.

In handheld computer user circles, the following quote is often used to highlight the trepidation with which most physicians view computer technology: "That it will ever come into general use, notwithstanding its value, is extremely doubtful because its beneficial application requires much time and gives a good bit of trouble, both to the patient and to the practitioner because its hue and character are foreign and opposed to all our habits and associations." Just look at the abysmal 5% of physicians who currrently use electronic medical records in their practice despite widespread availability for more than two decades.[1] However, this quote was actually made in an

1834 edition of the *London Times*, and was referring to the stethoscope, and not handheld computers. If the handheld's future is as bright as the stethoscope's was in 1834, watch out!

These handheld computers are coming to be known as "Medical Digital Assistants" or MDAs instead of the frequently used "Personal Digital Assistant" or PDA acronym of the business world. Nearly a quarter of physicians report using an MDA[2] and the numbers are growing rapidly, with more than two-thirds of family practice residencies reporting that they are using handheld computers in their training programs.[3] These devices are becoming so popular that physicians like Chris Vincent, MD, a clinical associate professor of family medicine at the University of Washington and Swedish Family Medicine Residency, proclaimed, "We think the PDA is the stethoscope of tomorrow. Within five years, everyone is going to have one."[4]

Will these technological marvels improve the quality of care? Do they hold the promise of making physicians more efficient, informed, and less error-prone? Can they help patients and physicians manage chronic diseases more effectively? These provocative questions, and many more, are currently the subjects of researchers' inquiries across the country and throughout the world. While MDAs are rapidly gaining acceptance in medical practice, designing the best interfaces (interfaces are how we interact with the computer) and eliminating error-prone or buggy devices and software will be critical. Additionally, designing handheld-based systems that patients can use to keep their physicians up-to-date on their latest peak flow readings or blood glucose trends may change the way we treat chronic disease.

This book is not intended to be an exhaustive review of all available hardware and software options. Rather, it should serve as a brief overview of how practicing physicians can use these tools in their practices. The book is written by practicing physicians with handheld computer expertise and will illuminate various unique and useful ways to employ handheld computers in your practice. It is designed to be helpful for all kinds of users, from the novice through the computer wizard. In Section I, we will take you through choosing your first handheld, its basic uses, and how to download and install software on your new machine.

In Section II of this volume, the various types of medical software are introduced, including where to find them and how you can use them on a daily basis to enhance your practice. Types of software covered range from keeping track of your patients to medical references and calculators. Creating simple tools for tasks such as tracking your CME hours is also covered. Finally, the ever-important task of capturing your patient charge information deserves a chapter. Although the focus is on tools for practicing physicians in this section, we will also learn how nurses and physician assistants use handheld computers in practice.

Finally, Section III contains some food for more advanced users, so keep it for later if you are a beginner handheld enthusiast, or you might want to skip to this section if you are a *Star Trek* fan trying to emulate Dr. McCoy, carrying a handheld since the introduction of the Apple Newton in 1992! Here we cover advanced topics, including wireless networks, creating your own databases, and programming your own software. This section also has a chapter for the academics in the group who want more information on how to teach about the use of handhelds in their "ivory towers," and a chapter on server synchronization reviews advanced deployment and retrieval of formation over networks and servers.

This is the first book of its kind devoted to healthcare professionals, and we realize that this is a rapidly evolving field. Every effort to bring you the latest, most up-to-date information was made at the time of printing, but the details will change very fast. The framework for the book should be an excellent guide through this dynamic topic, and it is our intention to provide Web updates of certain tables and text and to produce future editions on a timely basis. Please go to www.handheldsinmedicine.com for updates.

The book is also organized so that if you learn by doing things you can skip to the "hand-on" exercises in nearly every chapter denoted by the icon . There are also "power users" tips throughout the book for advanced handheld users.

It is our hope that using a handheld computer in medical practice will improve your efficiency while enhancing the quality of care at the same time. Sharing the small handheld screen to illustrate a medical concept for your patient, showing them how quitting smoking will improve their cardiac risk profile, and quickly looking up a medication dose give you precious additional seconds in the exam room, improve the quality of care, and show your patients that you are on the cutting edge of medical technology.

Scott M. Strayer, MD, MPH
Peter L. Reynolds, MD
Mark H. Ebell, MD, MS

References

1. Stringer J. Broken Records. Red Herring. Retrieved from the World Wide Web at http://www.redherring.com, December 11, 2003.
2. HarrisInteractive. Physician's use of handhelds increases from 15% in 1999 to 26% in 2001. Harris interactive poll results. Vol. 1, Issue 25. Retrieved from the World Wide Web at http://www.rnpalm.com/harris.htm, August 15, 2001.
3. Criswell DF, Parchman ML. Handheld computer use in U.S. family practice residency programs. J Am Med Inform Assoc 2002;9(1):80–86.
4. Connaughton D. "Stethoscope of tomorrow" puts medical information at your fingertips. FP Report. October 2000.

Contents

Section I Getting to Know Your Handheld Computer

Section II Medical Software

Section III   Advanced Topics

Contributors

David R, Blair, MD
Major, United States Army, Staff Family Physician, Reynolds Army Community Hospital, Lawton, OK 73503, USA; Information Technology Committee Chairman, Uniformed Services Academy of Family Practice, USAFP Headquarters, Richmond, VA 23229, USA; and, Clinical Consultant to the Wireless Medical Enterprise Working Group to the Telemedicine, and Advanced Technology Research Center (TATRC), United States Army, Frederick, MD 21702, USA

Daniel S. Brian
Project Manager, VNA Home Health Systems, Santa Ana, CA 92705, USA

Jeneane A. Brian, RN, BSN, PHN, MBA
President and CEO, VNA Home Health Systems, Santa Ana, CA 92705, USA

Mark H. Ebell, MD, MS
Associate Professor, Department of Family Medicine, Michigan State University, East Lansing, MI 48824, USA

Gary N. Fox, MD
Mercy Health Partners Family Practice Residency Program, Toledo, OH 43624, USA

Laura Kosteva, MS, CCC
Speech-Language Pathology, University of Michigan Health System, Ann Arbor, MI 48109-0043, USA

Dale Patterson, MD
Major, United States Air Force Medical Corps, and Assistant Professor, Department of Community and Family Medicine, St. Louis University School of Medicine, Bellville, IL 62220, USA

Amy Price, MD
Clinical Instructor of Family Medicine, Department of Family Medicine, University of Virginia Health Sciences Center, Charlottesville, VA 22908, USA

Peter L. Reynolds, MD
Major, United States Air Force, Staff Family Physician, United States Medical Clinic, Geilenkirchen, 52511 Germany

Greg Schaller, MPA, PA-C
Correctional Managed Care, University of Texas Medical Branch, Richmond, TX 77469, USA

Louis Spikol, MD
Louis E. Spikol Family Medicine, Lehigh Valley Physicians Group, Whitehall, PA 18052, USA

Yvonne Stolworthy, RN, BScN, CCRP
Editor, PDA Cortex, and, Research Educator/Auditor, Capital Health Centre for Clinical Research, Halifax, Nova Scotia B3H 1V7, Canada

Scott M. Strayer, MD, MPH
Assistant Professor, Department of Family Medicine, UVA Health System, University of Virginia School of Medicine, Charlottesville, VA 22908, USA

Sylvia Suszka Hildebrandt, BS, MN, ARNP, CCNI
Editor, PDA Cortex, and Group Health Cooperative, Kent, WA 98032, USA

James M. Thompson, MD, CCFP(EM), FCFP
Associate Professor, Department of Emergency Medicine, Dalhousie University, Halifax, Nova Scotia, B3H 3J5, Canada; and, Chief of Emergency Medicine, Queen Elizabeth Hospital, Charlottetown, PEI, C1A 8T5, Canada

Registered, Trademarked, and Copyrighted Material

"Box"
"The times they are a changing" Copyright 1963, Bob Dylan
1984-George Orwell
2001: A Space Odyssey
5 Minute Clinical Consult

abcDB
Accu-Chek
ActiveSync
Adderall
Address Plus
Adobe PDF
Allscripts
Amaryl
AOL
Aportis
AppForge
Archimedes
Audiovox
AvantGo
AvantGo Auto Channels
Avelox
Axim

Bactrim/Septra
BBC TV
BDCity
BigClock
Blackberry
Bluetooth
Bonsai Outliner

Caremark
Casio
Cassiopeia
Celebrex
CETerm
ChargeKeeper
Cipro
City Time
Clie
CNet
CNetX
CNN
Cochrane Collaboration
CodeWarrior
CogniQ
Colorgraphic
Compact Flash
Compaq
Concerta
CPT
Cross

Data Anywhere
Data on the Run
DataViz
DateBk5
Db2Hand
DBAnywhere
DBNow
DDH Software
Defender
Dell

Deloitte Research
Diabeta
Documents-to-Go

Easy I ching
Enterprise Intellisync
ePocrates
ePocrates qID
ePocrates Rx
ePocrates Rx Pro
EveryCharge
EveryPlace
Extended Systems

FileMaker
FileMaker Mobile
Fire Viewer
Firepad
FoxPro
FreeForms
Fulcrum Analytics

GANDM
Glucophage
Glucotrol
Google
Graffiti

HAL
Handango
HanDBase
HandEra
Handheldmed
Handspring
Handpring Visor Platinum
Health News Digest
Healthcare Information and Management
   Systems Society (HIMSS)
HotSync
HP

IBM DB2
ICD-9
InfoDB
InfoPOEM

InfoRetriever
Installigent
Internet Explorer
iPaq
iScribe
iSilo
iSilo3
iSiloX

J File
Jornada
Jot
Journal of Family Practice

Lasix
Lexi-Complete
Lexi-Diagnostic Medicine
Lexi-Drugs
Lexi-Drugs for Pediatrics
Lexi-Drugs Platinum
Lexi-Infectious Diseases
Lexi-Interact
Lexi-Natural Products
Lexi-Poisoning & Toxicology
List
List Pro
Lotus Notes

Margi
Presenter-to-go
Marietta PDE
MDEverywhere
MedicalPocketPC
Medical Toolbox
MedMath
Memory Stick (Sony)
Merck
Microsoft
Microsoft Access
Microsoft ClearType
Microsoft Excel
Microsoft Exchange
Microsoft Internet Explorer (NOTE:
   "Internet Explorer" registered by
   someone else.)

Microsoft SQL Server
Microsoft Visual Basic
Mission Impossible
MMWR
Mobile MedData
Mobile PDR
MobileDB
My Yahoo!

Netscape
New York Times
Newton
NSBasic

ObTech
ON-CALL
One Touch
One Touch Ultra System Kit
Oracle
Oracle Lite
Outlook
Ovid
Ovid@Hand
Oxycontin
OxyIR

PalmOne
Palm III
Palm M505
Palm M515
Palm OS (NOTE: with space!)
PalmGear
PalmReader
Pamelor
Patient Tracker
PatientKeeper
PDA Toolbox
Pendragon Forms
Pendragon Software Corporation
PEPID
PhotoSuite
Physicians' Desk Reference
Pocket Access
Pocket Database
Pocket DB
Pocket Excel

Pocket PC (NOTE: "Pocket PC" is
    registered by a computer magazine.)
PocketBilling
PocketMed
PocketPractitioner
PocketScript
PowerPoint
PrintBoy

QuickMemo
QuickOffice
QuickWord

Red Book
Ritalin
RNDiseases
RNLabs
Rolodex

Satellite Forms
Secure Digital (NOTE: "Secure Digital" not
    trademarked; only with stylized "SD
    Secure Digital")
Skyscape
Sony
SOTI
SplashData
SplashID
Sprint DB
Star Corps
Starship Enterprise
Star Trek
Starbucks
StacWorks
Stat Cardiac Clearance
Stat Cholesterol
StatCoder
Stat E&M Coder
SuiteMD
Sybase UltraLite
SynCalc
Synergy Medical Informatics

Taber's
Tarascon Pocket Pharmacopoeia

Teal Doc
Teal Info
Teal Paint
Tetris
ThinkDB
Thomson Corporation
TomeRaider
Toshiba
TouchWorks Charge
TouchWorks RX+
Trans/Form
Treo
Tricoder
Tucows
Tungsten

Unbound Medicine
USBMIS

Visor
Visual CE
Voyager VGA

W.R. Hambrecht
Wall Street Journal, The
Washington Manual
Windex
Windows CE
WinZip
Wireless Database
Word

XTNDConnect Server

Yahoo

Zaditor
Zafirlukast

Zaleplon
Zanamivir
Zantac
ZapBill
ZapMed
Zarontin
Zaroxolyn
ZDNetZebeta
Zemplar
Zemuron
Zenapax
Zerit
Zero-sixty Corp.
Zestril
Ziac
Ziagen
Zinacef
Zinecard
Zire
Z-max
Zocor
Zofran
Zonalon
Zonegran
Zostrix
Zosyn
Zovia
Zovirax
Z-pak
Zyban
Zydone
Zyflo
Zyloprim
Zyprexa
Zyrtec

Section I

Getting to Know Your Handheld Computer

1

Choosing a Handheld Computer: PDAs, MDAs, and the Alphabet Soup of Handheld Computers

SCOTT M. STRAYER AND MARK H. EBELL

Handheld computers have exploded onto the medical scene. It's a time of transformation, in which PDA no longer means "public display of affection," but rather "personal digital assistant." Already, the processing power and information storage (hundreds of megabytes!) that can fit in your pocket is astounding. As the technology advances in leaps and bounds, so too advances the promise of handheld computers to revolutionize health care. And guess what? You can turn your handheld into a sophisticated clinical tool today. The reality of a pocket "medical digital assistant," or MDA, has arrived. In the pages that follow, you'll learn, step by step, just how to turn your PDA into an MDA. First, though, you have to make a purchase. . . .

When it comes to picking the handheld computer itself, many healthcare professionals suffer from "analysis paralysis." The options available are vast and growing daily. In this chapter, we give you a good overview of the handheld computers available and hope we can enable you to select one to fit your clinical needs and lifestyle (yes, you can track your golf scores and grocery lists with them as well).

"Handhelds," "mobile computing," and "portable computers" are the buzzwords of this fast-growing consumer and enterprise market. Many types of devices and computers are available that could be considered handheld computers. To simplify your selection, we concentrate on traditional handhelds; this means small, portable handheld computers that easily slip into your handbag, lab coat, or shirt pocket.

Choosing the Right Handheld for Your Needs

As in desktop computers, the operating system (OS) is the software guts of any handheld computer. Currently two versions of this software dominate the market—Palm OS and Pocket PC. Each has advantages and disadvantages for handheld computing (Note that Palm, the company, sells hand-held computers that run its operating system, Palm OS, but also licenses Palm OS to other hardware manufacturers, such as Sony and Handspring. Microsoft licenses the Pocket PC operating system, but does not currently sell its own hardware.) Palm OS devices usually have more software (for the Palm, there are more than 1000 medical titles to choose from); a more intuitive user interface; longer battery life; and a smaller, compact design.

Pocket PC's offer faster, more powerful processors; higher-end software; better screen resolutions (so more information can fit on a single screen); built-in audio and color in every device; better wireless capability; and increased security features (i.e., encryption for wireless). Both devices offer some degree of integration with Microsoft Word, Excel, and Outlook, although this integration is somewhat more seamless and is always included with the Pocket PC.

Although Palm devices have traditionally been less expensive, there is now considerable overlap in the price range. You can still find a stripped-down Palm OS device with a low-resolution black-and-white screen and no expansion card for under $100, but you can also spend nearly $600 on a high-resolution color device with expandability, built-in audio, and a camera. Although Pocket PC's are generally in the $450 to $550 range, the Toshiba E310 is a great value at under $300 from some online retailers, and Dell's new Axim line has an entry model for under $200. The competition is sure to heat up among Pocket PC manufacturers. A complete comparison of currently available Palm OS and Pocket PC devices can be found in the Appendix.

It is worth visiting your local electronics or office supply store to look at the screen of the models that you are considering before you buy. Don't forget to look at the screen outdoors in bright light if you plan to use it on the golf course!

TIPS FROM THE POWER USERS ON HANDHELD SCREENS

1. Color screens are nice, but are hard to read without the backlight on, which can drain batteries quickly.
2. Some screens are actually very small to begin with and hard to read (i.e., the Palm Zire and Zire 21 series).

How much memory is enough? We recommend at least 32 to 64 MB for Palm OS and 64 to 128 MB for the Pocket PC (Pocket PC programs are larger and use memory less efficiently than Palm programs). Whichever size internal memory you have, make sure you have the option of adding more memory using an expansion card. This way, you can keep dozens of medical applications on one card, music on another, and recorded books on a third. Having an expansion slot also lets you connect to a network or even the Internet with a wireless or wired modem. For example, for less than $400 you can set up a cable modem connecting to a router with wireless network cards for several laptops and a Pocket PC. Such an inexpensive network allows you to connect to the Internet with a high-speed connection from anywhere in your home or office.

 TIP FROM THE POWER USERS ON MEMORY

Software applications tend to run best in main memory, so getting the most to begin with (i.e., 64 MB for Palm models, and 64 to 128 MB for Pocket PC models) is highly encouraged to decrease your frustration levels.

Here are some final questions to ask yourself as you consider Palm OS versus Pocket PC: Does it feel good in your hand? Does it have a screen cover to protect it on the wards? Does it have a rechargeable battery? Can you share the expansion memory card with your digital camera? And, if you find that you are developing "PDA envy" you can always sell yours and buy the latest, greatest device next year!

Key Points

1. There are advantages and disadvantages for both Palm OS and Pocket PC handheld computers. Choose the one that best suits your needs. Either one beats index cards any day!
2. We recommend at least 32 to 64 MB for the Palm OS and 64 to 128 MB for Pocket PCs. Physicians need extra memory, so buy a model that has the option of expanding memory.
3. Palm OS models tend to be less expensive than comparable Pocket PC handheld computers; however, there is a trend toward price overlap with both companies adding the latest features such as wireless connectivity and security enhancements.
4. Make sure you look at handheld computer models at the nearest electronics or office supply store before you buy. You can compare screen resolutions, feel the instrument in your hand, and check out the options.

Batteries and Bytes: Handheld Computer Features

Handheld computers have many innovative features that make them amazingly useful at the point of care. Every time you reach for an obstetrical wheel (OB wheel), your prescription pad, or your Rolodex, imagine having instant access to this information in the palm of your hand. Think of every time you have to sit down at a desktop computer to look up your schedule in Outlook or find an important phone number. All this functionality is also currently available on handheld computers.

Batteries

The first thing that makes these devices so useful is the long battery life. Anyone who has tried to watch a DVD movie on his or her laptop on a cross-country flight quickly realizes that most batteries aren't made to last an entire day, let alone weeks in the clinic. Handheld computers distinguish themselves here, and some models, such as the Palm OS handhelds with a monochrome screen, can last up to a month without recharging or replacement. Even the most power-hungry handhelds usually can survive at least a day without being recharged. This simple engineering feat distinguishes handheld computers from their laptop and Tablet PC cousins . . . at least with the current state of technology.

There are several types of batteries, and this is one of the choices you must make in your purchasing decision. Although some of the earlier models relied on AAA size batteries, most are now converting to rechargeable lithium ion batteries. Of the rechargeable varieties, some have removable and replaceable batteries, and others are fixed. This point could be important if you are in Europe or Africa without a conventional power source, so take this into consideration.

 TIPS FROM THE POWER USERS ON BATTERIES

1. If you plan to be somewhere with no access to conventional power, buy a handheld computer with replaceable batteries.
2. Color screens and Pocket PC handhelds tend to drain batteries quickly. If you can recharge daily, don't worry about it. If you can't, consider buying a monochrome screen or Palm OS model.

Bytes: The Memory of an Elephant

The next amazing feature of these pint-sized computers is the amount of memory they have relative to the requirements of most software programs designed for them. If you're a physician, drift back to your intern year, a sleep-deprived experience where you struggled to keep up with your information needs in the hospital or clinic setting. Most of us rose to the challenge by stuffing every pocket in our white doctor's coat with handbooks, calculators, slide rules, calipers, and index cards crammed full of patient information in the tiniest writing we could manage.

Now imagine being able to carry your 5-minute Clinical Consult, Harrison's, Harriet Lane, *Washington Manual*, an OB wheel, the *Physicians Desk Reference*, and anything else you can think of all in one tiny computer weighing only a few ounces! That is the miracle of handheld computing . . . all that valuable information stored on chips, memory, and storage cards ready for use at a moment's notice. With at least 16MB available in most Palm OS models and 32 to 64MB in most Pocket PC models, all this—and more—is achievable. Many models can be expanded using Compact Flash

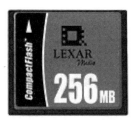

FIGURE 1.1. A Compact Flash card that adds 256 MB of memory (up to 1.0 GB available). (Reprinted with permission from CompactFlash.)

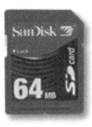

FIGURE 1.2. SD/MMC Card (up to 512 MB available). (Reprinted with permission from SanDisk.)

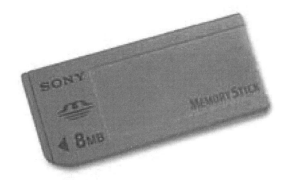

FIGURE 1.3. Sony Memory stick. (Reprinted with permission from Sony.)

cards (Figure 1.1), Secure Digital/MultiMedia cards (Figure 1.2), or Sony Memory Sticks (Figure 1.3). In some cases, this allows up to 1 GB of additional memory in a card the size of a book of matches (compact flash), and Secure Digital and Multimedia cards can provide an additional 512 MB in a tiny removable card the size of a postage stamp.

Just to put things in perspective, the full 5 Minute Clinical Consult takes up about 2 MB on the Palm operating system (without color images); on a Pocket PC, expect this to use about 17 MB with nice full-color case pictures. Although Pocket PC programs tend to use more memory, notice that they initially come with more memory to account for this. Simple programs such as an OB wheel take significantly less memory, using only about 50 KB on a Palm machine and 60 KB on the Pocket PC platform.

Synchronization

We're not talking about synchronized swimming here, but rather the ability of handheld computers to update and backup information to a desktop computer and vice versa. The details of synchronization and how to maximize this unique feature are described further in Chapter 2, but we want to give you a brief overview of this useful feature.

Let's say you've been rounding in the hospital before office hours, and you capture billing information on five hospitalized patients detailing their diagnoses and levels of service. To get that information to your office staff, all you need to do is synchronize your information to a desktop computer when you get to your office, and all the information will be accessible to the billing person. Also, if you lose your handheld or it malfunctions, all the data can be restored as of the last synchronization that you performed.

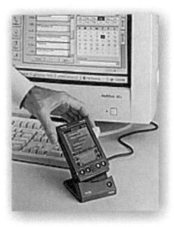

FIGURE 1.4. Palm OS HotSync Operation with a desktop computer. (Obtained from homepage.tinet.ie/~seadancer/ info.html.) (Reprinted with permission from palmOne, Inc.)

The mechanics are really quite simple. Most handhelds come with a cradle that connects to your desktop via a USB (universal serial bus) or serial cable. Information can be shared between the two computers with a push of the button (Figure 1.4). Palm calls their process HotSync, while Microsoft has labeled it ActiveSync. Palm OS products give you the option of synchronizing calendar information to their proprietary Palm Desktop (Figure 1.5) or to Microsoft Outlook program. Pocket PC simply integrates with your desktop Outlook program.

This feature can become extremely useful in helping you manage time. You can add appointments or important "to do" items while you are away from the office, and your assistant can enter data in your office-based Outlook or Palm Desktop at the same time. After a quick synchronization, all the items you and your assistant entered will be on both computers. You can even synchronize with your home PC so that you don't miss ballet recitals and swim meets entered by your spouse or significant other. What an incredible time-saver!

"Beam Me Up"

Handhelds have the unique feature of being able to beam information to another handheld within several feet (Figure 1.6). Users can beam everything from their business cards to the inpatient rounding list for weekend cross-coverage.

This feature is available on both Pocket PC and Palm OS handheld computers and operates similarly on either type. The only real difference is where the infrared beam port is located on different models; some have it located on the top of the machine while in others it is side-mounted. See a more detailed discussion of the beaming process in Chapter 2.

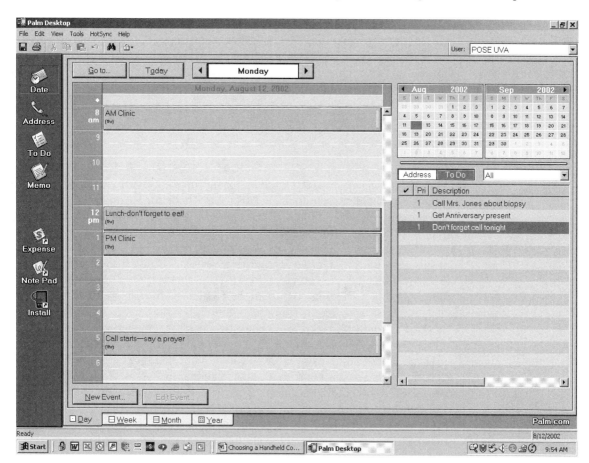

FIGURE 1.5. Palm Desktop Software. (Reprinted with permission from palmOne, Inc.)

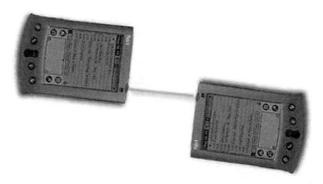

FIGURE 1.6. Beaming between two handheld computers. (Reprinted with permission from palmOne, Inc.)

Although this function is useful for beaming small amounts of information or conducting limited infrared synchronizations (yes, you can synchronize without a cable too), it hasn't been tested yet for actual teleporting. In addition to beaming patient lists and playing interactive games, this is yet another way to disseminate the all-important weekend home projects and errands list. Beware!

Handwriting Recognition

While this term may be considered an oxymoron for most physicians' handwriting, handheld computers have several methods for writing recognition that can actually make your writing legible. This feature makes handhelds more portable by leaving out a keyboard and is a unique way to enter data into a computer. Once you try it, you just might get hooked. Although entering large amounts of data, such as writing a book, is best left to a traditional keyboard (which can be attached to most handhelds if needed), entering a phone number, or tapping on a patient's diagnosis list using pick lists, can easily be done using handwriting recognition.

Both Palm and Microsoft offer their own versions of handwriting recognition. Graffiti, developed by Palm, is a simple and reliable method for entering limited amounts of information on your handheld. Pocket PC lets users choose between block recognizer (similar to Palm's Graffiti), letter recognizer, a keyboard, and another method called transcriber that takes your handwriting and converts it to typed text.

As already mentioned, you can always attach a keyboard if necessary, and both models of handhelds come with pop-up keyboards that can be used for on-screen text entry (Figures 1.7, 1.8). This topic is covered in additional detail in the next chapter.

As a side note, several new handheld models incorporate a tiny keyboard into the device. They're called thumb-boards, because (you guessed it) you press the buttons with your thumb. The speed of data entry compares

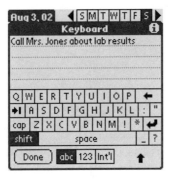

FIGURE 1.7. Palm pop-up keyboard. (Reprinted with permission from palmOne, Inc.)

FIGURE 1.8. Pocket PC's built-in keyboard. (Reprinted with permission from Microsoft, Inc.)

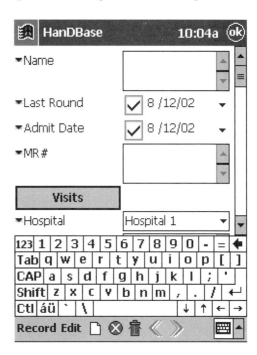

closely to Graffiti but, in their favor, you tend to make fewer mistakes. We'll have to wait and see how popular these thumb-boards become.

There are several unique keyboards that can be added to either Palm OS or Pocket PC handhelds. Some slip right over the machines themselves; others are collapsible and plug into the synchronization socket (Figures 1.9–1.11).

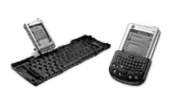

FIGURE 1.9. Two types of Palm add-on keyboards. (Reprinted with permission from Palm.)

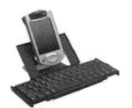

FIGURE 1.10. Pocket PC foldable keyboard. (Reprinted with permission from Microsoft, Inc.)

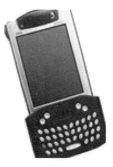

FIGURE 1.11. Pocket PC Micro Keyboard. (Reprinted with permission from Microsoft, Inc.)

Key Points

1. Most handhelds are now using rechargeable lithium ion batteries. Be sure to buy a handheld that has a battery life long enough for your particular situation.
2. We recommend buying a handheld with the most preinstalled memory; that's 32 to 64 MB with a Palm OS device or 64 to 128 MB on a Pocket PC. You should also purchase a handheld that can expand its memory to carry all the clinical information you will need.
3. Synchronization integrates items entered on the handheld computer and any desktop computer with which you synchronize so that both have the same appointments, addresses, and "to do" items. Never miss another birthday, ballet recital or "date night!"
4. Key bits of information can be beamed between handheld users standing within a few feet of each other using the infrared port found on either the side or top of most handheld computers. Watch out for additions to your private and personal information beamed to you when you least expect it!
5. There are several different ways to input data into handheld computers, including handwriting recognition, pop-up keyboards, and add-on keyboards.

Software Included "Out of the Box"

We've already alluded to many of the features you can begin using right away. An extensive software suite comes preinstalled on Pocket PC and Palm OS handhelds. This feature allows you, right out of the box, to track your appointments, keep your Rolodex electronically, and manage your to do list and the ever-multiplying index cards and "yellow stickies" throughout your office. You'll even have a calculator when you need it, and password protection comes built in as well.

There's not much difference between Palm OS and Pocket PC models here, other than Pocket PC synchronizes directly to Microsoft Outlook, and Palm OS users have the option of doing this through third-party software or with the Palm Desktop software. Let's take a brief look at the included software.

Appointments

Add appointments on the fly. Have your assistant enter them at work, and your spouse or significant other at home. Synchronize with desktop computers at home and at work, and like magic, all your appointments are on each computer. Say goodbye to your leather-bound organizer. Different views are available, including day, week and month. Figures 1.12 through 1.14 illustrate these views on a Palm OS device. Figures 1.15 through 1.17

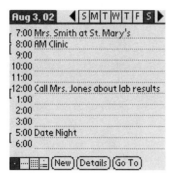

FIGURE 1.12. All your appointments in the day view of the Palm OS calendar software. (Reprinted with permission from palmOne, Inc.)

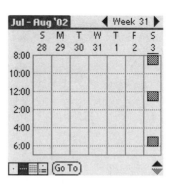

FIGURE 1.13. Week view with the Palm OS calendar software. (Reprinted with permission from palmOne, Inc.)

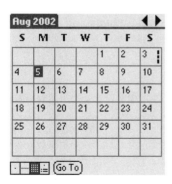

FIGURE 1.14. Month view with the Palm OS calendar software. (Reprinted with permission from palmOne, Inc.)

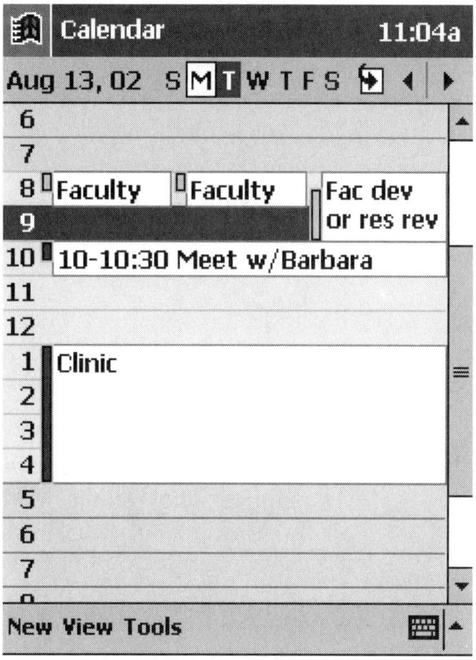

FIGURE 1.15. Pocket PC's built-in calendar function, day view. (Reprinted with permission from Microsoft, Inc.)

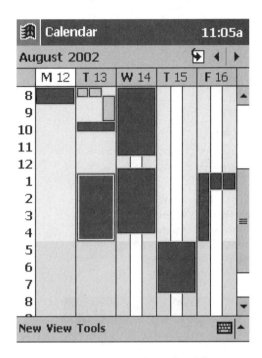

FIGURE 1.16. Week view in Pocket PC calendar. Tapping on the blue boxes tells you what is scheduled during that time. (Reprinted with permission from Microsoft, Inc.)

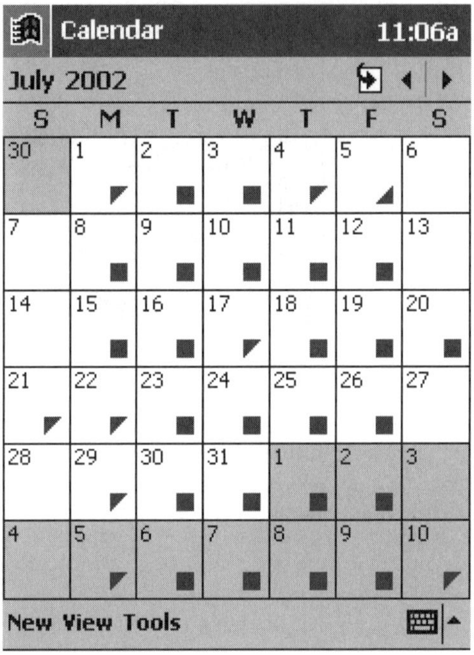

FIGURE 1.17. Pocket PC monthly view. (Reprinted with permission from Microsoft, Inc.)

illustrate the same on a Pocket PC device. Add-on software can give you additional functionality, such as icons for call nights and other features to turbo charge the basic software (Figures 1.18–1.20).

Address Book

The address book feature is probably the first one you'll use and is most likely to lead to early handheld dependency. Now you can have the numbers for every pharmacy in town, every clinic, and every hospital nursing station, not to mention your friends' and neighbors' numbers, all in one place. It's a physician's organizational dream come true. You can throw away your Rolodex and all those yellow stickies with numbers on them. This feature will also synchronize with your preferred desktop software (Figures 1.21, 1.22).

To Do List

Have you ever wanted to have a to do list that erased done items once they are checked, and can organize and prioritize by due date, or any other

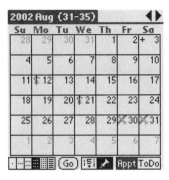

FIGURE 1.18. Turbocharge your Palm OS date book with Date Book 5. This program allows adding icons for call nights and vacation, for example. (Reprinted with permission from palmOne, Inc.)

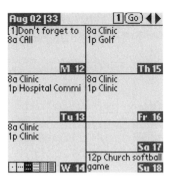

FIGURE 1.19. Week view display in Date Book 5 for Palm OS. (Reprinted with permission from palmOne, Inc.)

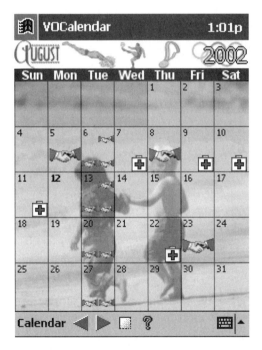

FIGURE 1.20. VOCalendar for Pocket PC (available at www.handango.com). (Reprinted with permission from Microsoft, Inc.)

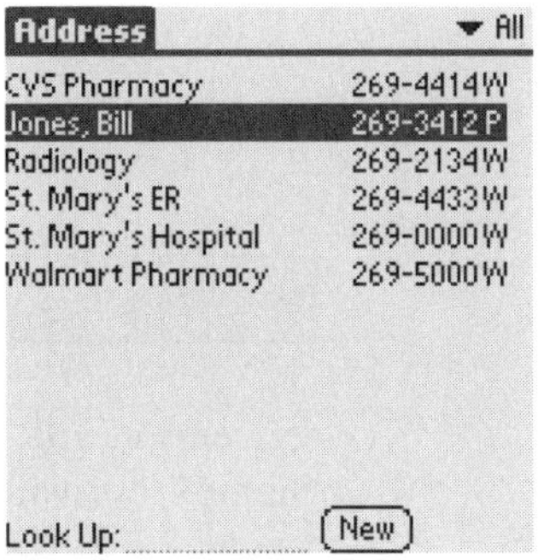

FIGURE 1.21. Palm OS address book. (Reprinted with permission from palmOne, Inc.)

FIGURE 1.22. Pocket PC contacts. (Reprinted with permission from Microsoft, Inc.)

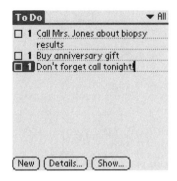

FIGURE 1.23. Palm OS to-do list. (Reprinted with permission from palmOne, Inc.)

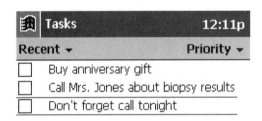

FIGURE 1.24. Pocket PC to do list. (Reprinted with permission from Microsoft, Inc.)

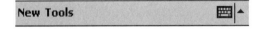

convention you choose? How about being able to categorize by "work," "home," "private and personal information," or any other organization scheme? If so, this will be your most often used feature (Figures 1.23, 1.24).

Memo Pad

The memo pad (Figures 1.25, 1.26) is another method for eliminating scraps of paper from your life. Anything that you would normally write down on

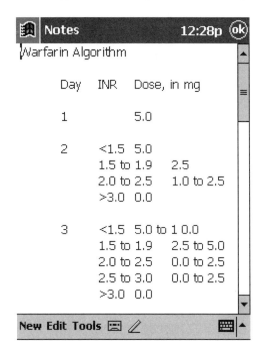

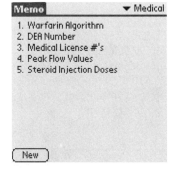

FIGURE 1.25. Palm OS Memo Pad. (Reprinted with permission from palmOne, Inc.)

FIGURE 1.26. Pocket PC showing memo for adjusting Coumadin dosage. (Reprinted with permission from Microsoft, Inc.)

an index card can be entered here. You can even convert entire word documents to store and organize them here on your handheld. There are many medical uses for the memo pad section as well (think "peripheral brain"). These uses are covered in more detail later.

Calculator

Don't leave calculating a drug dose to chance when you will have instant access to a calculator whenever you are carrying your handheld (Figures 1.27–1.30). This feature is especially useful for calculating pediatric medication doses after being up all night on call. Add-on software can turn the basic calculator into a scientific or programmable calculator, which is covered later in Sections II and III.

Password Protection

Leave it to the lawyers to make security of information on handheld computers clear as mud. The Health Insurance Portability and Accountability Act (HIPAA), passed in 1996, was supposed to simplify transactions and

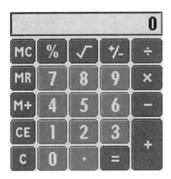

FIGURE 1.27. Basic Palm OS
Calculator. (Reprinted with
permission from palmOne,
Inc.)

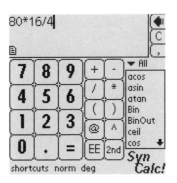

FIGURE 1.28. SynCalc
scientific calculator for Palm
OS (see subsequent chapters
for more on this type of
calculator). (Reprinted with
permission from Installigent
Team, a Zero-sixty corp.)

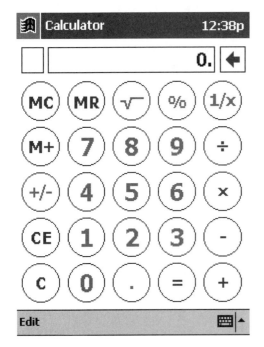

FIGURE 1.29. Basic Pocket PC Calculator.
(Reprinted with permission from Microsoft,
Inc.)

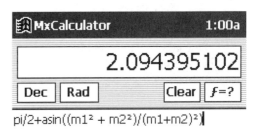

FIGURE 1.30. MX Calculator, a programmable
calculator for Pocket PC (available for
download at www.handango.com). (Reprinted
with permission from Microsoft, Inc.)

code sets, security, and privacy as these apply to electronic medical information. Of course, handheld computers were not being widely used at the time and are not directly addressed (i.e., is beaming an inpatient list a HIPAA violation?). A little common sense will go a long way with this new set of regulations as they go into effect.

With levels of hysteria regarding HIPAA rising, be sure you use the built-in password protection if you plan to carry patient information on your handheld computer. Lawyers are sure to have a field day with this one, but recognizing your handheld as a location for protected health information, and using the built-in password protection, is certainly a reasonable measure to protect confidential information. Several software developers offer higher levels of security that can be added, and companies are even making fingerprint and retinal scanners for handhelds.

If you decide to transmit data from your handheld over the Internet or a wireless network, you need to ensure that you are taking reasonable measures to provide for security of that information by using encryption and passwords as necessary. Many software vendors have products that perform these functions. For example, a quality wireless prescription or charge capture software product provides for encryption of sensitive data automatically. Just make sure that the solution you eventually choose is HIPAA-compliant so that your patient information is safe and secure. Then, don't lose sleep over being fined by the "HIPAA police."

HANDS-ON EXERCISE 1.1. SETTING A PASSWORD ON YOUR POCKET PC

Pocket PC's built-in password protection allows you to choose a four-digit number that must be entered every time you turn on the machine. It only takes a few seconds to enter the password. To set the password, click on "Start," "Settings," and "Personal." You will see a "Password" icon that should be tapped (Figure 1.31).

After tapping the password icon, you will see the screen shown in Figure 1.32. Enter your password, which in our example is "1–2–3–4." Make sure you also click the checkbox next to "Require password when device is turned on." After doing all this, tap on the "OK" button in the upper-right-hand corner of the screen. The next time you turn on your Pocket PC, you will see the screen prompting you to enter your password (Figure 1.33).

HANDS-ON EXERCISE 1.2. SETTING A PASSWORD ON YOUR PALM HAND-HELD COMPUTER

Setting a password on your Palm OS device is just as simple as doing it with a Pocket PC, and our "legal beagles" highly recommend it! The built-in Palm security feature lets you password-protect the entire handheld or only those records marked as "private." To enter the security function with Palm OS, tap on the "Security" icon seen on the main program menu (Figure 1.34).

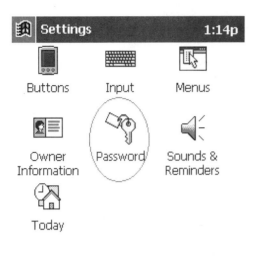

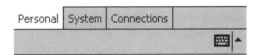

FIGURE 1.31. Location of built-in password program on Pocket PC. (Reprinted with permission from Microsoft Corporation and Pocket PC.)

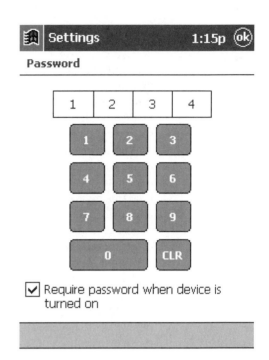

FIGURE 1.32. Setting password on Pocket PC.

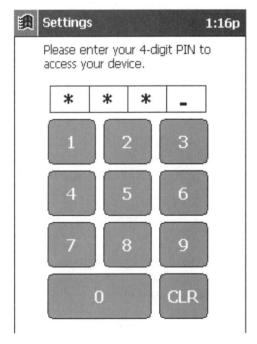

FIGURE 1.33. Pocket PC screen for entering password. (Reprinted with permission from Microsoft Corporation and Pocket PC.)

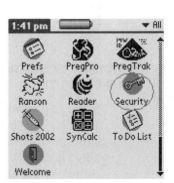

FIGURE 1.34. "Security" icon on Palm OS handheld. (Reprinted with permission from palmOne, Inc.)

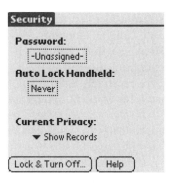

FIGURE 1.35. First password screen. (Reprinted with permission from palmOne, Inc.)

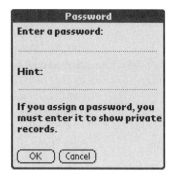

FIGURE 1.36. Password entry screen for Palm OS. (Reprinted with permission from palmOne, Inc.)

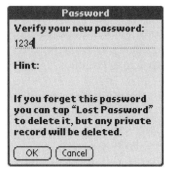

FIGURE 1.37. Password verification screen for Palm OS. (Reprinted with permission from palmOne, Inc.)

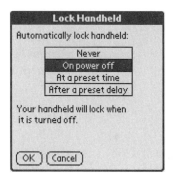

FIGURE 1.38. "Lock Handheld" selections. (Reprinted with permission from palmOne, Inc.)

After tapping on the security button, the next screen lets you enter the password and a "hint" just in case you forget it (Figures 1.35, 1.36), after you tap on "Unassigned." In our example, we use the password "1–2–3–4" (not recommended by the lawyers), and we won't enter a hint. After entering the password, tap on the "OK" button, which will bring you to a password verification screen (Figure 1.37), where you need to enter the password again and hit "OK."

Now that you have set the password, you can choose to lock either the whole machine or just private records. To lock the machine, click on "Autolock Handheld," which was set to "Never" in the first password screen; this will give you four selections (Figure 1.38). You can choose "Never," "On Power Off," "At a Preset Time," or "After a Preset Delay." We recommend "On Power Off," so that every time you turn your handheld off, a password is required to turn it back on. This approach offers maximum protection but can be annoying. Another good option is to choose "At a Preset Time," so that it turns off and becomes password-protected at a specified time at the end of each workday (such as 6 P.M.). In this way, your data are relatively safe if you inadvertently leave your handheld out in the open after work, but you spend less time entering your password.

A totally different approach is to mark certain records as private and hide them using the "Current Privacy" selector shown in the first password screen (see Figure 1.35). The disadvantage to this method is that you must change this setting to view hidden records, rather than getting access to the whole machine every time you enter the password.

Key Points

1. Both Palm OS and Pocket PC handheld computers come with built-in calendars that have day, week, month, and annual views. Kiss your "day planner" goodbye, especially with add-on software that turbocharges the native programs with icons, graphics, and better weekly and monthly views.
2. Using the address book on your new handheld will lead to immediate dependency on this feature. You can use this feature to store important numbers you use daily (and at night), and all the information will synchronize with your desktop.
3. The electronic To Do list will also lead quickly to handheld computer dependency.
4. The Memo Pad function is a useful way to get rid of index cards, scraps of paper, and "yellow stickies." This feature can also convert Word documents for display on your handheld.
5. The built-in calculator is great when you are struggling with simple calculations due to sleep deprivation. Add-on software such as SynCalc and MX calculator can turn your handheld computer into a powerful, programmable, scientific calculator (more on this in Sections II and III).

Summary

We sincerely hope that this chapter has helped you to understand the alphabet soup of handheld computers. By now, you should realize that PDA doesn't stand for "public displays of affection," and if you've been thinking about buying your first handheld computer or upgrading the old Newton, this chapter should help you do that.

Our discussion of batteries, memory, synchronizing, beaming, and handwriting recognition should give you a general idea of the features available on today's powerful handheld computers and should show you why they have become so popular and useful in the medical field.

Finally, the review of native software applications (i.e., address book, calendar, memo pad, to do list, calculator, and password protection) can help you make use of all these great features as soon as you start using your new handheld computer.

2

Getting to Know Your Handheld:
Palm OS and Pocket PC

PETER L. REYNOLDS AND MARK H. EBELL

Buying your first handheld computer is a blast—there's no doubt about it. It's the ultimate gadget for anyone who grew up watching *Star Trek* and *Mission Impossible*. And for the less nerdy crowd, handheld computers are the latest in a wave of must-have electronic performance enhancers. They're trendy—some models are even fashionable! Let's say, though, that you're not a gearhead, you're already organized, and you don't feel pressured to keep up with the Joneses (or the Jetsons, as the case may be). Maybe you still turn to the leatherbound address book you got in college to find phone numbers. What are you going to do with a handheld computer, really?

Case in point, the Apple Newton (an early handheld computer) was supposed to change your life, but the reality never materialized. So what's different about these handhelds today? What makes them worth your while? Three words: simplicity, reliability, and portability. Their simplicity invites a try by even the least computer savvy among us. For the "power users," it's a breath of fresh air in a world of 5-minute bootups. Consistent performance and reliability keeps them in your hands like a ballpoint pen. They perform as advertised. They get the job done. And let's not forget their sine qua non: portability. The first time you spend 30 minutes in an otherwise useless meeting organizing your schedule or surreptitiously reading an electronic book, the device has just about paid for itself!

Bells and whistles will come later. For now, as you get to know your handheld, keep things simple. Treat your handheld like a pager: keep a fresh battery installed, don't get it wet (the dreaded "bathroom kerplunk!"), and expect it to do a few things consistently well. You'll grow comfortable sooner than you think. Then, you'll be hooked. Play Tetris. Download family photos. Surf the World Wide Web. Read a novel. Or don't—the important thing is getting hooked.

The millions of handheld computer lovers out there use their new handhelds for many different things. Certain functions, however, are common to most users. These universally appealing features spell the key to your enjoyment of your handheld. We'll focus on the basics now.

Entering Information

Part of the fascination of handheld computers today is what's not there. They're different: there's no keyboard. If desktop computers, with all their operating systems and BIOS and drives and RAM and CPUs, weren't intimidating enough, now someone's gone and removed the one touch of home, the QWERTY keyboard. You may ask, "What kind of insanity is this?" Many do. To soothe immediate concerns, just about all handhelds do include a keyboard in the form of a pop-up window on the display screen. You can also enter lots of information via your desktop computer. We'll discuss those options in detail later. For now, think back, way back, to the first time you stood in front of a computer screen. What did you do? What was your first impulse? Take a look at the computer screen in the home of anyone with small children, and you'll remember. You can see them a mile away: fingerprints and smudges everywhere.

Truly, the natural instinct of every human being, when confronted with a new gadget, is to touch it.

Modern life has conditioned us not to touch computer screens. The fantastic thing about your handheld is that you can touch it. You're supposed to touch it. That's how you enter information. So forget that keyboard you think you're missing and have some fun.

The handheld screen is touch sensitive. The computer can feel pressure against the screen and detect the location where it is applied. On a basic level, the touch-sensitive screen can provide the same functionality as a computer mouse. On your desktop, you can position the mouse cursor over a program icon displayed on the screen, click the mouse button, and open the program. The mechanical mouse button is real. The program icon and mouse cursor are of course graphical, virtual images. In the same way, you can tap on the image of a program icon on your handheld screen with any blunt object, such as a finger, and also open the program. The computer feels the tap of your finger on the screen and forward the information to the handheld operating system to interpret.

Fingers are a bit fat compared to the size of most handheld computer screens. They do the job but only for large buttons. Fingers also leave smudges on the screen. There's nothing wrong with using your finger, but you may prefer using a stylus. A stylus is any device other than your finger used to tap on the screen. My personal handheld came with a nondescript black plastic stylus that attaches to the side of the device when not in use. The plastic tip is smaller and therefore more precise than a finger: that means it can tap smaller buttons. A word of caution: a ballpoint pen (or hair pin, or safety pin, or other pointed metal stick) does not make a good stylus because it leaves marks on the screen. You can ignore this fact for a while, but eventually stray ink marks on the screen become annoying. They're like finger smudges that don't come off.

Tips for the Power User on Screen Care

To clean a screen, I just spritz a little Windex into a tissue and wipe the screen gently. NEVER use acetone, ethanol, isopropyl alcohol, or toluene because these solvents can melt or damage the screen. You can also buy clear plastic screen covers that protect it from scratch marks.

Everything you can do with a mouse, you can do with a touch-sensitive screen using some kind of pointing device. (We'll call it a stylus instead of pointing devices from now on because it sounds less geeky.) Move scroll bars, highlight text, drag-and-drop—you can do it all. You can also do other functions that don't work well with a computer mouse. For example, there are several ways to turn on the backlight for reading your handheld screen in the dark. One way is to hold down the power button until the backlight comes on (Palm or Pocket PC). Let's do some exercises to customize your handheld computer.

HANDS-ON EXERCISE 2.1. A STROKE OF THE PEN (PALM OS)

Turn on your handheld. On devices made by Palm, Inc., you do so by pushing a mechanical green- or white-colored button at the bottom left or top right of the device. Other devices have similar mechanical power buttons. If you've just pulled your handheld out of the box, you'll have to follow the on-screen instructions to enter your user name and other setup information. Read the "Getting Started" booklet that comes in the box for more details. Now touch your stylus to the bottom-middle screen and slide it straight up to the top middle in one smooth stroke. What happens? Probably either your backlight comes on, a QWERTY keyboard pops up on the screen, or a help screen appears for handwriting recognition. To change what happens, go to the application launcher and tap on the Preferences icon (Figure 2.1a). Choose "Buttons" on the top-right-corner menu by tapping there and selecting from the drop-down list (Figure 2.1b). This

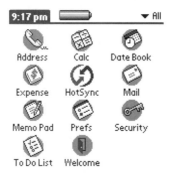

FIGURE 2.1a. Application launcher Preferences icon ("Prefs"). (Reprinted with permission from palmOne, Inc.)

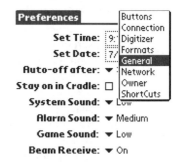

FIGURE 2.1b. Preferences menu. (Reprinted with permission from palmOne, Inc.)

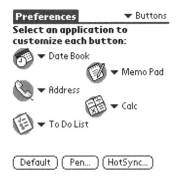

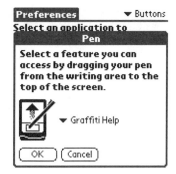

FIGURE 2.2. Screen for Button preferences. (Reprinted with permission from palmOne, Inc.)

FIGURE 2.3. "Pen . . ." preference menu. (Reprinted with permission from palmOne, Inc.)

screen allows you to customize the action of the permanent buttons on your handheld (Figure 2.2). Tap on the "Pen . . ." button at the bottom of the screen. Select the function you'd like from the menu that appears and tap "OK" (Figure 2.3). You'll discover that some of the possible functions work all the time, such as Backlight. Other functions are context dependent. If you pick Keyboard, for example, the keyboard only pops up when you are entering text; otherwise, nothing happens.

HANDS-ON EXERCISE 2.2. HOT KEYS (POCKET PC)

Turn on your Pocket PC—that's usually accomplished by pressing a small recessed button in the lower-left or upper-right corner of your device. Then, tap once on the little Windows flag in the upper-left corner and select "Settings" from the menu that appears. You will see a group of icons labeled "Buttons," "Input," "Menus," and so on (Figure 2.4). At the bottom of the screen are tabs that group the settings into three groups: Personal, System, and Connection. Tapping on a tab takes you to that group of settings. Tap on the "Buttons" icon, and you will see a list of "Hot Keys" (Figure 2.5). A Hot Key is an old fashioned computer term that refers to a key used to quickly run a program. On your Pocket PC, Hot Key 1 is the leftmost mechanical button near the bottom of your device, which probably has a little "Home" icon on it. The second from the left is Hot Key 2 and usually has a "Contacts" icon on it. Let's assign something important, such as the Solitaire game, to Hot Key 1. Tap it once to make sure it is highlighted, and then tap the downward-pointing arrow under "Button assignment" to reveal a list of programs (Figure 2.6). Scroll down the list using the arrows along the right side of the list, and tap once on Solitaire. Voila! Tap the "OK" button in the upper-right corner to confirm your selection, and try it out. How's that for handy! Want to go back to the way things were? We can't in real life, but we can on the Pocket PC. Just go to the

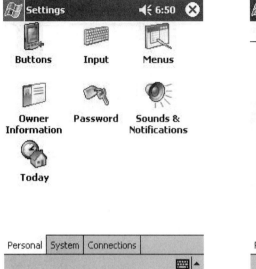

FIGURE 2.4. Pocket PC settings.
(Reprinted with permission from
Microsoft Corporation.)

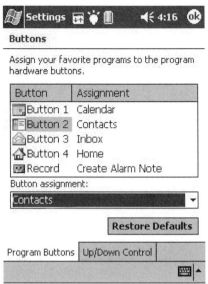

FIGURE 2.5. "Hot Key" button
assignments. (Reprinted with
permission from Microsoft
Corporation.)

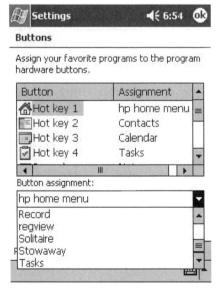

FIGURE 2.6. Programming "Hot Key"
button assignments. (Reprinted with
permission from Microsoft
Corporation.)

"Buttons" selection screen again (Figure 2.5) and press the "Restore defaults" button.

Key Points

1. The natural instinct of humans is to touch the computer screen. With handhelds, you can. In fact, you're supposed to.
2. Your handheld stylus does everything a mouse can and more.

Handwriting Recognition

A special function offered by handheld computers with touch-sensitive screens is handwriting recognition. In a perfect world, you would write with your stylus on the screen as you do on paper. This approach hasn't materialized in practice for many reasons. True handwriting recognition goes way beyond a 26-letter alphabet. It means interpreting the millions of variations possible for every letter. The kind of computing power needed is still much too bulky for handheld computers. Furthermore, small screens don't allow for natural left-to-right hand movement. Let's face it—if you or your patients can't read your handwriting, with a multibillion-cell parallel processing neural network at work, why should a computer be able to?

The challenge of handwriting recognition has understandably stumped electrical engineers and computer programmers alike. Then, in 1996, Jeff Hawkins and his development team introduced their first Palm Pilot handheld computer to the world and everything changed. The Palm Pilot applied a novel approach to handwriting recognition dubbed Graffiti. Graffiti required less processing power and worked fine with a small screen. And, unlike most previous attempts at handwriting recognition, it was an instant success. (Pocket PC owners, keep reading. Like most good ideas, Microsoft has its own version of Graffiti on the Pocket PC, called "Block Recognizer." Plus, it has some other options that we describe later.)

This is how it works. First, a stylized alphabet eliminates some of the ambiguity with certain letters, hence the name Graffiti. (How do you distinguish a "U" from a "V"? Write "U" forward—that's a "U"; write it backward—that's a "V.") Second, letters are written one on top of the other, as if in a stack.

If you're using a Palm OS, change the shortcut discussed in Hands-On Exercise 2.1 so that the Graffiti Help pop-up displays (Figure 2.7). If you're using a Pocket PC, open Pocket Word (tap on the Start menu, Programs, and Word) and then select "Block Recognizer" from the list that can pop up in the lower right-hand corner of the screen (Figure 2.8). Most people find the stylized letters surprisingly intuitive. Making a short upstroke of the pen in the text entry area works like the shift key on a typewriter

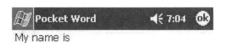

My name is

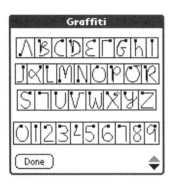

FIGURE 2.7. Palm OS Graffiti help. (Reprinted with permission from palmOne, Inc.)

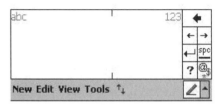

FIGURE 2.8. Pocket PC Block Recognizer. (Reprinted with permission from Microsoft Corporation.)

(Figure 2.9a). An up arrow appears at the bottom right of the screen to indicate the next letter entered will be capitalized. Make two short upstrokes, and the Caps Lock indicator appears, an up arrow with a line across it (Palm; Figure 2.9b) or the letters "ABC" instead of "abc" (Pocket PC). The Graffiti Help on the Palm OS devices is a bit incomplete. Some pen strokes are missing, such as the backward "U" just mentioned. Another is the alpha "α" pen stroke. Write it forward to make a "K." This is no surprise, but a backward alpha makes an "X" in one pen stroke instead of two.

Some people will never learn Graffiti, and that's OK. Although the learning curve is not too steep, it does require a little effort. You may find you

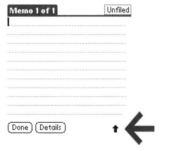

FIGURE 2.9a. Text entry area with "shift key" indicator. (Reprinted with permission from palmOne, Inc.)

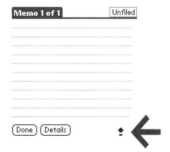

FIGURE 2.9b. Text entry area with "shift lock" indicator. (Reprinted with permission from palmOne, Inc.)

FIGURE 2.10. Example of program using pop-up menus for text entry. (Reprinted with permission from palmOne, Inc.)

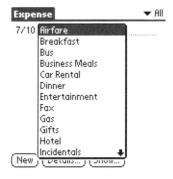

never have to input data on your handheld. The built-in software discussed next includes a comprehensive desktop component; you can input everything using your familiar desktop keyboard. Other programs are made to order for Graffiti. Most database programs for handhelds allow for text entry using pop-up menus. In this case, "writing" consists mostly of selecting text from menus. The Expenses program included with some versions of the Palm OS uses a pop-up list to enter expense categories (Figure 2.10). In the rare event that you do need to input a short blurb of text directly, Graffiti works very efficiently.

HANDS-ON EXERCISE 2.3. GRAFFITI SHORTCUTS (PALM OS)

Graffiti shortcuts make writing with Graffiti even faster. To create a shortcut, go again to the Preference program. This time, select "Shortcuts" from the top-right-corner menu (Figure 2.11). Tap the "New" button to write your own shortcut. The Shortcut Name should be something short, preferably a single letter, and easy to remember. Try "js" as the name, and then type in "Joe Smith" for the Shortcut Text (Figure 2.12). If "js" is already being used as a Shortcut Name, you can't use it again. Likewise, Shortcut Names are not case sensitive—"js" and "JS" count as one name, not two.

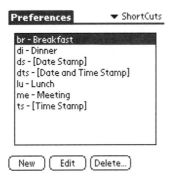

FIGURE 2.11. Shortcut preference menu. (Reprinted with permission from palmOne, Inc.)

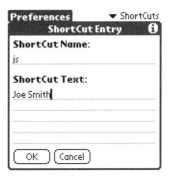

FIGURE 2.12. Creating new shortcut. (Reprinted with permission from palmOne, Inc.)

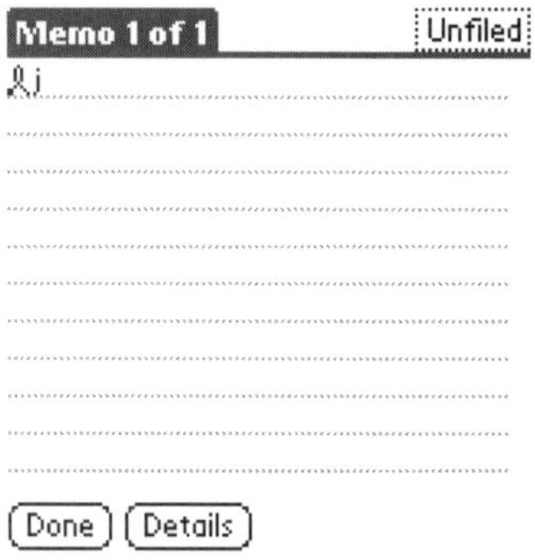

Memo 1 of 1 ⬛ Unfiled	Memo 1 of 1 ⬛ Unfiled
ℓj	Joe Smith‖
(Done) (Details)	(Done) (Details)

FIGURE 2.13a. Using a shortcut to enter text. (Reprinted with permission from palmOne, Inc.)

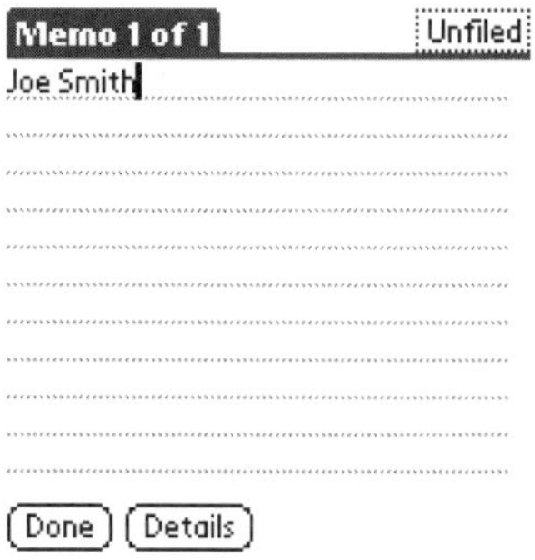

FIGURE 2.13b. Text substituted for shortage. (Reprinted with permission from palmOne, Inc.)

Once you've created a Shortcut, it's time to try it out. Go to any text entry area, such as the Memo Pad accessed by pressing the bottom-right mechanical button. Tap the New button to open a Memo, and, using Graffiti, draw a ℓ in the text entry area. Then write your Shortcut Name, and instantly, the Shortcut Text appears (Figure 2.13a, 13b).

You may find that the pop-up keyboard is the quickest way to enter text. Access the keyboard by tapping the small "abc" icon at the bottom-left corner of the text entry area. Type by tapping with your stylus on the screen (Figure 2.14). You can also position the cursor by tapping directly over the text and highlight text by dragging the stylus across it. Tap on the "Done" button at the bottom to close the pop-up keyboard and enter the text. Turn the keyboard into a numeric keypad by tapping the "123" button at the bottom center (Figure 2.15). Graffiti is sometimes too slow for quickly jotting down phone numbers. If you make one mistake along the way, that throws you off and you end up asking the person to repeat the number. The numeric keypad works well then.

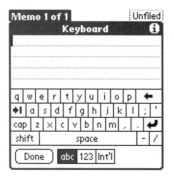

FIGURE 2.14. Pop-up keyboard. (Reprinted with permission from palmOne, Inc.)

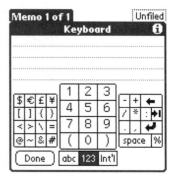

FIGURE 2.15. Pop-up numeric keyboard. (Reprinted with permission from palmOne, Inc.)

HANDS-ON EXERCISE 2.4. MORE DATA ENTRY TIPS (POCKET PC)

The Pocket PC also includes three other ways to enter data. Run Pocket Word by tapping on the Windows flag in the upper-left corner to open the Start menu, selecting Programs, and tapping once on the Pocket Word icon. In the bottom-right corner is a menu that pops up when you tap the upward-pointing arrow. Do that now (Figure 2.16) and select "Keyboard." This one's easy—just tap on it with your stylus. I find it best for entering text when there are lots of numbers and special symbols, like addresses. Now open the menu again, and select "Transcriber" (you may have to install this separately; see the CD-ROM that comes with your device for details). This is a version of the handwriting recognition software that came with the Newton—but don't let that turn you off. It is much more accurate now, and works quite well if your handwriting is neat. I find it very useful for scribbling quick notes, when I'm not too worried about an occasional transcription error (an error rate of about 1 in 30 letters with practice). With Transcriber, you can write anywhere on the screen, and your letters appear where the cursor is flashing. Make sure your letters are relatively neat and that each letter is s e p a r a t e d from the previous one. One hint about Transcriber—it is important to tell it how you make your letters, using the Letter Shapes tool (Figure 2.17). You can access this tool from the icon that looks like a Greek letter alpha, and then save your settings.

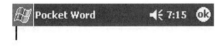

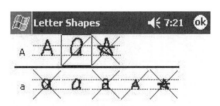

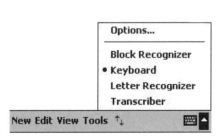

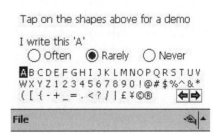

FIGURE 2.16. Select Pocket PC keyboard. (Reprinted with permission from Microsoft Corporation.)

FIGURE 2.17. Pocket PC letter shapes. (Reprinted with permission from Microsoft Corporation.)

Built-In Software (Palm OS)

Once you get the hang of the Palm OS user interface, mastering the built-in software is a breeze. The original Palm Pilot handheld computer of 1996 embodied the KISS principle ("Keep It Simple, Stupid") better than any commercial techno gadget since the first pocket calculator. Feature creep usually means more bells and whistles at the expense of performance and reliability. In the world of handheld computing, battery life and device size take priority, and feature creep can spell disaster. The Palm Pilot team did well to resist pressure to fatten up their software with other features. The resulting software package includes essential functions for a handheld digital organizer, no more and no less. The fact that Palm OS handheld devices are the most popular, least expensive such devices on the market (with the longest battery life!) goes to show that the KISS principle holds true.

So what functions are essential? The Palm OS includes the following components: (1) Address book, (2) Calendar with alarm function, (3) To Do list, (4) Memo pad, and (5) Calculator. Nothing too high tech, and nothing you haven't used before in a different form. Newer models include other built-in features including image viewers for personal photos and email programs for reading and authoring email messages on the go. Much to everyone's dismay, Solitaire, Tetris and, new on the scene, Bejeweled are not included in the Palm OS. While they are in fact essential programs and should be included, they are not. Nobody's perfect.

Using the built-in software is best experienced by trial and error. The functions mirror what you already do with Microsoft Outlook or the equivalent. Once you familiarize yourself with the touch-sensitive screen and stylus, the user interface proves straightforward to master. As a starting point, let's walk through an imaginary day with a handheld computer.

6:00 A.M.: Wake up, bathe, and get dressed slipping your handheld into a jacket pocket. As you walk out the door, a familiar beeping alarm gets your attention. You pull out your handheld and see a Reminder message on the screen, "Going away party—bring soda." Tapping "OK" with the stylus clears the message (Figure 2.18). You grab the soda from the basement and drive off to the office.

7:00 A.M.: Arriving at work, you sit down at your desk to review the day's schedule. Your secretary entered patient names and appointment times into the Palm Desktop software yesterday afternoon. You review the list on your desktop computer first (Figure 2.19). Then you perform a HotSync operation with the desktop computer to copy the schedule to your handheld device (discussed next). You must make an important phone call between patients at about 10 A.M., so you decide to set an alarm to remind you. Turning on the handheld, you press the bottom-left mechanical button to bring up the Calendar. Your schedule of appointments appears with today's date in the top-left corner of the screen

FIGURE 2.18. Alarm reminder message. (Reprinted with permission from palmOne, Inc.)

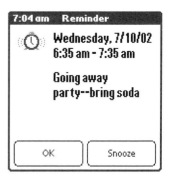

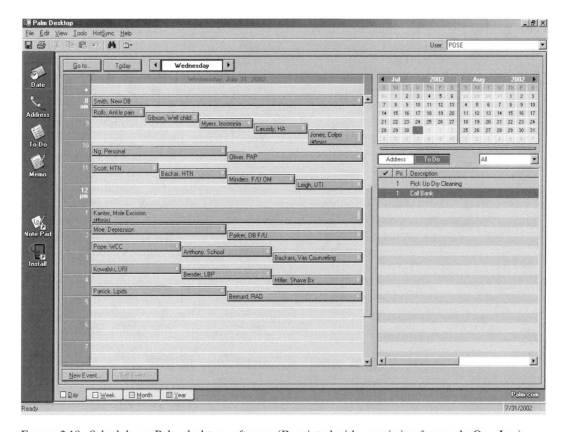

FIGURE 2.19. Schedule on Palm desktop software. (Reprinted with permission from palmOne, Inc.)

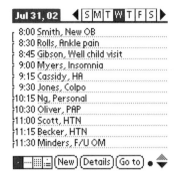

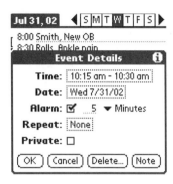

FIGURE 2.20. Schedule on handheld. (Reprinted with permission from palmOne, Inc.)

FIGURE 2.21. Setting alarm for event in calendar. (Reprinted with permission from palmOne, Inc.)

(Figure 2.20). Tap over the text entered at the "10:00" line to position the cursor there. Then tap the "Details" button centered at the bottom of the screen. Tap the "Alarm" checkbox to set the alarm. The default alarm occurs 5 minutes before the event, which is fine (Figure 2.21).

7:30 A.M.: It's time for your first patient. The day is rolling along nicely. Your 8:30 patient is moving soon to a new city. You have a good friend who practices in the area. Press the second mechanical button from the left to bring up the Address Book. The cursor is already positioned at the "Look Up" line centered at the bottom of the screen (Figure 2.22). Using Graffiti, you jot down the first two letters of your friend's name. Two different entries appear—one with his private address and the other with his professional information (Figure 2.23). Tapping on the second entry brings up the office address and phone number (Figure 2.24). You share this with your patient and say good-bye.

10:00 A.M.: Just when the day is getting very busy, an alarm goes off. Without looking at your handheld, you remember the phone call you need to make and hurry to your office. You need to call the bank to finalize a loan to buy new office furniture. The bank phone number is in your handheld

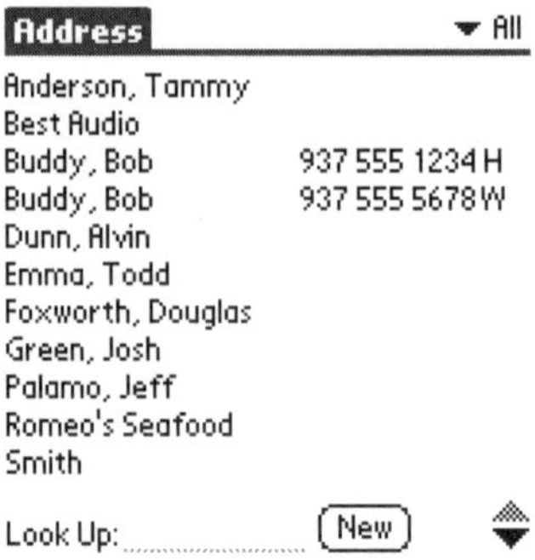

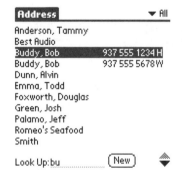

FIGURE 2.22. Address book. (Reprinted with permission from palmOne, Inc.)

FIGURE 2.23. Address book name lookup. (Reprinted with permission from palmOne, Inc.)

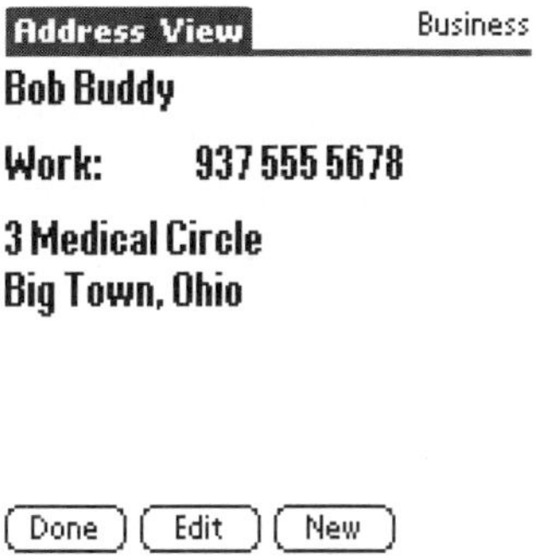

FIGURE 2.24. Address
book entry. (Reprinted
with permission from
palmOne, Inc.)

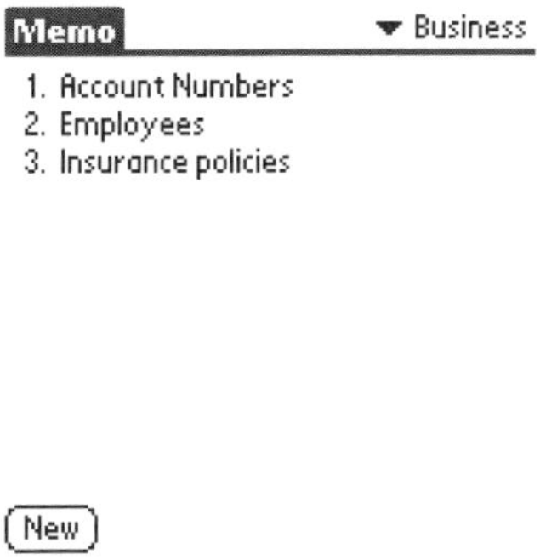

FIGURE 2.25. Memo pad.
(Reprinted with permission
from palmOne, Inc.)

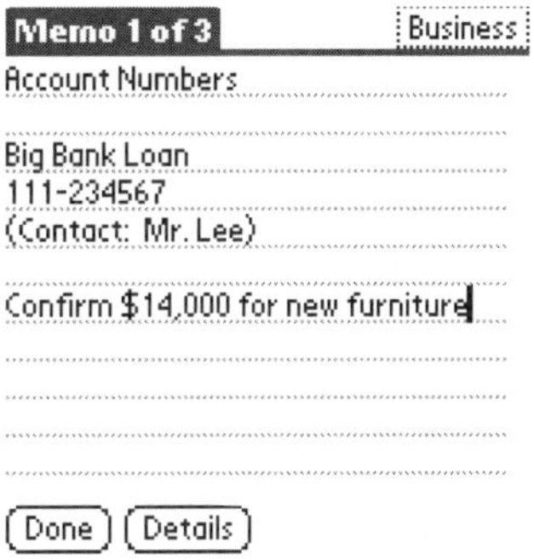

FIGURE 2.26. Memo pad
entry. (Reprinted with
permission from palmOne,
Inc.)

Address Book. When talking to the loan officer, he asks you to confirm
the account number and final amount. You keep that in the handheld
Memo Pad. Push the bottom-right mechanical button to open the Memo
Pad (Figure 2.25). Tap "Account Numbers" in the list of memos, and read
the account number off to the loan officer (Figure 2.26).

12:00 P.M.: You've now finished your morning clinic. There have been a
few reported cases of Lyme disease in your area. During your lunch
break, you take time to read a review article on diagnosis and treatment. You can type notes as a Memo on your Palm Desktop software
(Figure 2.27). When you perform another HotSync operation, the
Memo is transferred to your handheld for easy reference when seeing
patients (Figure 2.28).

2:00 P.M.: Several times during your afternoon clinic, the handheld calculator comes in handy to compute antibiotic dosages for children. The
calculator is accessed by tapping the permanent button at the top-right
corner of the Graffiti entry area at the bottom of the screen (Figure
2.29).

3:00 P.M.: You've also created a Memo with predicted Peak Flow Rates
according to age, sex, and height (Figure 2.30). (A friend e-mailed you
a text document with the info, and you easily copied and pasted this
into a Memo using your Palm Desktop software. How smart you are!)

5:30 P.M.: The last patient leaves the clinic. Before wrapping up, you check
the handheld To Do List and see "Pick up dry cleaning" at the top of
the list. You'll be able to get that on the way home, but don't check it
off yet in case you forget. "Call bank" is also on the list—you check
that off as completed (Figure 2.31). (The item disappears but will be
archived on your desktop the next time you HotSync.)

This example just skims the surface of how a handheld computer can
benefit a busy physician or other care provider. Third-party medical software does much more to optimize patient care directly. We discuss other
software in detail later.

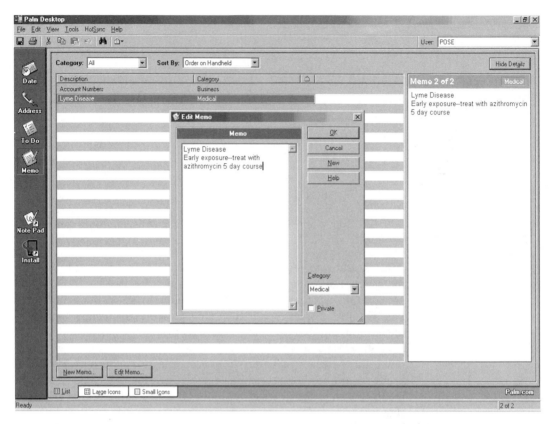

FIGURE 2.27. Memo pad on Palm desktop software. (Reprinted with permission from palmOne, Inc.)

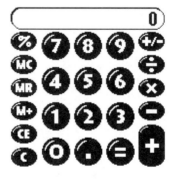

FIGURE 2.28. New Memo pad entry on handheld after HotSync. (Reprinted with permission from palmOne, Inc.)

FIGURE 2.29. Palm OS calculator. (Reprinted with permission from palmOne, Inc.)

FIGURE 2.30. Memo pad entry with Peak Flow rate. (Reprinted with permission from palmOne, Inc.)

FIGURE 2.31. To do list. (Reprinted with permission from palmOne, Inc.)

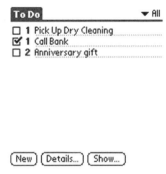

Built-In Software (Pocket PC)

When Microsoft designed the Pocket PC, they definitely had a "let's cram as much as possible in here" mentality. Your little 6- or 7-ounce Pocket PC comes with all the following:

- Calendar (date book)
- Contacts (address book)
- Tasks (to do list)
- Notes (note taker)
- Inbox (e-mail)
- Pocket Word (word processor)
- Pocket Excel (spreadsheet)
- Microsoft Reader (electronic book reader)
- Windows Media Player (plays music and movies)
- Internet Explorer (Web browser)
- File Explorer (file manager)
- And of course . . . Solitaire!

Wow! All this power means that you can do a lot more with your Pocket PC than with a simpler device. Their growing popularity (by the time this book appears in print, I hope to win my bet with Pete and Scott that they will be the best-selling handheld computers) means that people want to do more with their handheld computer than replace a date book. It also means that the learning curve is somewhat steeper—there are no free lunches. We'll step through a typical day, learning about the built-in software as we go along.

6:00 A.M.: A loud, insistent beeping wakes you. You fumble for the Pocket PC and turn it on. The bright screen guides you to the bathroom. After getting ready, feeding the dog, and grabbing some coffee, you turn on your handheld. The day's first appointment is shown on the

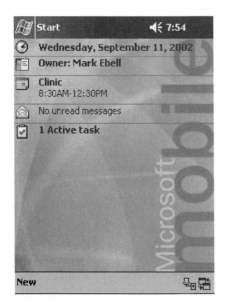

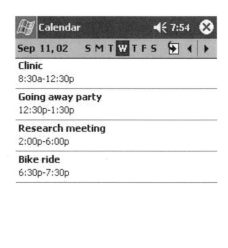

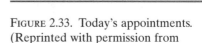

FIGURE 2.32. Pocket PC home page. (Reprinted with permission from Microsoft Corporation.)

FIGURE 2.33. Today's appointments. (Reprinted with permission from Microsoft Corporation.)

"Today" screen, sort of a home page for your Pocket PC (Figure 2.32). Tap on the calendar icon, and you are shown a list of all of the day's appointments (Figure 2.33). Cool, bike ride to finish the day.

7:00 A.M.: You get to the hospital a few minutes late for the monthly staff meeting . . . but as usual, you haven't missed much. Hmmm. You pull out your Pocket PC and load an electronic book, turning the pages with the "rocker button" and making the best of a stultifyingly boring meeting (Figure 2.34). Your partner nudges you, and asks if you'll cover his call on Saturday in exchange for a "call day to be named later." You press the mechanical "Calendar" button on the front of your Pocket PC, and tap the letter "S" near the top of the screen to show Saturday. No appointments. "Sure" you say, and select "New" to create a new appointment. A screen for entering information about your appointment appears, and you use Transcriber to write "Call," and then tap in the "Type" field and select "All day" (Figure 2.35). You set the alarm to remind you 1 day ahead of time, and you're done. Now, that day has a band with "Call" across the top to remind you of this all-day event (Figure 2.36). Tapping on the "monthly calendar" icon shows you the whole month, with the day of call indicated by the square in September 14th (Figure 2.37). There are other more polished planners, such as Pocket Informant, but you can do plenty with the plain vanilla calendar.

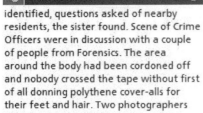

identified, questions asked of nearby residents, the sister found. Scene of Crime Officers were in discussion with a couple of people from Forensics. The area around the body had been cordoned off and nobody crossed the tape without first of all donning polythene cover-alls for their feet and hair. Two photographers were busy taking flash photographs under portable lighting powered by a nearby generator. And next to the generator stood an operations van, where another photographer was trying to fix his jammed video camera.

"It's these cheap tapes," he complained. "They look like a bargain when you buy

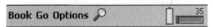

FIGURE 2.34. Electronic book example. (Reprinted with permission from Microsoft Corporation.)

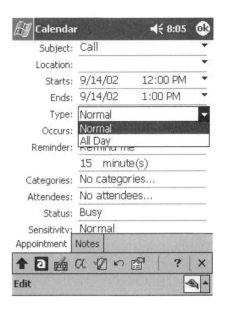

FIGURE 2.35. Appointment type. (Reprinted with permission from Microsoft Corporation.)

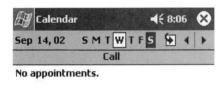

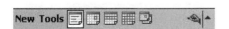

FIGURE 2.36. Event reminder. (Reprinted with permission from Microsoft Corporation.)

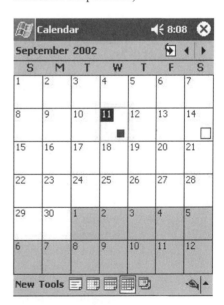

FIGURE 2.37. Monthly calendar. (Reprinted with permission from Microsoft Corporation.)

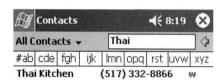

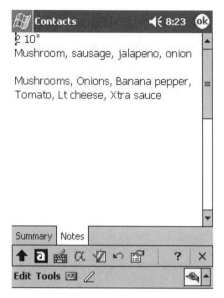

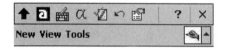

FIGURE 2.38. Search for "Thai Kitchen." (Reprinted with permission from Microsoft Corporation.)

FIGURE 2.39. Contact notes. (Reprinted with permission from Microsoft Corporation.)

12:30 P.M.: After a busy morning of clinic, you remember that you were supposed to call for dinner reservations at that Thai place—Thai Garden? Spice of Thai? what was the name? You tap on the Contacts button on the front of your Pocket PC and write "Thai" on the screen. The letters appear in the search windows, and the handheld computer quickly searches more than 1200 contacts to find the one with the word Thai in it: Thai Kitchen (Figure 2.38). Hey, this is handy! You decide to enter your favorite pizza joint, tap on the Notes tab, and enter your usual order (Figure 2.39).

4:00 P.M.: Your research meeting is going well. You've used your Stow-away folding keyboard, attached to your Pocket PC, to take detailed notes and develop an "Action plan" for your team. To share it with each member, you all pull out your Pocket PC's. On yours, which has the original document, you select "Beam Document . . ." from the Tools menu in Pocket Word (Figure 2.40). Your colleagues each select "Pro-grams" from the Start menu, and then "Infrared Receive" (Henry does a lot of this, so he's already assigned this program to one of his hard-ware buttons to speed things up). You point your devices at each other, each remembering your favorite Star Trek episode, and watch the file beam via infrared to each of the other devices (Figure 2.41).

7:30 P.M.: Great ride! Now it's time to add it to my log, which I keep in a Pocket Excel spreadsheet (Figure 2.42). The spreadsheet even syn-chronizes with a copy on my desktop. Now, I've got to save up for a GPS card and mapping software for that next bike tour!

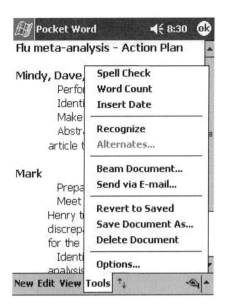

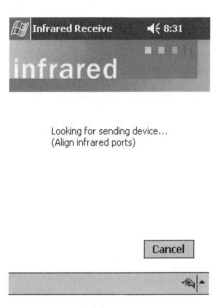

FIGURE 2.40. Pocket PC word processing. (Reprinted with permission from Microsoft Corporation.)

FIGURE 2.41. Beaming files. (Reprinted with permission from Microsoft Corporation.)

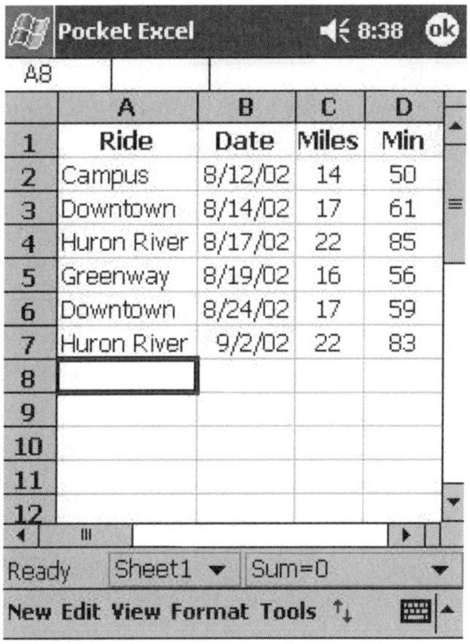

FIGURE 2.42. Using a Pocket PC spreadsheet. (Reprinted with permission from Microsoft Corporation.)

Key Points

1. Palm OS devices include all the essential software needed in a personal organizer. The intuitive user interface is quickly mastered by most users.
2. Pocket PC devices come with more extensive software that reproduces many functions of desktop computers. The learning curve is steep, but less so if you already use Microsoft Office.

Connecting and Synchronizing

An unsynchronized handheld is like one hand clapping; synchronization is the defining element that made the Palm Pilot, its progeny, and Pocket PC's the successes they are today. Without synchronization, we all may have fallen in and out of love with handheld computers the same way we did with other digital address books and organizers on the market. You know the drill. Enter all your names, phone numbers, and addresses. Gradually gain confidence that the alarm will work and you won't miss your meetings. Boldly declare, "I've bought the last address book I'll ever need to buy!" Then, "Oh, @##$! Where are my data?" The moment of revelation is nauseating. Dropped in the toilet, batteries fell out, memory wiped clean by a diabolical cosmic ray—it doesn't matter how—you are out of luck. Back you go to your desk drawer full of old address books, calendars, and sticky notes. "Why did I ever go digital?" you ask yourself. You breathe a sigh of acceptance and make a heartfelt vow, "Never again."

The Palm and Pocket PC handhelds, however, shine for this one all-important reason. Your data are backed up on your desktop computer every time you synchronize. Although doom may strike your handheld, you'll live to see another day. All you do is place your new or repaired handheld device in the cradle (and push the HotSync button if it is a Palm OS device). The whole process takes from seconds to several minutes, and you're covered. Unless some catastrophe takes out both your desktop and your handheld computer simultaneously, you can always restore one from the other.

HotSyncing Your Palm Device

During the HotSync process, one of four actions can occur with each program running on the handheld device, including the built-in programs. The possible actions are as follows: (1) nothing happens; (2) the desktop data overwrite the handheld data (all handheld data are lost); (3) the handheld data overwrite the desktop data (all desktop data are lost); or (4) data are synchronized between the desktop and handheld software. You can change what happens with each program via the HotSync Manager software installed together with the Palm Desktop software. Double-click the

HotSync Manager icon on your system tray (usually at the bottom right of your Windows desktop next to the clock) (Figure 2.43). A menu will appear. Click "Custom . . ." to see the current action selected for each program (Figure 2.44). Select a program, and click the "Change" button to change the current action (Figure 2.45).

Thus, "performing a HotSync operation" and "synchronizing your handheld" can mean two different things. Sometimes the HotSync operation will overwrite information from one device to the other; sometimes files will be actually synchronized. True synchronization entails one of two processes, FastSync or SlowSync, that occur invisibly to the user. The difference are unimportant if you only HotSync on one computer. However, you may choose to HotSync on multiple computers, such as one at work and one at home, or across a network. In this case, the difference may be significant.

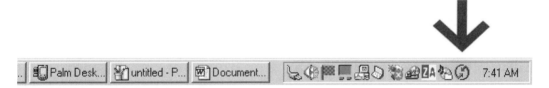

FIGURE 2.43. HotSync Manager icon. (Reprinted with permission from palmOne, Inc.)

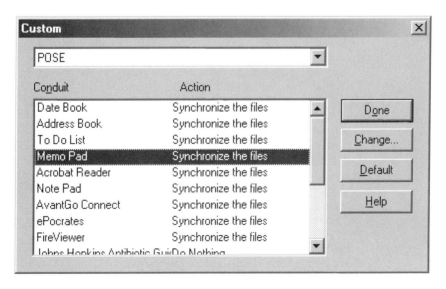

FIGURE 2.44. HotSync Manager on desktop. (Reprinted with permission from palmOne, Inc.)

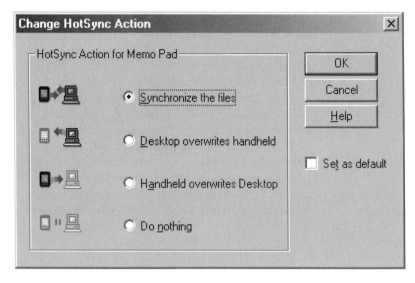

FIGURE 2.45. Changing HotSync action for Palm OS Memo Pad. (Reprinted with permission from palmOne, Inc.)

Advanced Topic: Fast and Slow Synchronization

To understand the different types of synchronization, you need to first know how data are stored in the handheld memory. With Palm OS handhelds, all data are stored in the Palm Database format. On your desktop, these files carry the corresponding ".PDB" file extension. Program files, on the other hand, carry the ".PRC" files extension. Within each file, information is further divided into records. For example, the Palm OS Memo Pad resides in the file "Memo.PDB." Each Memo is stored as a record within this file. Each PDB file includes header info that lists, among other things, the record number, record length, and whether or not each record is "Dirty." Records are marked as "Dirty" if modified since the last HotSync Operation.

Palm OS supports two types of synchronization. Standard synchronization is termed FastSync. During FastSync, file header information is queried first. Only "Dirty" records are transferred to the desktop computer for further comparison to corresponding desktop records. (All newly created records are by default marked "Dirty.") If neither the handheld nor the desktop record in a given database file is "Dirty," nothing happens. Otherwise, the date/time last modified is compared, and the most recently modified record is saved to both the handheld and the desktop.

FastSync is elegant and proceeds very quickly when most records in a database have not been modified, as is often the case. FastSync fails however when synchronizing your handheld on multiple desktop computers.

Continued

Consider this example. Let's say you have a record in your Address Book with the telephone number for Mr. Lincoln. This record exists on your hand-held as well as Desktop Computer A at home and Desktop Computer B at work. As it happens, you edit the record at different times at all three loca-tions, and all three records are marked "Dirty." Next, you perform a HotSync operation with Desktop Computer A. The handheld record for Mr. Lincoln is marked "Dirty" and is compared to the equivalent desktop record as expected. The record that was most recently modified is saved to both the Desktop Computer A and the handheld, and the "Dirty" attribute is removed. OK, all is well. Now, perform a HotSync operation with Desktop Computer B. With FastSync, confusion occurs because, whether or not the handheld record contains the most recent information, it is no longer marked "Dirty." The record on Desktop Computer B is still marked "Dirty" and may over-write the handheld record regardless of date/time last modified.

SlowSync solves the problem of corrupted data when synchronizing with more than one desktop computer. With its built-in applications, such as the Address Book and Memo Pad, Palm OS reliably implements SlowSync when-ever the HotSync Manager detects that the handheld was last synchronized with a different desktop computer.

In this case, the "Dirty" status for handheld records is determined de novo. Each record is compare to a backup copy saved on that particular desktop during the last HotSync operation. (This backup copy is separate from the Palm desktop database files and is not modified between HotSync events.) A handheld record with a time/date last modified later than that of its backup equivalent is considered "Dirty" and is compared, in turn, to its desktop equiv-alents as described above for FastSync synchronization.

With SlowSync, every single record is transferred between the handheld and desktop at least once. This guarantees the integrity of your data but also makes for significantly slower synchronization times.

Importantly, not all handheld applications support both types of synchro-nization, FastSync and SlowSync. Palm recommends strongly that they do, but some software developers take the easy way out. The choice between Fast-Sync and SlowSync occurs without user input and, for the most part, you can only guess how synchronization takes place for a given application. You'll notice that some programs synchronize very slowly every time—they proba-bly take a SlowSync approach and compare every record in all situations. The delay is unnecessary and annoying, but at least data integrity is maintained.

Other handheld applications will synchronize using a FastSync approach even when synchronization occurs among different desktop computers. This can be extremely dangerous if you are managing critical data such as patient and other medical information on your handheld!

Simply put, **don't synchronize sensitive medical data between different desktop computers unless you're sure data integrity is maintained**. If you plan to synchronize medical applications in this way, first check with the software developer or, better yet, test out yourself, whether your data will synchronize reliably.

Some software applications handle well the challenge of synchronizing with multiple desktop computers. Others do not and ultimately lead to corrupted or lost data. A safe solution, when synchronizing with two desktop computers, is to set up one computer to synchronize and the other to overwrite. For example, if you keep your schedule on your office computer, you should synchronize your handheld there at work. Then, the Palm Desktop software will reflect changes you make on your handheld, and your handheld will reflect changes made on the desktop, perhaps by a secretary or assistant. On your home computer, edit your HotSync Manager settings so the "Handheld Overwrites Desktop." When you HotSync at home, all info will be copied from handheld to desktop by default. You can view your schedule at home, access phone numbers and memos, etc.

If you make changes that you'd like to add to your work computer, you can temporarily set the HotSync Manager for "Desktop Overwrites Handheld," perform a HotSync operation, and then change back to your default settings of "Handheld Overwrites Desktop."

Pocket PC Synchronization

The Pocket PC synchronizes very much like Palm OS. It uses software called "Microsoft ActiveSync." You can always download a free copy from www.microsoft.com/pocketpc: click on the link to "Downloads." The first time you place your device in the cradle, it will take up to 5 or 10 minutes to synchronize your information. After that, it only takes about 1 minute or less. You can check or uncheck boxes next to an item (such as Calendar or InBox) to determine whether it is synchronized. Go to www.avantgo.com to set up an account if you want to use this feature.

A great feature is the ability to synchronize files. ActiveSync creates a folder on your desktop that allows you to synchronize word processor files, spreadsheets, maps, or whatever else you want to keep on your desktop computer and Pocket PC (Figure 2.46). Just drag and drop a file into this folder, and the next time you synch, it will be converted and copied to the Pocket PC. Then, any changes made to the file on your Pocket PC will also show up in the synchronized file in the desktop folder. One caveat: because Pocket Word and Pocket Excel do not support some of the desktop program's features

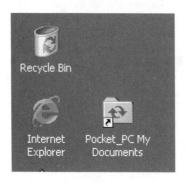

FIGURE 2.46. Pocket PC ActiveSync folder icon on desktop computer. (Reprinted with permission from Microsoft Corporation.)

(notably tables in Pocket Word), you can lose some formatting. Therefore, this works best with relatively simple documents and spreadsheets.

If you are having problems, make sure you open "Connection Settings" from the "File" menu, and that the "Allow USB connection with this desktop computer" box is checked. That assumes that you are using USB, which most of us do. Also, note that you can customize the rules controlling which version of a file or date or address "wins" when there is a conflict, and whether files are converted to and from the Pocket PC format.

Beam Me Up, Mr. Scott!* Communicating with Other Handhelds

Some people have a strong natural aversion to electronic gizmos. Beaming, however, always attracts attention, even from the most diehard antitechnology types. Why exactly is a mystery; wireless communication occurs all around us, all the time, without much applause. Most people under 40 take such things as satellite TV and cell phones for granted. But beam a Memo or Address Book between two handhelds and a crowd gathers.

Beaming uses the same type of infrared (IR) technology found in home stereo remote controls. Unlike radio frequency transmission, IR transmission is line of sight only. It does not travel around corners or through walls. All the Palm OS and Pocket PC built-in programs support beaming. You can easily beam Address Book and Memo Pad entries, for example. Physicians often use beaming to transfer patient lists when going on and off call. The maximal beaming distance depends on ambient lighting conditions. Strong sunlight can interrupt beaming altogether. Beaming is also slow: it isn't a great way to transfer files large than 100 to 200 KB.

Line-of-sight transmission is inherently secure. If you can't see someone standing nearby with another handheld device, they shouldn't be able to intercept your transmission. Theoretically, a program could request and verify an identification code before beaming (an electronic handshake). The built-in Palm OS and Pocket PC programs, however, do not incorporate any such additional security measures. You can actually beam to several devices at the same time. Each person receives the transmission and has the option to accept or reject it.

Automatic receipt of beamed transmissions can be disabled via the Palm OS Preferences program already discussed. Few computer viruses exist for handhelds, but there is potential for beamed computer viruses.

All in all, beaming has pluses and minuses. Beaming an address is definitely faster than writing it down and saves the extra step of data entry later. It's also a good way to swap trial versions of software, as we discuss later. Of note, you can perform an infrared ActiveSync (Pocket PC) or HotSync (Palm) operation with a properly equipped desktop or notebook computer. It goes very slowly, however, taking much longer than even a serial connection.

*Kirk never actually says "Beam me up, Scotty"—he says "Mr. Scott." Often misquoted.

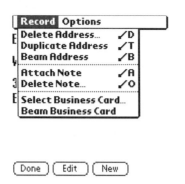

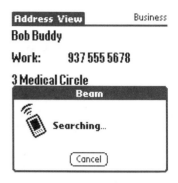

FIGURE 2.47. Selecting "Beam" from menu options. (Reprinted with permission from palmOne, Inc.)

FIGURE 2.48. Accepting beamed data from other handheld user. (Reprinted with permission from palmOne, Inc.)

Many programs incorporate some type of beaming function. Try beaming from the handheld Address book. For a Palm OS device, open the Address book and select a name as you did in the "7:30 A.M." example earlier. Then tap on the permanent Menu button at the bottom-left corner of the screen. A menu will appear across the top of the screen. Tap "Record" and then "Beam Address" from the pop-down menu (Figure 2.47). A status window will appear on your handheld with messages indicated that it is searching for another handheld, beaming the address, and has completed beaming (Figure 2.48). A similar status window will appear on the receiving handheld anytime an IR signal is sensed. You can turn off automatic receipt of beamed messages. Go the Preferences program already discussed and select "General" from the top-right corner menu. "Beam Receive" is the last option on the screen.

It works much the same way on the Pocket PC. Just select "Beam contacts" from the Tools menu of the Contacts, Calendar, or other IR-enabled application. To receive a contact, select "Start | Programs | Infrared receive." If you regularly beam back and forth with people, I'd recommend adding that little program to your start menu. Just select "Start | Settings | Menus," scroll down till you find "Infrared receive," and check the box next to it.

Summary

We've introduced you to touch-sensitive screens, use of a stylus, and handwriting recognition capability for both Palm OS and Pocket PC devices. You've walked through a typical day using the built-in handheld software and learned to synchronize data between your handheld and a desktop computer. You've even learned to beam data wirelessly from one handheld to another.

So now you're getting to know your handheld and the question becomes, "Are you hooked?" We hope you are. In the following sections, we'll delve more into medical-specific software and clinical applications of handheld computers.

3

Getting Software from Cyberspace to the Palm of Your Hand: Downloading and Installing Software on Your Palm OS or Pocket PC Handheld

Scott M. Strayer and Mark H. Ebell

By now, you have probably rushed out to your favorite handheld computer retail outlet, and taken the plunge to buy your first handheld computer. Trust me, you won't be disappointed. The fun is just about to begin!

In this chapter we detail the process of downloading and installing all the great medical software from the Internet that is described in Section II. I personally struggled with downloading and installing software for 2 weeks until a generous fellow handheld user explained the process to me. It really isn't that hard, so long as you stick to the basics of file management on your PC or Mac computer and follow these simple step-by-step instructions.

One of the great things you will learn about handheld software is that it usually comes as a very small file (normally less than 1 MB). Even better, most of the software programmers must have learned a thing or two from drug reps, because many programs are free, and even the commercial versions usually have a free 30-day demo. Thus, you can stock your handheld with excellent medical software at no cost, and you can trial just about any other software available through the Internet. On the other hand, as with the information from drug reps, there is sometimes a catch with the free software. Creating high-quality software, keeping it up-to-date, and responding to the needs of users is a full-time job, so don't hesitate to part with a little green to support your local computer programmer!

Getting all these great medical resources from cyberspace into the palm of your hand really involves three simple steps. First, you have to identify the software you want, which we cover in detail in the next section of the book. Second, you have to download and sometimes "uncompress" the software package. Finally, you have to install it to your Palm OS or Pocket PC handheld computer.

Downloading the Software from Cyberspace

The first step in downloading software is identifying the software you want to use. We highly recommend checking out all the Web sites listed in Chapter 4, as well as the Web sites of the applications listed in subsequent chapters.

HANDS-ON EXERCISE 3.1. GETTING THE SOFTWARE FROM CYBERSPACE

Let's begin with the example of downloading PocketBilling, a popular charge capture program developed by yours truly (SMS) and available at www.pocketmed.org on the Internet. If you have a Pocket PC, don't worry—the steps are exactly the same for downloading and uncompressing software. You may want to go to www.handango.com and download the Pocket PC "program of the day" from their home page.

To complete the exercise described in this chapter, you need:

1. A desktop computer with Internet access.
2. A Palm OS handheld computer that is charged and has been HotSync'd at least once to the desktop (or laptop) computer that you will be using to download the software or a Pocket PC that is charged, sitting in its cradle, and synchronized with the desktop using "ActiveSync."
3. The latest version of the Palm Desktop (Palm) or ActiveSync (Pocket PC) software installed on your desktop or laptop computer.

Now, begin the exercise. Log on to the Internet as you normally would with your desktop or laptop computer, and use your browser (either Microsoft's Internet Explorer or Netscape) to locate this site: http://www.pocketmed.org/ PocketMed%20Products.htm. You can also go to www.pocketmed.org, click on "products," and then under "PocketBilling," select the "download demo" link. When you click on this or any site's download link, you should immediately see a box notifying you that you are downloading something (Figure 3.1).

Internet Explorer usually gives you the "File Download" box, and you should select "Save" (Figure 3.1). Netscape's browser may either give you a "File Download" box, or an "Unknown File Type" box (Figure 3.2). Depending on which box appears, select either "OK" or the "Save File" button to proceed with downloading the software to your desktop computer.

After selecting to download the file, you are prompted to specify where you would like to save it (Figure 3.3). This is an important step, and you should set up a folder on your computer where you consistently save your downloaded software. In this exercise, we have chosen a folder called "Downloads," which you can easily create on your desktop computer by following the instructions that come with your operating system. One of the

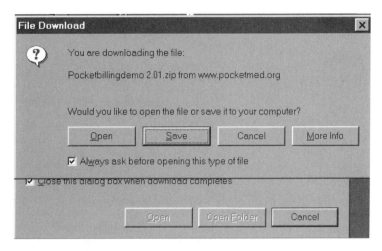

FIGURE 3.1. File Download box in Internet Explorer. (Reprinted with permission from Microsoft Corporation and PocketMed.)

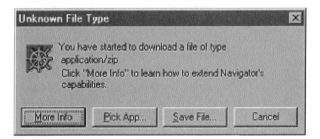

FIGURE 3.2. Unknown File Type download box in Netscape. (Reprinted with permission from Netscape.)

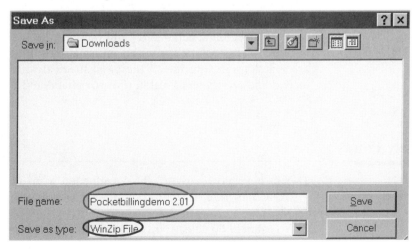

FIGURE 3.3. "Save As" box. (Reprinted with permission from Microsoft Corporation and PocketMed.)

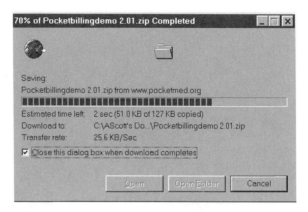

FIGURE 3.4. "File Download" box. (Reprinted with permission from Microsoft Corporation and PocketMed.)

most common mistakes for beginners is forgetting where they downloaded their software. Having a consistent location is very helpful in the long run. The more compulsive among us even create a subfolder within the Downloads folder for each new software package, especially when our lithium levels get a little low.

After you have determined where to download the file, click the "Save" button. A file download status box will appear, and a blue "progress bar" will show you the status of your download (Figure 3.4). At the end of the download, you should see a "Download complete" box; clicking on "Close" will clear your computer screen.

While the file is downloading (see Figure 3.3), be sure to make a note of the file name and also the file type (see light colored circle for file name and dark circle for file type in Figure 3.3). In this example, the name of the file is "PocketBillingdemo 2.01" and the file type is a "WinZip" file, which is in the "Save As Type" box. This information will be important when you are searching in vain for all the great medical software you have downloaded and are trying to install it to your handheld.

Key Points

1. You have now successfully downloaded a medical software program from the Internet using either Microsoft's Internet Explorer or Netscape's browser.
2. You should download software to a consistent location. In this example, we downloaded PocketBillingdemo 2.01 to the C:\Download file we created on the desktop.

3. Make sure you remember the name of the files you download, otherwise they are likely to get lost in computer land!

HANDS-ON EXERCISE 3.2. TO UNCOMPRESS OR NOT

As we mentioned in the previous section, noting the type of file helps you know whether uncompression is needed. Many files are compressed in either "zip" format or "sit" format and require uncompression before you can install the program to your handheld. Compression ("zip" and "sit" files) is simply a method of making software smaller for e-mailing and downloading. It also allows users to put many files into one big compressed file. If the file you downloaded was a ".prc," ".pdb," or ".exe" file, decompression won't be necessary as these files will either automatically install to the Palm OS (.prc files or .pdb files) if they are double-clicked, or will run automatically once they are double-clicked (.exe files) on the desktop. Most Pocket PC programs come in a ".exe" file.

Uncompression software programs are readily available on the Internet or might have already been installed on your computer when you bought it. If you double-click on the downloaded file and nothing happens, this is usually an indication that you need to download the utility. For example, in this exercise, we would browse to C:\downloads, and look for the file we just downloaded there (Figure 3.5).

If we double-click on the program and nothing happens, or a message warns you about an "Unknown file type", then you will need to download uncompression software. We like WinZip (www.winzip.com) for ZIP files and Stuffit (www.stuffit.com) for SIT files, but there are other good shareware programs that do the same thing. Most of these programs also come with a free trial, but you might want to register it if you plan on downloading a lot of software.

After you have the proper decompression software in place, simply double-click on the program, and you will see a window similar to Figure 3.6. In this window, you can see all the files that are included in the zip file along with information on the file sizes and compression ratios. You might notice that there are different types of files included in most downloads. In our example, there is a Palm file depicted by this icon ▣, along with a user manual in Word format depicted by this icon ▥. Even in this window, double-clicking on the Palm files will put them in the Palm installation tool so that they install on your next HotSync. Also, double-clicking on the user's manual or "Read me" text will open it for immediate viewing (assuming you have Word installed on your main computer).

Most users will want to select the "Extract" button on the top of the WinZip window (circled in Figure 3.6). After doing this, another window will pop up that asks you where you would like to save the uncompressed files (Figure 3.7). Of course, you can put the files anywhere you would like, but to simplify your life, I would highly recommend using a specific folder

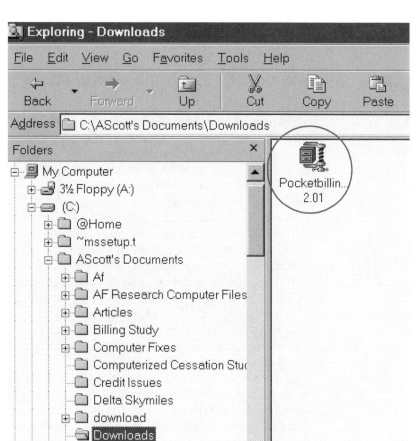

FIGURE 3.5. Downloaded file in Windows Explorer. (Reprinted with permission from Microsoft Corporation and PocketMed.)

similar to the "Download" folder created in the previous exercise. As noted earlier, you can even create a folder for your program within the Downloads folder.

In this exercise, let's create a new folder for just this set of files by clicking on "New Folder" (circle in Figure 3.7). We will call the new folder

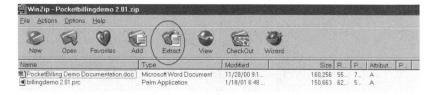

FIGURE 3.6. WinZip window showing decompressed software contained in zip file. (Reprinted with permission from Microsoft Corporation and PocketMed.)

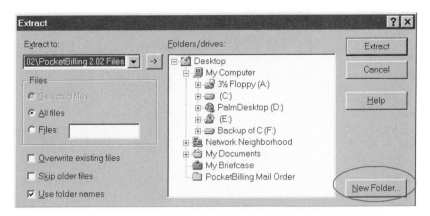

FIGURE 3.7. Winzip extraction window. (Reprinted with permission from Microsoft Corporation and PocketMed.)

"C:\PocketBilling Demo" in this example (Figure 3.8). Select "OK" after you have named the new folder. Next, select "Extract" to complete the uncompression process.

You can check on your progress by using the file manager on your computer and browsing to the location where everything was uncompressed. In our example, you would browse to C:\Downloads\PocketBilling Demo and "presto!" all the files are there (Figure 3.9). At this point you can decide whether you want to keep the compressed file in addition to the uncompressed files. If disk space isn't an issue, we would recommend keeping both. For organizational purposes, it might be a good idea to keep all the compressed files under the C:\Downloads directory and all the uncompressed files in folders named after each program. Use any naming and storage loca-

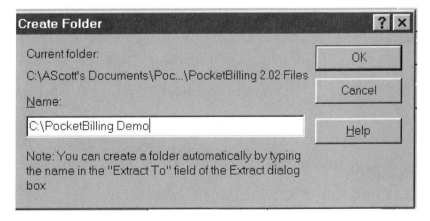

FIGURE 3.8. Creating a new folder in Winzip. (Reprinted with permission from Microsoft Corporation and PocketMed.)

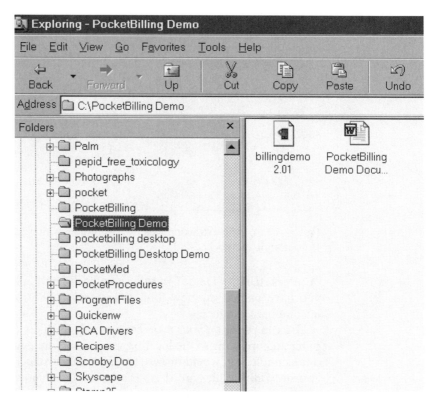

FIGURE 3.9. PocketBilling Demo folder in Windows Explorer with extracted files. (Reprinted with permission from Microsoft Corporation and PocketMed.)

tion that makes sense to you so that you don't forget where all this valuable software is stored.

Key Points

1. If the file you download is a "ZIP" file or "SIT" file, you will need to uncompress it using special uncompression software.
2. We recommend using either Winzip or Stuffit Expander for decompression. Some computers already have this software installed, but if you double-click on one of these files and nothing happens, you need to download it from the Internet.
3. Remember where you put the files after decompression!

The Final Step: Putting It on Your Handheld Computer

Congratulations! You have now successfully downloaded and decompressed your first medical software program from cyberspace. It's on your desktop computer, and in a few more steps, it will be ready for use on your

Palm or Pocket PC. At this point, our instructions diverge for the two major operating systems: Palm or Pocket PC.

Installing Software on a Palm Handheld Computer

Once the software is on your desktop, you have two easy solutions for adding the software to your handheld computer—either double-clicking on the software files with the "Palm icon" ⬛ or opening the Palm desktop and "adding files" through the desktop interface. Let's go over these two simple methods.

HANDS-ON EXERCISE 3.3. DOUBLE-CLICKING THE "PALM ICON"

Most software programs will be added to the Palm desktop installation tool seamlessly by double-clicking on the Palm icon. In this example, after uncompressing the "PocketBillingdemo 2.01.zip" files into the C:\PocketBilling Demo folder, browse to that folder as described earlier, and notice that there is one "Palm icon" file named "billingdemo 2.01" (see Figure 3.9). Please note that some Palm programs require installation of more than one file to run. You can usually tell this if you uncompress the software and see multiple Palm icons. It is essential to read the manual or "Read me" documentation that comes along with most good Palm software to find out if this is the case.

In the present example, you would just double-click (using your computer mouse's left button) on the file. After that, the Palm desktop installation dialog should appear (Figure 3.10), and you would simply click on "OK" after making sure that the correct Palm username is selected (using the down arrow to the right of the username).

After you have clicked "OK," another install tool window should open, showing the program you have selected to be installed (Figure 3.11). Make sure you click on "Done" at this point, and don't make the common beginner's mistake of clicking on "Add." Of course you have the option of changing the username and destination at this point, but most likely the default location will be fine.

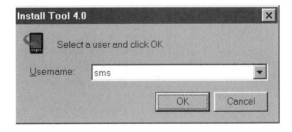

FIGURE 3.10. Install Tool Dialog box. (Reprinted with permission from palmOne, Inc.)

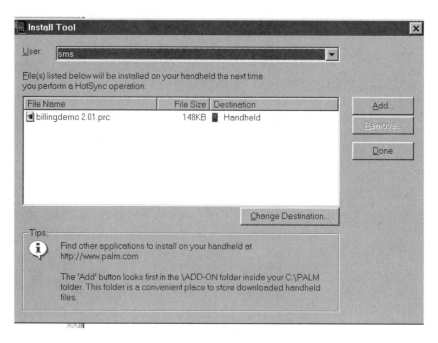

FIGURE 3.11. Second Install dialog box. (Reprinted with permission from palmOne, Inc.)

After clicking on "Done," a final dialog box appears (Figure 3.12). All you have to do is click on "OK" for this last message, and, because this is sometimes a nuisance step, you may want to put a check in the box that says, "Do not show this message again."

After you have double-clicked on the file, simply insert your Palm into its cradle and press the HotSync button on the cradle. So long as the cradle is properly attached and your Palm desktop software is correctly installed, you should see a message saying "Installing handheld application" on the desktop as the installation and backup process occurs (Figure 3.13). Make sure that it is also installing to the right handheld username. In addition to the desktop "HotSync Progress" box, your handheld screen itself should show the program being installed. In this case it is called "Billing" (Figure 3.14).

If you don't see these messages, or your Palm doesn't appear to communicate well with your desktop PC, it would be advisable to get support from the manufacturer of your handheld computer, as this is a critical process to be able to access all the functionality described in this book.

At this point you should be able to turn your Palm handheld on, and the "PocketBill" icon should appear in your programs list (Figure 3.15). Tapping on the icon should open the program and allow you to run it.

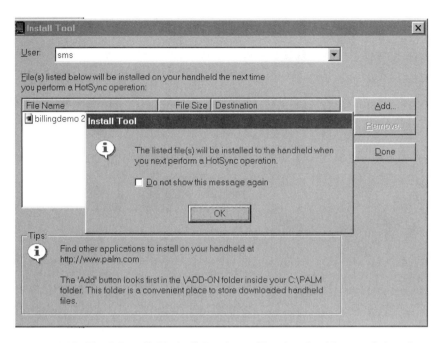

FIGURE 3.12. Final Install Tool dialog box. (Reprinted with permission from palmOne, Inc.)

Key Points

1. Most of the time, double-clicking on any software with the Palm icon 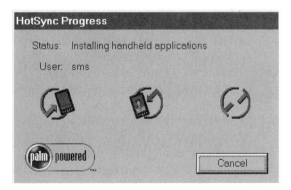 will install it on your handheld.
2. Make sure you choose the right username so that the software gets installed on your handheld.

FIGURE 3.13. Installing handheld applications box. (Reprinted with permission from palmOne, Inc.)

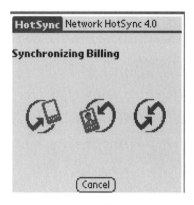

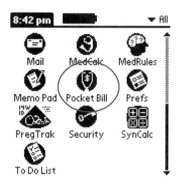

FIGURE 3.14. Palm screen showing "Billing" being installed. (Reprinted with permission from palmOne, Inc.)

FIGURE 3.15. Palm with program successfully installed. (Reprinted with permission from palmOne, Inc.)

3. After a successful HotSync operation, you should see the new software icon on your handheld screen. Make sure the "All" selector is picked in the upper-right-hand corner as shown in Figure 3.15.

HANDS-ON EXERCISE 3.4. AN ALTERNATIVE METHOD: USING THE PALM DESKTOP TO INSTALL SOFTWARE

If your downloaded software isn't automatically added to the desktop installation software when you double-click it, or if you have multiple software files to install in different locations of your hard drive, you may want to use the Palm Desktop to install your software.

Open the Palm Desktop software by clicking on either the icon on your desktop or the name of the program in your "Start Menu," and then click on the "Install Tool" icon (Figure 3.16; circled). Once the installation tool is open (see Figure 3.11), make sure that your username is selected in the "User:" box (see Figure 3.10) and then click the "Add" button (Figure 3.17; circled).

You will see a file directory box in Windows (Figure 3.18) that allows you to select the location where the files were downloaded or decompressed. In our example, simply select C:\PocketBilling Demo, and you should see the files to be installed. At this point, simply left-click the "billingdemo 2.01" file, choose "Open" on the file directory box, and click on "Done" on the Palm Install tool. To finish the installation process, insert your handheld computer into the cradle, and select the "HotSync" button to install the software. See the final instructions on troubleshooting this process in the previous description. If you were successful and the HotSync operation has finished, you will see the PocketBill icon (see Figure 3.15) on your handheld. Tapping this icon should open the program and allow you to use it.

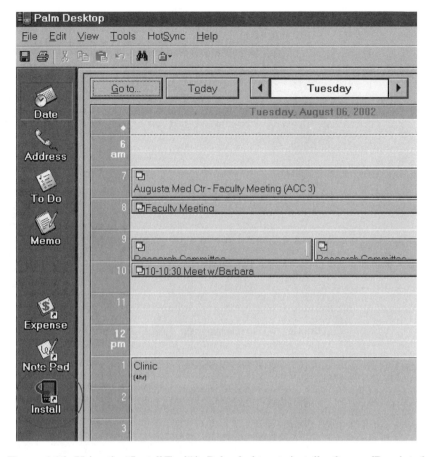

FIGURE 3.16. Using the "Install Tool" in Palm desktop to install software. (Reprinted with permission from palmOne, Inc.)

Key Points

1. Another way to install Palm software is by opening the Palm Install tool from the Palm Desktop software.
2. This method can be helpful if you have multiple programs to install.

Installing Programs on a Pocket PC Handheld Computer

Pocket PC's generally have more features and capabilities than their Palm brethren, but they are also more complex. Software installation is no exception, but the following hands-on exercise will make you an expert. Let's take it step by step.

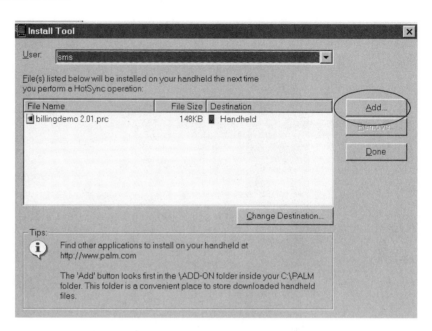

FIGURE 3.17. Selecting the "Add" button in the Install Tool. (Reprinted with permission from palmOne, Inc. and PocketMed.)

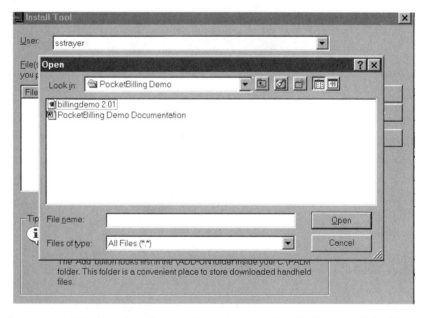

FIGURE 3.18. Windows file directory box after selecting "Add" from Palm Install Tool. (Reprinted with permission from palmOne, Inc. and PocketMed.)

HANDS-ON EXERCISE 3.5. INSTALLING A PROGRAM ON A POCKET PC HANDHELD

I'll assume that you have a program you want to install. As an example, I'm going to install the InfoRetriever program that I wrote (MHE). A demo version of this program can be downloaded from www.medicalinforetriever. com (select "Downloads," and then "InfoRetriever 4.X for Pocket PC"). Make sure you select the correct processor type. Depending on which handheld you have, it may be the Strong Arm, MIPS, or SH3 processor. Consult your user's manual to verify which one is the correct version for your handheld computer. If you are unfamiliar with downloading software from the Internet, see Hands-On Exercise 3.1.

1. First, make sure your Pocket PC is in its cradle and connected to your desktop computer using ActiveSync. For more on ActiveSync, please visit the Microsoft website at http://www.microsoft.com/Pocket PC, or read the user's manual that came with your handheld. Then, on your desktop computer run the inforetrieversa.exe, inforetrievermips.exe, or inforetrieversh3.exe file that you just downloaded by double-clicking on it (Figure 3.19).
2. Press "Next" and proceed to the following screen (Figure 3.20).
3. Press "Next" again, and the licensing agreement will be displayed (Figure 3.21). (Does anyone really read these?)

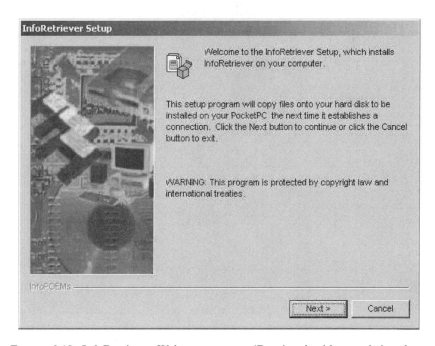

FIGURE 3.19. InfoRetriever Welcome screen. (Reprinted with permission from InfoPOEM, Inc.)

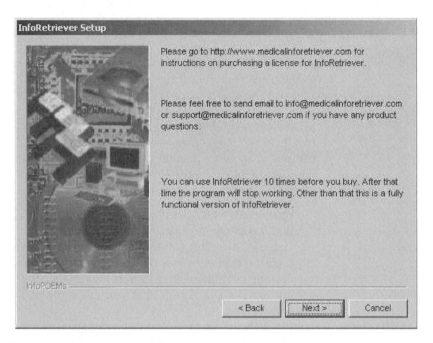

FIGURE 3.20. InfoRetriever Setup screen. (Reprinted with permission from InfoPOEM, Inc.)

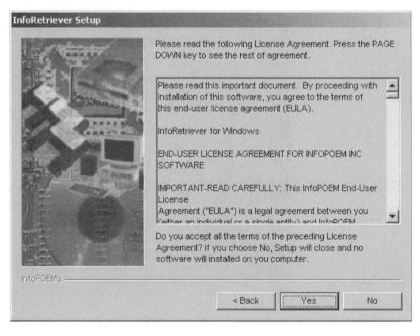

FIGURE 3.21. Licensing agreement screen on InfoRetriever. (Reprinted with permission from InfoPOEM, Inc.)

4. Assuming that you are not an attorney, press "Yes" to accept the license terms and proceed to the destination directory screen (Figure 3.22).
5. Press "Next" to accept the default location. This is the place where the setup files are stored on your desktop computer. Pressing "Next" on the following screen (Figure 3.23) will install InfoRetriever on your Pocket PC handheld computer.
6. After pressing "Next" on the final installation confirmation screen (Figure 3.23), you will see another confirmation button (Figure 3.24). If you want to install the base files in internal memory, press "Yes." If you want to install them to a compact flash card, press "No."
7. Pressing "No" in the final confirmation box (Figure 3.24) will allow you to select between main memory or a storage card (Figure 3.25). This is an important point, as it isn't very obvious in the ActiveSync program.
8. Use the downward-pointing arrow to choose the location for installation (Figure 3.26).
9. I'll leave it as "Main memory," which refers to the memory inside your device. To install to the storage card, choose "Storage card" from that menu. Next, you may see a "not enough space" warning if you have a 32-MB device (Figure 3.27).
10. This message is often erroneous, go ahead and try the installation anyway. If it fails, or your program doesn't work, you can always

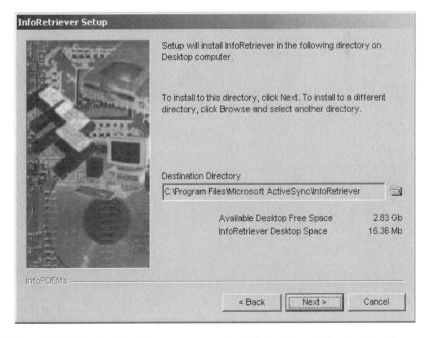

FIGURE 3.22. Destination directory screen for InfoRetriever. (Reprinted with permission from InfoPOEM, Inc.)

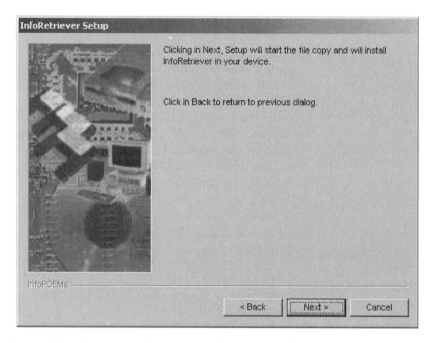

FIGURE 3.23. Final installation confirmation screen. (Reprinted with permission from InfoPOEM, Inc.)

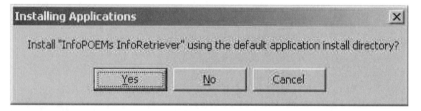

FIGURE 3.24. Final confirmation button. (Reprinted with permission from InfoPOEM, Inc.)

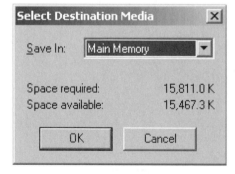

FIGURE 3.25. Destination selector in ActiveSync. (Reprinted with permission from InfoPOEM, Inc.)

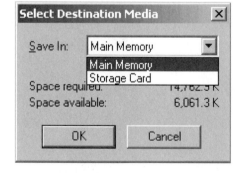

FIGURE 3.26. Using the down arrow to select installation destination. (Reprinted with permission from InfoPOEM, Inc.)

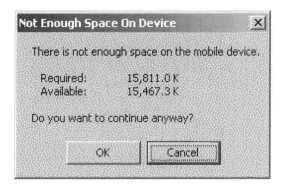

FIGURE 3.27. Space limitation warning. (Reprinted with permission from InfoPOEM, Inc.)

uninstall using the "Remove programs" under Start Menu | Settings | System and install to a compact flash card or make room in the internal memory. Press "OK" to proceed and ignore the warning, and an installation bar will appear (Figure 3.28).

11. At this point, the setup file is being copied to your device. It could take several minutes for a large program like InfoRetriever. Be patient. Drink a cup of coffee. Pet your dog. When it is done, you will see an installation completion message (Figure 3.29).

12. Press "OK" and you will see the final dialog box (Figure 3.30).

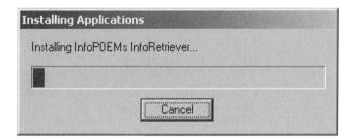

FIGURE 3.28. Installation bar. (Reprinted with permission from InfoPOEM, Inc.)

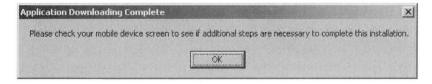

FIGURE 3.29. Installation completion box. (Reprinted with permission from palmOne, Inc.)

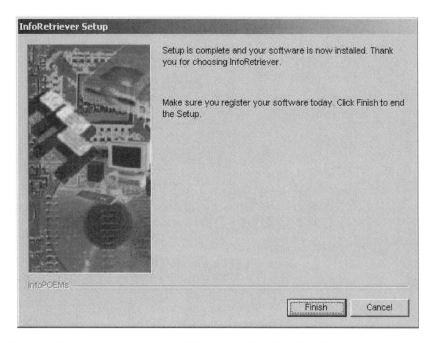

FIGURE 3.30. Final installation dialog box. (Reprinted with permission from InfoPOEM, Inc.)

13. Press "Finish" and turn your attention to your device, where you will see the message shown in Figure 3.31.
14. This is a scary screen for many people, and for good reason; copy over a newer file with an older version and you can "break" some software that is innocently sitting on your Pocket PC already. For InfoRetriever, we recommend selecting "Yes to all." If you choose "No to all" and your program won't run, repeat the process and select "Yes to all."
15. You'll now see the program install a bunch of files to your Pocket PC (Figure 3.32). In some cases the screen may appear to freeze, as happens with InfoRetriever. However, it isn't frozen, it's just madly trying to copy more than 550 photos to your device! Be patient . . . it takes 5 or so minutes.

That's it! You'll now see InfoRetriever 4.x (or whatever the latest number is) in your Start Menu (Figure 3.33).

Sometimes you want to directly copy a file to your handheld, such as a Word document, a map, or a photo. It's easy: just drag and drop. First, double-click on the ActiveSync icon (it looks like a little green yin-yang symbol in the tray in the lower-right-hand corner of your desktop) and press the "Explore" button. In Figure 3.34, I have done this and opened a folder on my desktop. In this example, I have transferred our faculty call

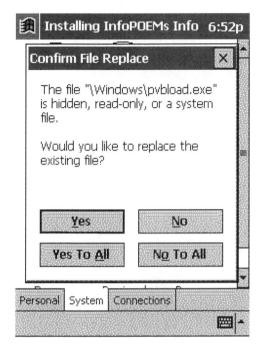

FIGURE 3.31. Installation messages on Pocket PC device. (Reprinted with permission from Microsoft Corporation and InfoPOEM, Inc.)

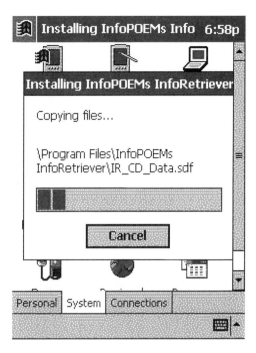

FIGURE 3.32. Installation progress bar on Pocket PC device. (Reprinted with permission from Microsoft Corporation and InfoPOEM, Inc.)

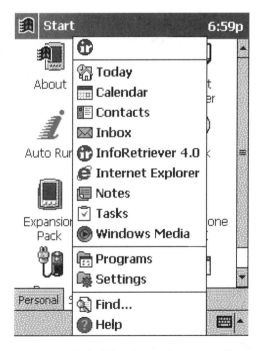

FIGURE 3.33. InfoRetriever in your "Start menu" on a Pocket PC device. (Reprinted with permission from Microsoft Corporation and InfoPOEM, Inc.)

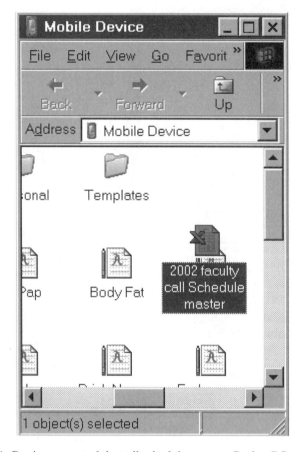

FIGURE 3.34. Putting a copy of the call schedule on your Pocket PC.

schedule in Excel to the Pocket PC. Now you can carry the schedule with you wherever you go!

Then, just click on the file you want to copy and hold the button down, drag the file over the "Explore" folder from ActiveSync, and drop it. That's it! You can choose where to put it on the Pocket PC by navigating up or down the folders in the Explore window.

Key Points

1. Installing software can be a little trickier on Pocket PC's, but if you follow these instructions you shouldn't get lost.

2. You will need the latest version of Microsoft's ActiveSync software installed on your desktop, and the handheld computer should be able to communicate with your desktop; if not, get help!
3. You can also drag any software or files to your handheld by opening "Explore" from ActiveSync.

Summary

We've covered a lot of ground in this chapter. At the very least, you should now realize how you can download specialized medical software from the Internet. Without this additional software, your handheld computer will never realize its full potential!

In the first hands-on exercise, we showed you how easy it is to download the software to your desktop. You can do this using either Internet Explorer or Netscape browsers. We also made a few suggestions on how to keep track of your downloads. In the second hands-on exercise we showed you how to uncompress software so that it can be installed on your handheld. We also showed you ways to manage all the files that you will accumulate after uncompressing software.

In the third and fourth exercises, two ways of installing Palm software to your handheld were illustrated step by step. If you don't have the Palm Desktop (for Palm users) or the Microsoft ActiveSync software (for Pocket PC users) installed on your desktop, it's time to do this now. Also, make sure that your handheld and desktop are communicating nicely; otherwise, the rest of this book will not be very helpful to you!

Finally, in the last exercise, we showed you two ways to install software on a Pocket PC handheld computer. It's important to make sure you download the software for the right processor (check your user's manual). We also showed you the "trick" for installing software to your additional memory or main memory.

Now that you see how simple it is to download and install software on your handheld computer, all the uses and applications that we describe in the following chapters will be usable with your Palm OS or Pocket PC device. The nebulous mystery of getting software from cyberspace to the palm of your hand is solved once and for all, and you can join the growing numbers of health care professionals who use handheld computers at the point of care on a daily basis. Whatever you do, don't forget to take time out to play a quick game of Tetris or Defender!

Section II

Medical Software

4

"Where in the World Wide Web Do I Find All This Stuff?" Finding Medical Software and Information on the Web for Handheld Computers

PETER L. REYNOLDS AND SCOTT M. STRAYER

So far we have given you an overview of why handheld computers are becoming so popular in medicine and how to choose one for yourself. We have gone over the basics of using your handheld computer and showed you how to download software from the Internet. Are you still hanging on? There's much more you can do in the medical field with a handheld computer, but before we continue, we thought an overview of Web sites might be helpful.

This chapter is devoted to reviewing some of the top medical sites for handheld software and information on the Internet. For the very basics of handheld use, we refer you to Kent Willyard's top-notch site "ectopicbrain" (http://pbrain.hypermart.net). This site offers a wealth of information on using Palm OS handheld computers and references many of the websites reviewed (Figure 4.1). It is a great site to visit if you are just starting out with a Palm handheld and need answers to basic questions such as "How long can I go between battery charges?" and "How many times can I drop my new Palm in the toilet?" (The answer to that last question is "Usually, only once!")

An equivalent, all-purpose Web site for Pocket PC's comes to us gratis from the generous people at Microsoft at www.pocketpc.com (Figure 4.2). This site is equally useful, with everything needed by the beginning handheld user. You'll find free downloads, information on hardware and software, accessories, reviews, tutorials, and even a club you can join to share thoughts with other users. (If you're wondering about the question "How many times can you drop a Pocket PC in the toilet?," the answer is pretty much the same . . . usually one time does the trick, unless it's in a waterproof case.)

Another thing to keep in mind is that every hardware manufacturer has its own Web site, and these are usually useful regarding technical support, updates, and general information. Check out the following sites for more information on hardware and accessories:

www.palmone.com
www.handspring.com
www.sony.com
www.toshiba.com
www.hp.com
www.compaq.com
www.dell.com
www.casio.com
www.audiovox.com

Also, try searching for manufacturers' names using an Internet search engine such as Yahoo or Google.

Over time, you'll develop your own list of favorite Web sites. We hope our straightforward review format and discerning eye will provide you with a useful reference as you forge ahead into this new frontier of handhelds in medicine!

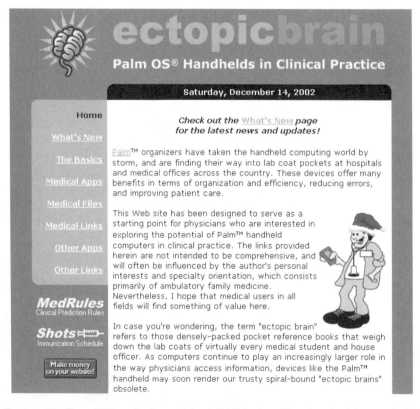

FIGURE 4.1. Kent Willyard's "ectopicbrain" Web site. (Reprinted with permission from palmOne, Inc.)

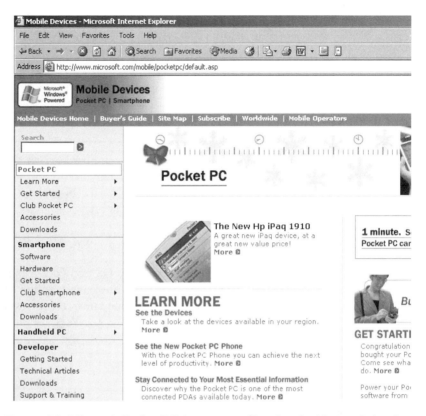

FIGURE 4.2. Microsoft Pocket PC home page. (Reprinted with permission from Microsoft Corporation.)

How We Reviewed Web Sites

We tried to take a consistent approach to reviewing sites, with "5 out of 5" stethoscopes being our top rating. Of course, every site about handhelds is, by definition, a great site, and our overall ratings are inflated accordingly. Table 4.1 defines types of content as used in our reviews. By nature, Internet content is dynamic, and the quality of a given site varies from week to

TABLE 4.1. Content categories.

Type	Content
News	Press releases and news articles about handhelds
Reviews	Reviews of software and hardware
Advice	How-to advice for new and advanced users
Online forum	Online user conversations on various handheld topics (includes e-mail list servers)
Software downloads	Downloadable freeware and shareware software
Online store	Sale of hardware and software online
User reviews	Unsolicited reviews of software and hardware by independent users

week. We can't guarantee that you'll agree with every review but encourage you to visit the sites and judge for yourself. Within categories, sites are listed in alphabetical order unless otherwise noted.

Commercial Web Sites

Although understandably biased, commercial sites are usually well maintained and easy to navigate. Frequent visitors mean quick feedback and more consistent quality. These sites are both a good starting place for novices and popular destinations for advanced users.

1. www.CollectiveMed.com

Target: Health professionals, Palm OS and Pocket PC.
Content: Reviews, advice, software downloads, online store.
    Pros: Software titles nicely grouped into categories (includes "Free Software"), as shown in Figure 4.3. Very useful Buyer's Guide. Has AvantGo Auto-Channel for site.
    Cons: No user reviews.
Overall: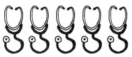

2. www.Handango.com

Target: All users, Palm OS and Pocket PC.
Content: Software downloads, online store (up to 100 medical titles and thousands of nonmedical titles), user reviews.
    Pros: Unsolicited user reviews very helpful. Several well-rated medical software suites.
    Cons: Specific software titles sometimes are hard to find. Medical titles not as well organized as on medical-only sites.
Overall: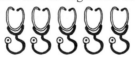

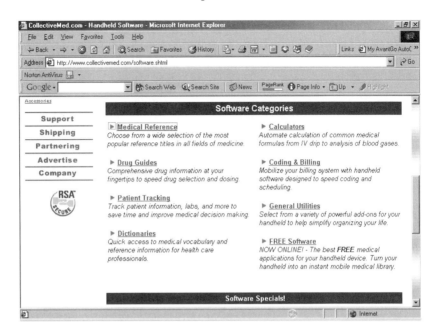

FIGURE 4.3. CollectiveMed.Com software categories. (Reprinted with permission from http://www.CollectiveMed.com.)

3. www.HandheldMed.com

Target: Health professionals, Palm OS and Pocket PC.
Content: Software downloads, online store
Pros: Excellent reputation for clinical reference software.
Cons: Must create account to access some features. No user reviews. Online forum and advice areas under construction at time of review.
Overall:

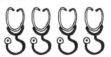

4. www.MedicalPocketPC.com

Target: Health professionals, Pocket PC only.
Content: Reviews, advice, online forum (reviewed separately below), software downloads, online store.
Pros: Extensive tutorials and great links for Pocket PC users. Software grouped by specialty.
Cons: No user reviews. Layout not as easy to navigate as some.
Overall:

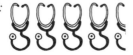

5. www.MedsPDA.com

Target: Health professionals, Palm OS and Pocket PC.

Content: Reviews, advice, software downloads, online store.

Pros: Search for software by platform, including Macintosh desktop, and by specialty, such as nursing. Interesting articles.

Cons: No user reviews. Software selection less comprehensive than some other sites.

Overall: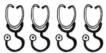

6. www.Palmone.com
(http://www.palm.com/us/solutions/healthcare/)

Target: Health professionals, Palm OS only.

Content: Comprehensive healthcare page from the developers of Palm OS (news, reviews, advice, software downloads, online store, user reviews).

Pros: Unique content including software, calendar of upcoming healthcare conferences and events, and information on Palm OS success stories in health care. Good resource for large groups investigating enterprise solutions.

Cons: Possible biased information; sometimes not as comprehensive as other sites.

Overall: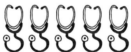

7. www.PalmGear.com

Target: All users, Palm OS only.

Content: Software downloads, online store (up to 400 medical titles and thousands of nonmedical titles), user reviews.

Pros: Unsolicited user reviews very helpful. "Essentials" list of recommended general software highly regarded.

Cons: Medical titles not as well organized as on medical-only sites. Site sometimes slow.

Overall: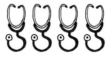

8. www.PDAcortex.com (formerly www.RNPalm.com)

Target: Health professionals, Palm OS and Pocket PC.

Content: News, reviews, advice, online forum (reviewed separately below), software downloads, online store.

Pros: Great list of free applications for Palm OS and Pocket PC, helpful reviews written by practicing providers, several active e-mail lists including those for nurses and emergency care providers.

Cons: No user reviews. Up-and-coming site.

Overall: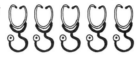

9. www.pdaMD.com

Target: Health professionals, Palm OS and Pocket PC.

Content: Reviews, advice, online forum (reviewed separately below), software downloads, online store.

Pros: One-stop research and shopping; active online forums.

Cons: No user reviews.

Overall: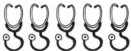

10. www.PocketGear.com

Target: All users, Pocket PC only.

Content: News, software downloads, online store.

Pros: Up to 50 medical titles for Pocket PC; nice section on Pocket PC news.

Cons: Navigation only fair.

Overall: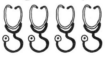

If you still can't find the title for which you're searching, the following are other popular sites for downloading handheld software:

www.tucows.com
www.cnet.com
www.freewarepalm.com
www.zdnet.com

In particular, www.tucows.com (pronounced "two cows") brings together an enormous library of handheld and desktop software, while making it easy to search for medical titles by type of handheld, Palm OS or Pocket PC.

Talking with Other Health Professionals About PDAs: Handheld Computer Medical Forums and E-Mail Lists

There is a lot of information on the Internet regarding uses of handheld computers. It's nice to find forums and e-mail lists that are solely devoted to health professionals because this saves you from "information overload." These forums and e-mail lists are excellent places to discuss software, hardware, accessories, and creative uses of handheld computers with like-minded health professionals. Many of them link to great websites with additional software reviews, downloads, and how-to articles available.

1. Doctor Palm

http://groups.yahoo.com/group/DoctorPalm/

Target: Physicians, Palm OS only. Good for other health professionals also.

Content: Online forum (messages, chat, polls, links, files, and photos).

Pros: Simple and easy to use, yet has a lot of nice features that are built in to Yahoo! groups. Find out what other physicians are using. The polls are great when considering a specific type of software or hardware that you would like to purchase.

Cons: Another e-mail to add to your already crowded inbox, but easy to turn off if desired.

Overall: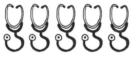

2. MedicalPocketPC.com

http://www.medicalpocketpc.com/cgi-bin/ubb/ultimatebb.cgi

Target: Health Professionals, Pocket PC only.

Content: Online forum (basic forum with discussions about Pocket PCs in medicine).

Pros: Simple and easy to use.

Cons: Pretty basic; Web site reviewed above.

Overall: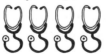

3. PDACortex

http://www.rnpalm.com/phpBB/

Target: Health professionals (including nurses, emergency workers, and veterinarians), Palm OS and Pocket PC.

Content: Online forum

Pros: Simple and easy to use. Moderated by well-respected physician and nursing handheld users.

Cons: Pretty basic forum; good content on Web site as reviewed above.

Overall: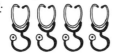

4. PDAMD.com

http://www.pdamd.com/vertical/forums/index.php

Target: Health professionals, Palm OS and Pocket PC.

Content: Online forum (PDAs in health care, student issues, support questions, article discussion, and classifieds).

Pros: Nice breakdown of the different forums. Interface is easy to use.

Cons: Basic forums, but great Web site, as reviewed above.

Overall: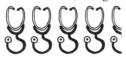

5. Wireless Medical Applications

http://groups.yahoo.com/group/WirelessMedicalApplications/

Target: Health professionals with an interest in wireless applications (but not limited to wireless topics).

Content: Online forum (messages, chat, polls, links, files, and photos).

Pros: Excellent group that is well moderated. Has full features, and a fairly active discussion (but not too active).

Cons: Not always about wireless, but this added content may be one of its strengths.

Overall: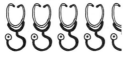

6. Palm-Med Listserver

http://listserver.itd.umich.edu/cgi-bin/lyris.pl?enter=palm-med&
text_mode=0

Target: Health professionals, Palm OS only.

Content: Online forum (basic mailing list discussion of Palm handheld uses in medicine).

Pros: Low volume and moderated by an informatics-trained physician at the University of Michigan.

Cons: Subscribing and unsubscribing can be difficult, but the moderator is always helpful.

Overall: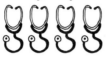

News from the "Ivory Towers:" Sites from Educational Institutions

Educational sites come in a few basic flavors. Many of these Web sites are hosted by a small group of medical students or other handheld user group. They may be limited in scope with nothing more than a list of links to various other handheld sites. Another type of educational Web site has information on the handheld computer policies at the hosting institution. You may find this interesting if you are trying to set up a program in an educational setting. The more useful sites, from our point of view, include types of software used and, better yet, reviews about the software from the end-user perspective. Some sites even have software developed at that institution and available for free downloading. A few have great bibliographies of published journal articles on handheld computers. Although most of these sites are geared toward Palm OS users, we have tried to present good sites with Pocket PC information as well. We reviewed the top sites and listed others if you have time for more.

1. Handheld Recommendations

http://www.medicine.dal.ca/palm/
Dalhousie University.

Target: Healthcare professionals, Palm OS and Pocket PC.

Content: Reviews, advice.

Pros: One of the most comprehensive lists of reviewed software, with a great comparison between Palm and Pocket PC handheld computers. This site is very well organized.

Cons: Software selections are mostly geared toward Palm users (although not exclusively).

Overall: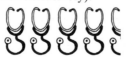

2. JEFFLINE-Palm/Handheld Support for Clinicians

http://jeffline.tju.edu/Clinicians/palm.html
Thomas Jefferson University.

Target: Healthcare professionals, mostly Palm OS with some Pocket PC content.

Content: Reviews, advice (with online presentation), software downloads.

Pros: This site is particularly notable for its homegrown software, including Alticopeia (an herbal database), a lab test differential diagnosis program, an internal medicine admissions program, and two Q&A programs for pathology and microscopic anatomy. There is also a good list of Palm OS medical software with reviews.

Cons: Some of the homegrown software will run only on Palm handhelds.

Overall: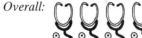

3. Palm Pilot Page

http://www.bcm.tmc.edu/medpeds/palm.html
Medicine-Pediatrics Residency Program at Baylor College of Medicine.

Target: Health professionals, Palm OS only.

Content: Reviews, advice (with "how-to" section).

Pros: A great list with reviews of Palm medical applications.

Cons: Chat room and manuals are only for Baylor residents.

Overall: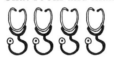

4. PDAs for Health Care Providers

http://educ.ahsl.arizona.edu/pda/index.htm
University of Arizona.

Target: Health professionals (including separate pharmacy, nursing, and veterinary sections), Palm OS and Pocket PC.

Content: Reviews (extensive list for hardware and software with the best reviews highlighted) (many from published journals or other Web sites), advice (with tips and tricks section), bibliography.

Pros: This site is impressive for its comprehensiveness and the PDA bibliography, which is one of the most extensive available (and is updated regularly). One of the coolest features is a link (under "living in the future") to media where handheld computers were featured before their commercial availability, such as Star Trek's Tricoder and "Box" from the BBC TV series "Star Cops."

Cons: This is one of the best sites out there. No real complaints.

Overall: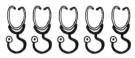

5. PDAs in Family Practice

http://www.urmc.rochester.edu/FamMed/PDAatFMC.htm
University of Rochester Department of Family Medicine.

Target: Health Professionals, Palm OS with minimal Pocket PC content.

Content: Reviews (software and hardware), advice.

Pros: Nicely written description of the PDA program in this family medicine department. Offers great ideas for residency program applications.

Cons: Does not appear to have been updated recently.

Overall: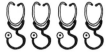

6. Pediatrics On Hand

http://www.pediatricsonhand.com/
Children's National Medical Center and Pediatrics On Hand.

Target: Pediatric health professionals and parents, Palm OS and Pocket PC.

Content: Reviews, advice (with online presentation, new user guide, "how-to" files, and software for parents!), software downloads (with original software titles).

Pros: This is a very well organized Web site that should be seen by anyone practicing pediatrics, and by parents who own a handheld computer . . . what a great idea!

Cons: No real complaints here.

Overall: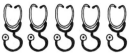

7. UCSF's E-Brain

http://missinglink.ucsf.edu/sitefinder/XcDirViewInCat.asp?ID:80
University of California-San Francisco.

Target: Health professionals, Palm OS only.

Content: News, reviews, advice (with frequently asked questions, tutorials, and tips and tricks section).

Pros: Well organized, with a good set of reviews of Palm software. The tutorials are also well done.

Cons: A few of the links were broken, and the online forums were only for UCSF students. "Latest" news was out of date.

Overall: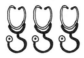

8. University of MN Medical School Palm Pilot Page

http://www.student.med.umn.edu/palmpilot/index.html
University of Minnesota.

Target: Health professionals, Palm OS and Pocket PC.

Content: News, reviews, advice (including "Top Handhelds for Medical Students" and "Top Software for Medical Students").

Pros: One of the best listings of software around (great rating system, costs, reviews, and links all in one table). Nice tables of top handhelds and software for medical students; gives you an idea of what others are using.

Cons: Out-of-date "latest" news, but somewhat balanced by a daily update from Palm InfoCenter.com.

Overall: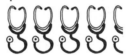

9. WardRounds

http://www.wardrounds.com/
Commercial site for medical students.

Target: Health professionals, especially medical students, mostly Palm OS with minimal Pocket PC content.

Content: Reviews, advice (with tips and tricks section), online forum, software downloads.

Pros: The interactive software searcher is one of the best. You can search by specialty, or by type of software, and if it is freeware, there are links to download the software. One of the best discussions of patient-tracking software; especially helpful for medical students and residents.

Cons: Would love to have Pocket PC software included.

Overall: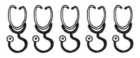

Other Educational Sites

- **Creighton University**
  http://www.creighton.edu/~dyoung/palm.htm
  Mostly links to several commercial sites.
- **Crozer-Keystone PDA**
  http://www.ckfprinformatics.org/pda.html
  Mostly links to tutorials, Internet sites, and a Palm model comparison for the basic models.
- **East Carolina University**
  http://www.ecu.edu/handheld/
  Details on a corporate–academic partnership between ECU and various hardware/software vendors.
- **Electronic Resources for PDA Users**
  http://www.wfubmc.edu/library/pda.html
  Good catalogue of medical sites, manufacturer sites, and software sites.
- **Evidence-Based Medicine Tools for the PDA**
  http://www.ils.unc.edu/~caham/ebmtools/ebmtools.html
  From the University of North Carolina School of Information and Library Science, this site focuses on EBM-related handheld services and applications, including links to news and abstract services.
- **Handheld Computers in Family Medicine**
  http://www.fammed.wisc.edu/education/res/PilotWeb.htm
  Collection of links especially notable for a good collection of free medical documents and databases. The music can be a little annoying, though.
- **Intro to Palm**
  http://dmi-www.mc.duke.edu/oem/palm.htm
  Decent collection of links to hardware and software.
- **MCV's Med/Peds Program PDA Links**
  http://views.vcu.edu/medpeds/pda.html
  Just the links.
- **New York Medical College**
  http://www.nymc.edu/fammed/palmproject/index.htm
  For Palm OS handhelds in a fourth-year clerkship program. A few links available.
- **OHSU Internal Medicine Residency Program**
  http://www.ohsu.edu/som-Medicine/residency/handheld.html
  Short list of basic links.
- **Palm Organizer @ NYU School of Medicine**
  http://endeavor.med.nyu.edu/research/pda/pilot/
  Good links and a homegrown diagnosis tracker for peds and ambulatory care.
- **Palm Paradise**
  http://www.medsch.wisc.edu/studgrps/palm_paradise.htm
  Basic links with a "what do I use" list for medical students.

- **Palmtop Medicine**
  http://www.cbil.vcu.edu/pda/
  Basic links.
- **PDA Requirement**
  http://www.medstudent.ucla.edu/pdareq/
  Some good general advice on recommended software with decent links.
- **Stanford University School of Medicine Palm Project**
  http://palm.stanford.edu/index.html
  Decent list of software with reviews.
- **UCCOM PDA Resource Page**
  http://www.medsch.ucla.edu/som/fammed/PALMWEB/intro.htm
  List of links.
- **University of Cincinnati PDA Resource Page**
  http://www.med.uc.edu/medical/pda/
  Links for software, hardware, and such for Pocket PC and Palm.
- **University of Kentucky College of Medicine**
  http://www.uky.edu/StudentOrgs/KMA/pda.htm
  Pretty basic list of links for Palm and Pocket PC.
- **University of Louisville-Handheld PCs**
  http://www.medschool.louisville.edu/palm/index.htm
  Links for support and software.
- **UNC-CH School of Medicine: PDA Initiative**
  http://www.med.unc.edu/pda/welcome.htm
  Nice site with hardware, software, UNC software, and a good list of links.
- **University of Virginia SOM-Palm Pilots**
  http://www.med.virginia.edu/medicine/student-affairs/book-h3.html
  Hardware, software, advice on general software, and links to medical and general sites for Palm.
- **University of Virginia School of Nursing**
  http://www.nursing.virginia.edu/its/handhelds/Recommendations.html
  A few software programs and sites.
- **University of Washington Family Practice Residency**
  http://faculty.washington.edu/dacosta/palm.html
  Mostly for UW students. Has how to document procedures and deliveries in their residency.
- **USDSM Palm Program Site**
  http://med.usd.edu/palm/index.html
  Mostly list of links. Sites are reviewed.
- **Washington University Medical Pam Initiative**
  http://medicine.wustl.edu/~wumpi/
  Nicely organized list of links with software and hardware as well.
- **WSUIM Palm Pilot Page**
  http://wsuim.org/PDA/
  Comprehensive list of medical software with short reviews.

- **Yale ITS-Med**
  http://its.med.yale.edu/pda/
  Nicely organized list of links, with bonus drop-down jump feature.

Top Ten Miscellaneous Web Sites

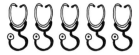

The following sites were judged to be best in their class, especially well constructed, or offer unique content not to be missed.

1. **Best Internal Medicine Site**
   ACP-ASIM PDA Portal
   http://www.acponline.org/pda/
   From the American College of Physicians-American Society of Internal Medicine, this site offers several free downloads including a list of commonly used ICD-9 codes and a bioterrorism diagnosis and treatment tool for Palm OS.

2. **Best Family Practice Site**
   DocSpence.com
   http://www.docspence.com/
   From Dr. Steven Spence, the director of the Blackstone Family Practice Residency in Virginia, this site includes links for Palm OS and Pocket PC as well as other medical related sites including electronic medical records and telemedicine.

3. **Best Dentist Site**
   DMD-Palm-DDS
   http://www.palmdmd.com/
   A site devoted to handheld news and software for dentists.

4. **Best EMS Site**
   Firehouse.com
   http://www.firehouse.com/tech/pda.html
   Great site for firefighters and other emergency responders. Mostly Palm OS.

5. **Best Medical Links Site (Figure 4.4)**
   Handheld Healthcare
   http://www.himss.org/webguides/handheld/index.asp
   Well-engineered collection of links compiled by the Healthcare Information and Management Systems Society (HIMSS).

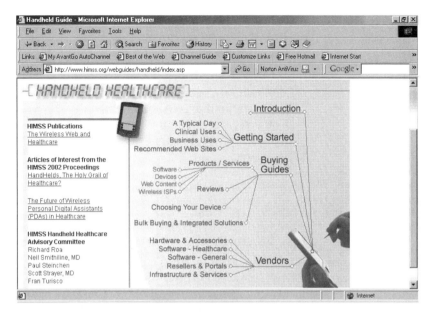

FIGURE 4.4. Healthcare Information and Management Systems Society (HIMSS) handheld healthcare links. (Reprinted with permission from HIMSS.)

6. Best Pharmacist Site
Handheld Information for Pharmacists
http://www.alittletoolate.com/pda/
Handheld info for pharmacists. Long list of drug information software, but with links only, no reviews.

7. Best Health Resources Site
Healthy Palm Pilot
http://www.healthypalmpilot.com/
Nearly 800 Palm OS resources available for download; updated frequently.

8. Best Anesthesiologist Site
PDA Anaesthetic
http://www.pdaanaesthetic.com/
Dedicated site for anesthesiologists and anesthetists with Palm OS and Pocket PC handhelds.

9. Best Pediatrician Site
PedsPalm.com
http://www.pedspalm.com/

Excellent site for pediatricians with Palm OS handhelds. Notable for a "Top Ten" software for section pediatricians as well as a software section for parents.

10. **Best Handheld Medical Enthusiast Site**
    Jim Thompson's Pilot Pages
    http://www.jimthompson.net/palmpda/
    Highly regarded Palm OS resource maintained by Canadian ER physician and longtime handheld computing enthusiast Jim Thompson.

Other Miscellaneous Web Sites

- **BiomedicalPDA** (maps to Wiley Interscience)
  http://www.biomedicalpda.com/
  Peer-reviewed biomedical databases for Palm OS with facts and figures needed by researchers. Adhesion molecules, cytokine receptors, restriction enzymes, gel filtration, etc.
- **Burdie's Medical Palm Site**
  http://www.angelfire.com/oh3/burdette/palm.htm
  Lots of links and downloads from Steve Burdette at Wright State School of Medicine.
- **Doctor's Gadgets**
  http://www.newmediamedicine.com/doctorsgadgets/
  Some interesting articles, but most links go offsite and reviews are simplistic.
- **Dr. B's PDA**
  http://mtf115.50megs.com/pdasoftware.htm
  Several freeware Palm OS applications and well-chosen medical links. However, aggressive pop-up ads at this site.
- **GasPalm**
  http://www.gaspalm.co.uk/
  Anesthesia software for Palm OS and Pocket PC handhelds.
- **GuineaSOFT**
  http://www.guineasoft.net/
  Several inexpensive software applications for physicians including GuineaPeds, a specialized patient tracker program for pediatrics.
- **Handheld Medical Resources**
  http://www.users.fast.net/~cascomp/
  A collection of links related to Palm OS and Windows CE handhelds; includes list of development tools.
- **Handhelds For Doctors**
  http://www.handheldsfordoctors.com/
  Useful information for beginners recently condensed into book form.

- **Malaysian Medical Palm Pilot Page**
  http://medpilot.cjb.net/
  One physician's opinion of how to choose a handheld and preferred programs.
- **The Matt Delaney Page**
  http://www.geocities.com/docpanama/
  Freeware for iSilo including references for interpreting chest X-rays and EKGs.
- **Medical iSilo Depot**
  http://meistermed.com/isilodepot/
  Well-indexed depository of iSilo documents.
- **MedLists.net**
  http://www.medlists.net/
  Free databases of medical abbreviations (requires list.prc, a freeware database program).
- **medrevu.com**
  http://www.medrevu.com/products/pda.asp
  Purchase selections from the popular "Recall" series for your Palm OS or Pocket PC handheld.
- **Medscout Palm Medical Links**
  http://www.medscout.com/palm_pilot/
  More Palm OS links.
- **MeisterMed**
  http://www.meistermed.com/
  Well-known medical reference company with excellent ICD-9 and CPT references for Palm OS and Pocket PC handhelds.
- **Nephro To Go**
  http://www.nephrotogo.com/
  Palm OS handbook of nephrology.
- **PalmDocs**
  http://www.palmdocs.org/
  Great site if you're looking for more iSilo documents. Also offers several well-done tutorials.
- **palmpsychiatrist.com**
  http://www.palmpsychiatrist.com/
  Dedicated site for mental health professionals, but being redesigned and currently under construction.
- **PDASurgery.com**
  http://pdasurgery.com/
  Good to check out if you're a surgeon. Also offers up-to-date handheld news.
- **The Pediatric Pilot Page**
  http://www.keepkidshealthy.com/pedipilot.html
  Good first stop for pediatricians looking for Palm OS software.
- **Pilot First Aid Page**
  http://www.dogpatch.org/firstaid.html

Comprehensive listing of first-aid files converted into the Palm DOC format (provided by the Irish Emergency Ambulance Services Resource).

- **Pocket DVM**
  http://www.pocketdvm.com/
  First electronic textbook for veterinarians—uses iSilo on either platform.
- **PocketPsych**
  http://www.pocketpsych.com/
  Dedicated site for mental health professionals; includes Palm OS software downloads and frequently asked questions.
- **Matt Price's Links**
  http://plaza.ufl.edu/mgprice/Links.htm
  Downloadable iSilo files including ECG Palm Brain and Arrhythmia/ACLS Palm Brain, both by Dr. Ken Grauer, and study guides for first- and second-year medical students from the University of Kansas.
- **Raja's Palm Library**
  http://abusharr.net/palm.html
  More links to Palm OS medical resources.
- **Andrew Yee's Palm Pilot Page**
  http://eponyms.net/
  Includes a free database of 1300 medical eponyms, now downloadable for both Palm OS and Pocket PC, as well as a comprehensive list of Palm OS links.

Summary

So there you have it—every handheld healthcare Web site we could find. We've covered everything from huge commercial behemoths to one-page personal home pages ("labors of love"). If we missed your favorite, please accept our sincere apologies and let us know. Until then, happy Web surfing!

Acknowledgment. Our special thanks to Kent Willyard, MD.

5

What Floor Is Mrs. Jones on, and What Does Her CBC Look Like Today? Patient Records on Handheld Computers

AMY PRICE

All of us have experienced the frustration of arriving at the hospital to make early-morning rounds and spending considerable time trying to find where a patient is located and what their latest lab work shows. Of course, if it's the weekend, this may be compounded by the fact that your partner's checkout list is completely illegible or, worse, lost somewhere in your trunk or laundry basket. Now imagine doing all this without the assistance of caffeine, as of course, the coffee cart is closed on Saturday mornings.

As a patient care provider, nothing seems more desirable than a handheld computer that manages all the data collection, note writing, and paperwork hassles. Now, imagine being able to do all this while walking into the hospital from the parking lot (this might allow time to stop somewhere for a cup of coffee). Indeed, current handheld technology begins to chip away at the current inefficiencies of medical record keeping, and lays the groundwork for what is rapidly becoming a reliable, secure, timesaving development. Certainly, as institutional capabilities advance, using these record-keeping devices will be natural extensions of the electronic medical record. There are programs for nearly every specialty, and all the basic programs can be tailored to individual practice preferences. The range of capacity goes from a simple census and "To Do" list to widely configurable platforms with multiple preset pull-down menus. The specialty-specific software often includes a combination of coding and tracking as well.

Palm OS and Pocket PC units have many similar offerings. For the purposes of this discussion, we'll look at one premade program for the Palm OS that is currently one of the most widely used. It is freeware, which is not an indication of its value; in fact, it seems to be among the most versatile programs available at this time. We also show you a roundup of all the various programs available for Palm and Pocket PC handhelds so that you can get rid of your index cards and start tracking patients using your handheld computer.

97

The Basics of Keeping Track of Mrs. Jones: Formats for Patient Trackers

There are two kinds of software for patient tracking: stand-alone programs or database templates. The database templates are exactly what they sound like—veritable tabulae rasae that require some work on the front end to make them what you want. HanDBase is one of the easiest database programs to use for this type of project. The software is available for both Palm and Pocket PC platforms and can be downloaded at www.handbase.com. We show you in Chapter 17 how to build a simple procedures log using this program, and you can also build your own patient tracker using the same basic skills. Other database programs are covered in more detail in Chapter 11.

The stand-alone programs also run the gamut of flexibility and capacity for customization, but are ready to use out of the box. Many are specific to a certain specialty, thus requiring little in the way of input for basic record keeping. The more general patient-tracking programs out there have similar format:

- A patient census
- Individual patient data
- Location
- Medications, labs, vital signs, studies, problem list, notes
- "To do" list

Depending on the other interfaces your handheld has, and the hospital information technology infrastructure where you practice, patient tracking on handhelds can range from complete manual input to generally "pushed" data that come magically from central databases every time you synchronize or enter the hospital's wireless network (if you're lucky enough to have one). Many of these programs can be linked into any hospital's legacy information databases (for a small fee, of course). Table 5.1 lists some common handheld programs for patient tracking, for Pocket PC and Palm handhelds.

Palm OS Software

PatientKeeper Personal is a Palm application that is a fun and fairly straightforward system for managing your patient list. It is one of the most versatile systems, and the most complex! It uses an open platform centered around a patient list that allows you to add programs from other developers. It comes with "modules" that run databases for labs, tests, notes, etc. The personal version is a free download available at the PatientKeeper website, www.patientkeeper.com. Look for the demos: they are a good introduction to the desktop systems that augment these packages tremen-

	Desktop version	Palm OS	Pocket PC		
TABLE 5.1. Palm OS and Pocket PC Programs for patient record keeping.					
Software name				Cost	Site
PatientKeeper	+	+		Free	patientkeeper.com
PocketPractitioner 2002	+	+		$69.00	PalmGear.com
WardWatch		+		$29.95	pdaMD.com
Patient Tracker	+	+	+	Free	handheldmed.com
Mobile MedData Charts	+	+	+	$49.00 for handheld; $599.00 for desktop	medcomsys.com
DOXUITE			+	$49.00	Handango.com
Quick Rounds			+	$19.95	medicalpocketpc.com
Noteworthy Clinical Companion 2.2			+	$69.00	medicalpocketpc.com

dously. There is also a user manual that is downloadable in PDF format; the following discussion should clarify much of their text.

Getting Started: Logon Screens and the Mobile Patient Index

Select the PatientKeeper icon from the application/launch screen of your Palm (Figure 5.1). The main page in PatientKeeper is called the mobile patient index, or mPI, which is your patient census (Figure 5.2). From here, you enter or select an individual patient and start rolling. This is also the

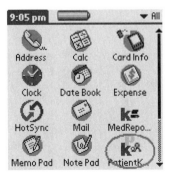

FIGURE 5.1. PatientKeeper icon, Palm home page. (Reprinted with permission from patientKeeper, Inc.)

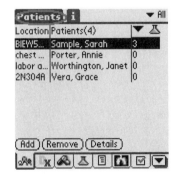

FIGURE 5.2. Mobile patient index screen (patient census). Tap on the menu bar at the top to access pull-down menus. (Reprinted with permission from patientKeeper, Inc.)

screen from which patient information is shared with other users via beaming or printing. Filters can be applied to the patient list so that only certain populations pop up for a given selection, and patients can be sorted from this screen into various categories. PatientKeeper is based on several modules centered around each patient, from notes to labs to demographic data. Everything is accessed from this mPI page.

Hands Off! Logon Security

With all the Health Insurance Portability and Accountability Act (HIPAA) regulations and confidentiality needs of medical record keeping, it's a good idea to make the use of your device secure. PatientKeeper has a security code option. From the mPI screen, tap on the menu bar at the top (Figure 5.2, circled) to access the pull-down menus (Figure 5.3). Under "Configure," go to "User Settings" and type in your username. You'll be "queried" about setting a password on next startup; say "yes," and then the next time you boot up PatientKeeper, you will enter a PIN that you need to remember. PatientKeeper has a few additional preferences for programming and memory use.

Memory Use

PatientKeeper has an optional Cache Framework component that maintains information from the program in memory even when the program itself is not being used; this increases the speed of starting the program, but requires extra memory. To use the feature, access the Menu pulldown as above. Under "Configure," go to "Framework Preferences" (Figure 5.4), and select "Cache Framework."

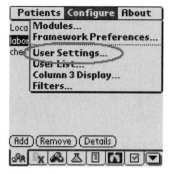

FIGURE 5.3. User Settings. (Reprinted with permission from patientKeeper, Inc.)

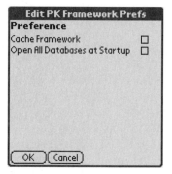

FIGURE 5.4. Preferences for memory use. (Reprinted with permission from patientKeeper, Inc.)

Power Users Tip

This feature must be unchecked if you need to install a new version onto your Palm at a later time, or if you want to add new modules as they come out. The other selection in this screen allows all the modules to be booted up at startup, making it faster to use the program once you are in it (but slower to start). This feature cannot be used if Cache Framework is enabled.

Power Users Tip

If you toggle frequently between programs on your Palm during the day, use the Cache Framework setting, but if you get into PatientKeeper and stay there while you're rounding, the extra time on the front end to boot up the modules saves you a lot of time while you're in the program.

Programming Preferences

This feature allows you to make advanced programming options in the NoteKeeper module, linking data from individual modules such as vitals or test results to daily notes. Access this from the NoteKeeper screen (Figure 5.5). Use the Menu Pulldown (Figure 5.6), and choose "Options," then "Preferences." Select the box for Advanced Mode (Figure 5.7) then tap OK.

For the hands-on exercises in the rest of this chapter, we highly recommend that you download a demo version of Patientkeeper (if you have a Palm handheld, of course), and try these tasks yourself.

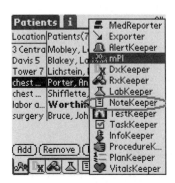

FIGURE 5.5. Programming in advanced mode. Access this feature via the NoteKeeper module. (Reprinted with permission from patientKeeper, Inc.)

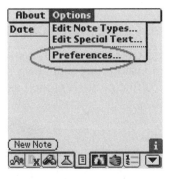

FIGURE 5.6. In NoteKeeper mode, choose Preferences. (Reprinted with permission from patientKeeper, Inc.)

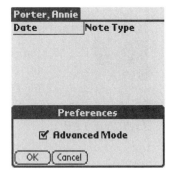

FIGURE 5.7. Preferences: Advanced mode. (Reprinted with permission from patient-Keeper, Inc.)

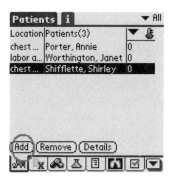

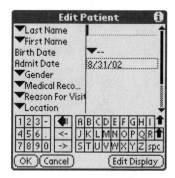

FIGURE 5.8. Mobile Patient Index: Add a new patient. (Reprinted with permission from patientKeeper, Inc.)

FIGURE 5.9. mPI: Edit patient screen. (Reprinted with permission from patientKeeper, Inc.)

HANDS-ON EXERCISE 5.1. FROM NOTECARDS TO THE PALM OF YOUR HAND

Your patient list is displayed in three columns: location, name, and a customizable column that you can change by using the pull-down arrow (this helps to avoid that "confused where-are-my-patients" physician look). After we try entering a patient, we'll get to the more fun stuff. Let's walk through adding a new patient first.

From the main screen of PatientKeeper, select "Add" to begin adding a new patient to your list (Figure 5.8). The "Edit Patient" screen appears (Figure 5.9), where you can either type data in or use drop-down menus that you have customized to enter patient information.

HANDS-ON EXERCISE 5.2. HIERARCHICAL PICKER

PatientKeeper uses the interestingly named Hierarchical Picker as the basis for editing and customizing pull-down menus for each field. In entering patient data, you first notice it in the Last Name field.

Getting There

Let's try using it to customize the Reason For Visit field. As you enter a patient's information, select "Edit" from the Reason for Visit pull-down menu (Figure 5.10). The Hierarchical Picker screen is displayed, which gives you several options (Figure 5.11). For all customization, the Hierarchical Picker allows both "branches" and "leaves." This field already comes with some preset "leaves," but we can try adding a branch and then some leaves of a common admission diagnosis. Tap "New Branch," and use the free text site to enter a branch (Figure 5.12). Pneumonia then shows up in the main Hierarchical Picker screen with an arrow to the right. This arrow allows you

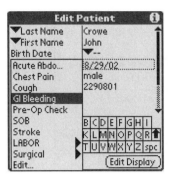

FIGURE 5.10. mPI: Edit reason for visit. (Reprinted with permission from patientKeeper, Inc.)

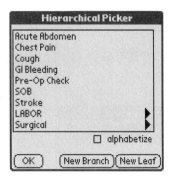

FIGURE 5.11. mPI: Hierarchical Picker: Customize your data entry fields. (Reprinted with permission from patientKeeper, Inc.)

to access the "Leaves." Tap Pneumonia again, and then open, and let's add some leaves (Figures 5.13, 5.14). Tap "New Leaf" from the main screen to enter a common diagnosis without subheadings, such as Fever of Unknown Origin.

Each of the drop-down menus for patient data entry has the capacity for customization. An initial investment of thought and time will make later patient entry much quicker. As you are getting started, go through each of the fields and set it up according to your preference, if you have the time.

You can now "clean up" your patient information display by selecting "Edit Display" to change the fields that are presented (Figure 5.15). Let's change it to reflect what we really want to know. By unselecting the fields, you decrease unnecessary information and fields you have to scroll through (Figure 5.16). Finally, tapping OK on the Edit Patient display gets you back to the mPI where you see your list (growing!).

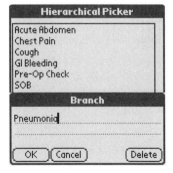

FIGURE 5.12. Hierarchical Picker: New branch. (Reprinted with permission from patientKeeper, Inc.)

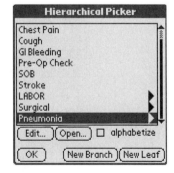

FIGURE 5.13. Hierarchical Picker: New leaf. (Reprinted with permission from patientKeeper, Inc.)

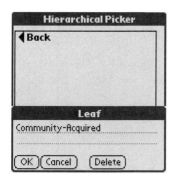

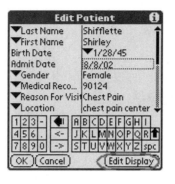

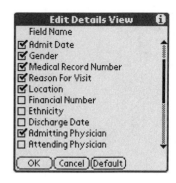

FIGURE 5.14. Hierarchical Picker: New leaf. (Reprinted with permission from patient-Keeper, Inc.)

FIGURE 5.15. mPI: Edit display. (Reprinted with permission from patientKeeper, Inc.)

FIGURE 5.16. mPI: Edit details view. (Reprinted with permission from patientKeeper, Inc.)

HANDS-ON EXERCISE 5.3. FURTHER CUSTOMIZATION OF THE MPI (FURTHER REFINEMENT OF THE "CONFUSED-WHERE-ARE-MY-PATIENTS" AVOIDANCE SYSTEM)

There are a few other ways to customize the mPI screen. You can hide patients who you might have discharged but know might "bounce back" (Figure 5.17). From the mPI screen, highlight the patient you want to hide, and then tap the Patients dropdown. Select "Un/Hide Selection," and that patient will be stored on a hidden list. To recover them to the main screen, go to the upper-right dropdown (Figure 5.18) and select Hidden. While in the Hidden mPI screen, selecting the Un/Hide Selection will put that patient back in your active list.

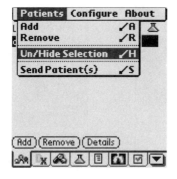

FIGURE 5.17. mPI: Un/Hide patients. (Reprinted with permission from patientKeeper, Inc.)

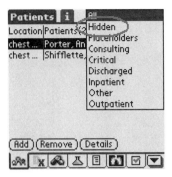

FIGURE 5.18. mPI: Recover hidden patient. (Reprinted with permission from patient-Keeper, Inc.)

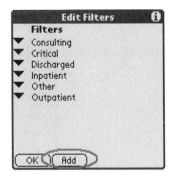

FIGURE 5.19. mPI: Add a filter. (Reprinted with permission from patientKeeper, Inc.)

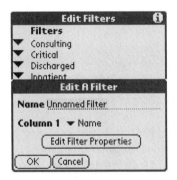

FIGURE 5.20. mPI: Editing filters. (Reprinted with permission from patientKeeper, Inc.)

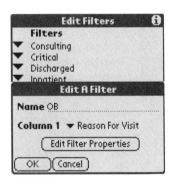

FIGURE 5.21. mPI: Editing filters. (Reprinted with permission from patientKeeper, Inc.)

You can use the Filters option under the Configure dropdown (see Figure 5.3) to change how you view your patient list. Let's say you have a busy obstetric practice in addition to all your critically ill patients, and you'd occasionally like to see only your OB list. From "Edit Filters," tap "Add" (Figure 5.19) and then, on the "Edit a Filter" screen, highlight "Unnamed Filter" and type OB (Figures 5.20, 5.21). By editing the filter properties, you can identify OB patients by calling them *inpatient* and *other* (Figure 5.22) under the "Patient Type" drop-down menu. In the "Edit Patient" screen from the mPI, all your OB patients can be entered as *inpatient* and *other* and they will be filtered as OB patients (Figure 5.23).

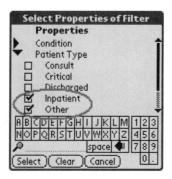

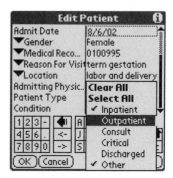

FIGURE 5.22. mPI: Identifying patients for a new Filter. (Reprinted with permission from patientKeeper, Inc.)

FIGURE 5.23. mPI: When entering patient data in the mPI, use the identifiers shown to select them for your new filter. (Reprinted with permission from patientKeeper, Inc.)

HANDS-ON EXERCISE 5.4. EXPLORING MODULES: WHAT, WHERE, AND WHEN SANS PAPER

The modules in PatientKeeper are a smorgasbord of data. There are 14 possible features that you can display, 8 of which can be accessed at any time from the toolbar at the bottom of the mPI. Learning the symbols is fairly intuitive. Edit the modules on the toolbar by visiting the "Configure" dropdown menu (Figure 5.24). Learn what the individual icons in this display mean (Figure 5.25) by tapping the "Information" button (i) at the upper right corner of the screen (Figure 5.26).

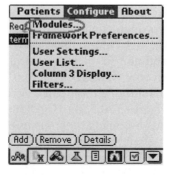

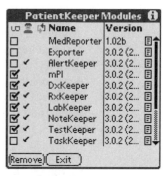

FIGURE 5.24. mPI: Edit module display. (Reprinted with permission from patientKeeper, Inc.)

FIGURE 5.25. mPI: Edit module display. (Reprinted with permission from patientKeeper, Inc.)

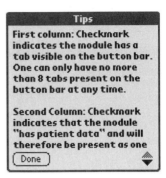

FIGURE 5.26. mPI: Information about the icons in the Edit module display. Access from the icon in the upper right corner of the screen. (Reprinted with permission from patientKeeper, Inc.)

Power Users Tip

Be careful when you're in this editing site: the "Remove" feature deletes modules from the program, and will clear the contents of any stored patient data in that module! You can add the module back, but this requires rebooting the whole program.

HANDS-ON EXERCISE 5.5. DIAGNOSISKEEPER: THE PROBLEM LIST

Sally "I-think-I'm-in-labor-again" Smith is finally admitted and is in active labor. As you admit her, use the DiagnosisKeeper to house an active problem list and link to tasks (Figure 5.27). DiagnosisKeeper allows you to enter free text or to select from drop-down menus (Figure 5.28). For this

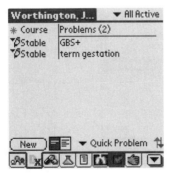

FIGURE 5.27. DiagnosisKeeper main screen. (Reprinted with permission from patientKeeper, Inc.)

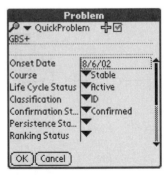

FIGURE 5.28. New diagnosis: Tap "New," then enter free text. (Reprinted with permission from patientKeeper, Inc.)

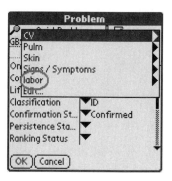

FIGURE 5.29. Diagno-
sisKeeper: QuickProblems.
(Reprinted with permission
from patientKeeper, Inc.)

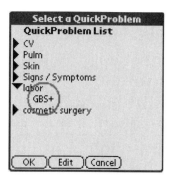

FIGURE 5.30. Hierarchical
Picker of QuickProblems.
(Reprinted with permission
from patientKeeper, Inc.)

patient in labor, an additional problem is her previously diagnosed Group
B Strep (GBS) infection. This factor can be added as free text, or can be
accessed from a customized QuickProblem drop-down menu, under labor
(Figures 5.29, 5.30). A great feature of this module is the ability to link to
TaskKeeper. Use the box to identify tasks, which then can be accessed from
either TaskKeeper or DxKeeper (Figures 5.31, 5.32). To save a free text
entry as a QuickProblem, enter it (Figure 5.33) and then click on the "plus"
icon (Figure 5.34). You'll be prompted to select a branch under which to
store the new QuickProblem leaf (Figure 5.35).

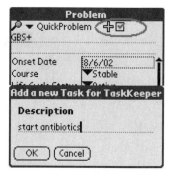

FIGURE 5.31. Link to
TaskKeeper using the check
box in the Problem Edit
screen. (Reprinted with permission from patientKeeper,
Inc.)

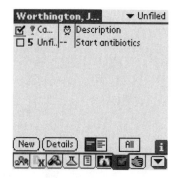

FIGURE 5.32. View tasks from
TaskKeeper module, as
entered in DxKeeper.
(Reprinted with permission
from patientKeeper, Inc.)

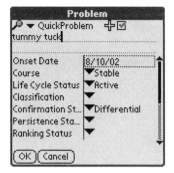

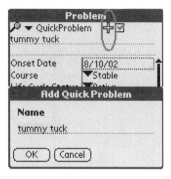

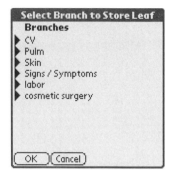

FIGURE 5.33. Store free
text as a QuickProblem.
(Reprinted with permission
from patientKeeper, Inc.)

FIGURE 5.34. Store free
text as a QuickProblem.
(Reprinted with permission
from patientKeeper, Inc.)

FIGURE 5.35. Store free
text as a QuickProblem.
(Reprinted with permission
from patientKeeper, Inc.)

HANDS-ON EXERCISE 5.6. PRESCRIPTIONKEEPER

Billy-everything-is-wrong, who was just discharged from his most recent
200+-day inpatient hospitalization, is on the phone. As the funny sinking
feeling in your chest mounts, he relates the story of how his overjoyed
dog slobbered on the 30 written prescriptions you gave him and he needs
them redone. Smiling to yourself, you open your handheld and remember
how much you hated these calls 6 months ago: "Where do you want me to
call these in?"

This is a neat module that allows you to track meds, link them to problem
lists, write prescriptions, and record events such as when meds are stopped
or started or when you last wrote a prescription.

Getting There

From the mPI, tap the RxKeeper icon (circled) and you come to the main
page, where all the medications are listed (Figure 5.36).

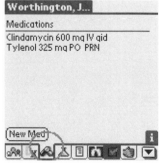

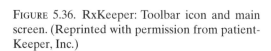

FIGURE 5.36. RxKeeper: Toolbar icon and main
screen. (Reprinted with permission from patient-
Keeper, Inc.)

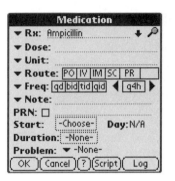

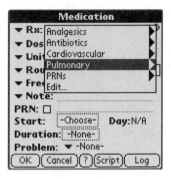

FIGURE 5.37. RxKeeper: Adding meds. Note the magnifying glass in the upper right. Use that to get to the macro (see Figure 5.39). (Reprinted with permission from patientKeeper, Inc.)

FIGURE 5.38. RxKeeper: Pulldown menus of common meds. (Reprinted with permission from patientKeeper, Inc.)

Adding New Meds

To add a new med, tap "New Med," and an edit screen appears. Patient-Keeper has a great database of medications. As you type, several medication names will try to fill in your Rx field. Just typing "Amp" gets you Ampicillin (Figure 5.37). There is a drop-down menu as well for common meds (Figure 5.38). From the medication edit screen, a searchable macro is accessed from the magnifying glass at the upper right. Enter the med name to access the alphabetical list (Figure 5.39a). This is a handy dosing guide for many common medications. You cannot add medications to the list, but you can alter the dosing regimen to suit your style. Let's say you generally order acetaminophen as a PRN for patients. Under the standard listing, the dose is 325 mg. To change this to 650 mg, go to the macro (see Figure 5.39a), and select acetaminophen. Acetaminophen will appear in the medication screen; from here, tap the menu button. Select "Update Current Med Macro" (Figure 5.39b). You then get a screen of categories to choose from that you can edit (Figure 5.39c). Select PRNs, Tylenol (Figure 5.39d). The screen will revert to the Medication screen; type in the dose you prefer in the highlighted dose field (Figure 5.40) and this will be saved as your new acetaminophen PRN dose.

Deleting a Med

Delete a current medication by selecting "Delete Med Record" from the screen in Figure 5.39b. The program will ask you to confirm the deletion (Figure 5.41).

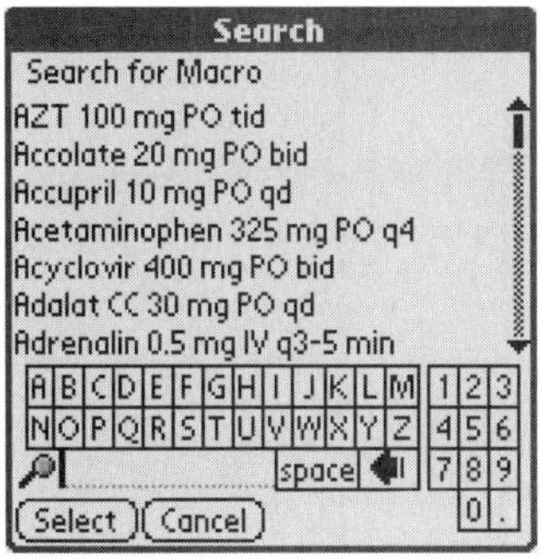

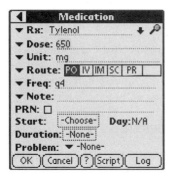

FIGURE 5.39a. RxKeeper:
Search medications with a
dosing guideline. (Reprinted
with permission from patient-
Keeper, Inc.)

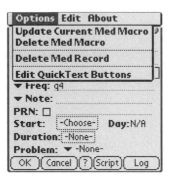

FIGURE 5.39b. RxKeeper:
Select Update Med Macro.
(Reprinted with permission
from patientKeeper, Inc.)

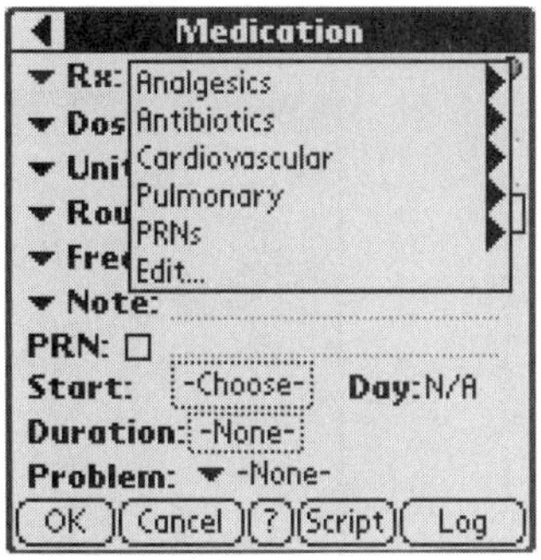

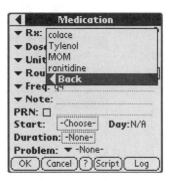

FIGURE 5.39c. RxKeeper:
Update Med Macro. Cus-
tomize PRN order set.
(Reprinted with permission
from patientKeeper, Inc.)

FIGURE 5.39d. RxKeeper:
Update Med Macro. Choose
PRNs. (Reprinted with per-
mission from patientKeeper,
Inc.)

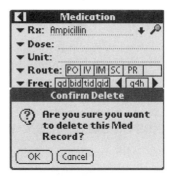

FIGURE 5.40. RxKeeper:
Screen reverts to Medication
screen. Customize highlighted
dose. (Reprinted with permission from patientKeeper, Inc.)

FIGURE 5.41. RxKeeper:
Delete med from Macro.
(Reprinted with permission
from patientKeeper, Inc.)

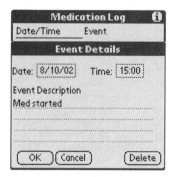

FIGURE 5.42. RxKeeper: Event log for medications. Access using the Log icon in the lower right of the Medication edit screen. (Reprinted with permission from patient-Keeper, Inc.)

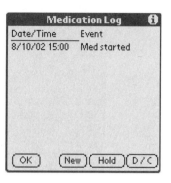

FIGURE 5.43. RxKeeper: Medication Log screen. (Reprinted with permission from patientKeeper, Inc.)

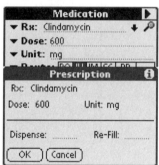

FIGURE 5.44. RxKeeper: Prescription feature. (Reprinted with permission from patient-Keeper, Inc.)

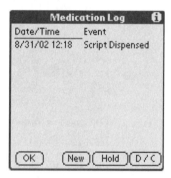

FIGURE 5.45. RxKeeper: Event log of an Rx dispensation. (Reprinted with permission from patientKeeper, Inc.)

Event Recording

RxKeeper also has a log feature to record events such as prescription dispensation or hold times (Figures 5.42, 5.43). The prescription feature (Figure 5.44) lets you record when you've given a prescription to a patient. It then automatically stores this as an event (Figure 5.45).

HANDS-ON EXERCISE 5.7. VITALSKEEPER

Although most practicing physicians rely on bedside charts and nurse's reports for vital signs, hark back to your days as a medical student when not having the excruciating details of each and every vital would be your downfall during "Dr. Jones-the-nasty-attending-pimping-rounds."

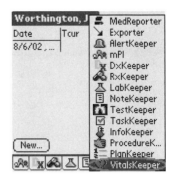

FIGURE 5.46. VitalsKeeper.
(Reprinted with permission
from patientKeeper, Inc.)

Although you may not want to hand enter vitals in the program, synchronizing with a hospital information system to get this information is possible. Recording vitals for your patients in this program serves many functions. Once this information is stored, it can be accessed by the note-writing program and directly linked to your text.

Getting There

The data entry page is found after tapping the "New" icon. From the main vitals screen, the date and data can be accessed by scrolling with the arrows (Figure 5.46).

Recording Vitals

Tap "New" in the VitalsKeeper main module screen (Figure 5.47), or tap on a recorded item to edit it in the "Detail" view (Figure 5.48).

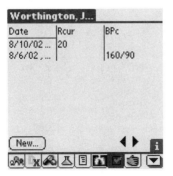

FIGURE 5.47. Scroll with the
arrows in VitalsKeeper.
(Reprinted with permission
from patientKeeper, Inc.)

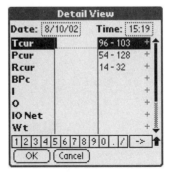

FIGURE 5.48. VitalsKeeper:
Edit in the Detail View.
(Reprinted with permission
from patientKeeper, Inc.)

HANDS-ON EXERCISE 5.8. LABKEEPER: HAVING FUN BEING A GEEK

Similar to VitalsKeeper, this is one feature that will certainly delight the most obsessive-compulsive medical students. Of course, if these data were uploaded automatically, any physician would welcome it with open arms.

In the LabKeeper module, patient labs can be entered into standardized panels, which are then displayed by date from the main screen of the module. Once again, the information from this module will be accessible for the note-writing function, so you never have to write things twice!

Getting There

From the mPI, access LabKeeper from the pull-down menu. In the main screen, labs can be viewed in simple list form (Figure 5.49), or a more detailed view can be accessed from this screen (Figure 5.50). This is a feature similar to the DxKeeper main screen. To toggle between these, simply click the box in the lower-left corner of the screen (Figure 5.50).

New Patient Entry

Data entry is very straightforward. From the New Panel pulldown in the main screen of LabKeeper, select the type of lab to be added (Figure 5.51). Enter the data either by tapping on the part of the stick diagram where the information goes or by using the written prompts (Figure 5.52). Once entry is complete, click "Done" to return to the main screen.

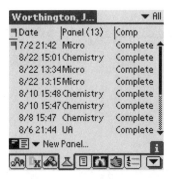

FIGURE 5.49. LabKeeper: Main module screen. (Reprinted with permission from patientKeeper, Inc.)

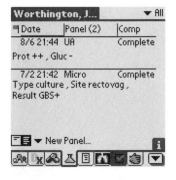

FIGURE 5.50. Details View of LabKeeper. Toggle using the icon in the lower left corner of the screen. (Reprinted with permission from patient-Keeper, Inc.)

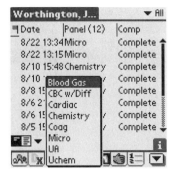

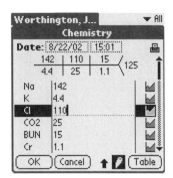

Figure 5.51. LabKeeper: Add a new lab. (Reprinted with permission from patient-Keeper, Inc.)

Figure 5.52. LabKeeper: Enter lab values on the stick figure or on the line. (Reprinted with permission from patientKeeper, Inc.)

Editing Patient Data

Once data are recorded, editing is possible by selecting the lab to be edited from the main LabKeeper screen. Once you are in the panel view, click on the pencil icon at the bottom of the screen (Figure 5.53) so that the red line is not apparent in the box; this transforms the lab from a read-only screen to one that can be edited.

Highlighting Important Labs

While still in the panel view, you can highlight or annotate labs that will make it obvious in the main LabKeeper screen. To do this, you can't be in edit mode, so make sure that the pencil icon at the bottom of the screen has the red line through it. From the Panel view, click on the result you want to highlight (Figure 5.54); this will take you to a *Result* page in which you

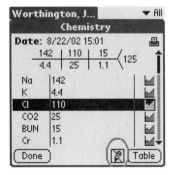

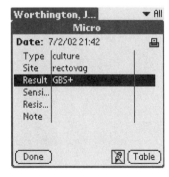

Figure 5.53. LabKeeper: Pencil icon. Change from read-only to edit mode. (Reprinted with permission from patientKeeper, Inc.)

Figure 5.54. LabKeeper: Flagging important labs by highlighting the lab. (Reprinted with permission from patientKeeper, Inc.)

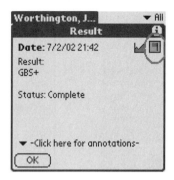

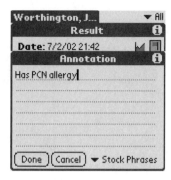

FIGURE 5.55. LabKeeper: Click on the flag to mark it as important. (Reprinted with permission from patient-Keeper, Inc.)

FIGURE 5.56. LabKeeper: Use the annotation pulldown to make notes. (Reprinted with permission from patient-Keeper, Inc.)

can click on the flag to note importance, or use the pulldown at the bottom to enter any pertinent data (Figures 5.55, 5.56). Any lab highlighted as important will then move to the top of the list (Figure 5.57).

Deleting Patient Data

Labs are also deleted from the panel view. Click on the menu button (Figure 5.58) to a pulldown where you can select *Delete Panel*.

Graphing Patient Data

This module's most respectable feature is graphing, but it also has a table form for those of you who remain unimpressed. Can you believe it? You can look at the sodium rise and fall in fantastic detail. To use the graphing

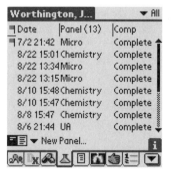

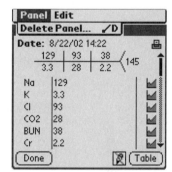

FIGURE 5.57. LabKeeper: Main screen view with important lab flagged. (Reprinted with permission from patient-Keeper, Inc.)

FIGURE 5.58. LabKeeper: Delete a lab from the list. (Reprinted with permission from patientKeeper, Inc.)

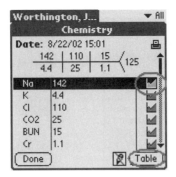

FIGURE 5.59. LabKeeper:
Graph icon (upper circle)
accesses graphing function, or
click on Table to view table
form (lower circle).
(Reprinted with permission
from patientKeeper, Inc.)

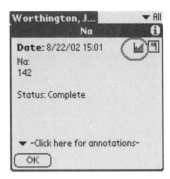

FIGURE 5.60. LabKeeper:
Access graphing function
from individual result view.
(Reprinted with permission
from patientKeeper, Inc.)

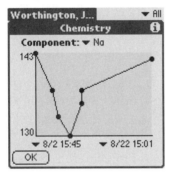

FIGURE 5.61. LabKeeper:
Graph view. (Reprinted with
permission from patient-
Keeper, Inc.)

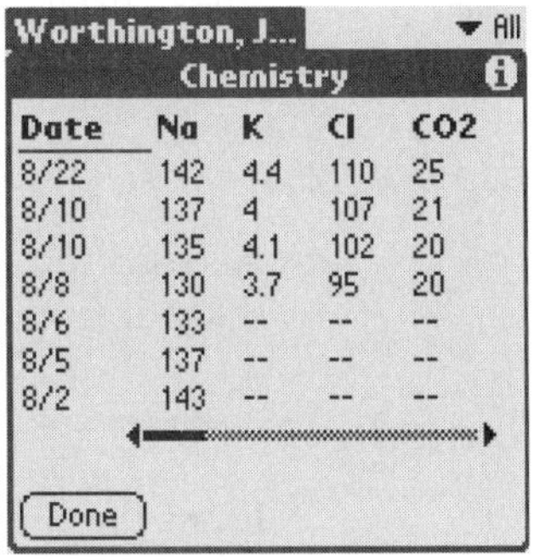

FIGURE 5.62. LabKeeper:
Table view. (Reprinted with
permission from patient-
Keeper, Inc.)

function, click on the graph icon from the panel view (Figure 5.59). You can
also view the graphing feature by clicking on the result itself (the same page
where you can highlight information and make annotations) (Figure 5.60).
Finally, the graph is booted up and Voila! Impressive, eh? (Figure 5.61).
Table view, accessed from the panel view, will load a table with dates and
results (Figure 5.62). Even the "infogeeks" are impressed now, right?

Printing Patient Data

Print individual labs from the printer icon in the upper right of the panels.
     By now, all your colleagues may think you've been reduced to a giddy hand-
held computer-addicted fiend, but wait until they see these other features!

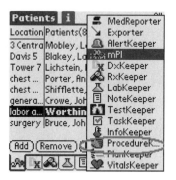

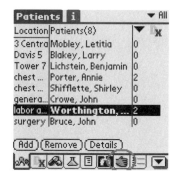

FIGURE 5.63. Procedure-Keeper: Access from the mPI pulldown. (Reprinted with permission from patient-Keeper, Inc.)

FIGURE 5.64. Access ProcedureKeeper from the Toolbar. (Reprinted with permission from patientKeeper, Inc.)

HANDS-ON EXERCISE 5.9. PROCEDUREKEEPER

ProcedureKeeper is a really useful module for those of you who need to keep track of your procedures. It is customizable and can store a lot of detail.

Getting There

Access ProcedureKeeper from the mPI screen (Figure 5.63). Alternatively, select it from the Toolbar at the bottom of the screen (Figure 5.64).

Customizing

From the main screen of ProcedureKeeper, tap "New," and select "Edit Procs." (Figure 5.65). Tap "New," and use the free text entry line to enter the procedure (Figure 5.66). Tap "Add," and then you will be asked to enter

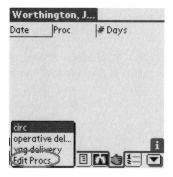

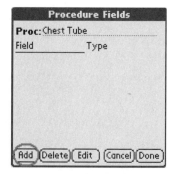

FIGURE 5.65. Procedure-Keeper: To Edit Procedures from the main screen, tap "New." (Reprinted with permission from patientKeeper, Inc.)

FIGURE 5.66. Procedure-Keeper: Use "Add" enter a new procedure in the Proc. Field. (Reprinted with permission from patientKeeper, Inc.)

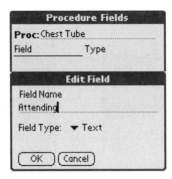
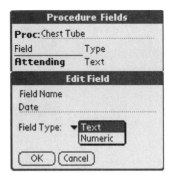

FIGURE 5.67. Procedure-Keeper: Enter Fields regarding procedure that you want to track. (Reprinted with permission from patientKeeper, Inc.)

FIGURE 5.68. Procedure-Keeper: Also track numeric fields. (Reprinted with permission from patientKeeper, Inc.)

a field, which is any information about the procedure that you wish to record, such as Attending physician, which is a Text entry (Figure 5.67), or Date, which is a Numeric entry (Figure 5.68). Although you are editing your procedure list within an individual patient area, the list is available for any patient in your census.

Entering Procedures

Once you have entered your procedures and fields, select the patient for whom you will record a procedure. Tap "New," and select the procedure you've done. The screen will then come up with the name of the procedure and the fields that you already entered (Figure 5.69). From here, you can either manually enter data in a free text screen, by tapping the + sign to the right of the center column, or you can access a Hierarchical Picker and enter

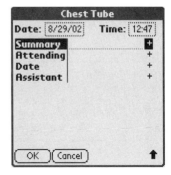

FIGURE 5.69. ProcedureKeeper: Screen view of the newly entered procedure. (Reprinted with permission from patientKeeper, Inc.)

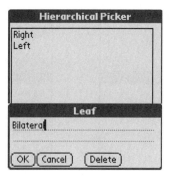

FIGURE 5.70. Procedure-Keeper: Tap Summary to enter details of the procedure in a Hierarchical Picker. (Reprinted with permission from patientKeeper, Inc.)

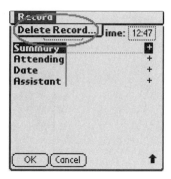

FIGURE 5.71. Procedure-Keeper: Delete a procedure. (Reprinted with permission from patientKeeper, Inc.)

common themes (Figure 5.70). See the tutorial for the Hierarchical Picker (Hands-on Exercise 5.2) for more information.

Deleting Procedures

Delete a procedure from the patient's list by selecting it from the main screen in ProcedureKeeper. Tap the Menu pulldown, then choose "Delete Record" (Figure 5.71).

TestKeeper

TestKeeper is straightforward and allows you to input data that can be viewed in list format with a brief summary of results. It can also be linked to your notes.

Getting There

Select from the mPI toolbar or the pulldown menu to the bottom right of the mPI screen (Figure 5.72).

Customizing Tests

Select "New" from the main TestKeeper screen, and then select "Edit Tests" (Figure 5.73). In the Tests screen, you can add a new test and specify other fields of information pertinent to that test.

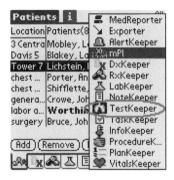

FIGURE 5.72. TestKeeper: Access from the mPI pull-down. (Reprinted with permission from patientKeeper, Inc.)

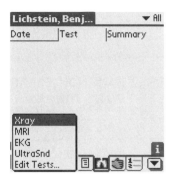

FIGURE 5.73. TestKeeper: Edit a test. (Reprinted with permission from patientKeeper, Inc.)

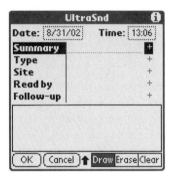

FIGURE 5.74. TestKeeper: Add a new test and access the drawing feature. (Reprinted with permission from patient-Keeper, Inc.)

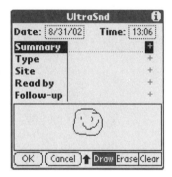

FIGURE 5.75. TestKeeper: Use the drawing feature. (Reprinted with permission from patientKeeper, Inc.)

Adding Tests

From the main module screen of TestKeeper, select "New," and then pick a test from the pull-down menu (Figure 5.74). What follows is another of those features in this software that will delight the gadget geeks: the drawing feature (Figure 5.75).

Power Users Tip

Remember that as in the ProcedureKeeper module, once the Test is added, there will be a Summary field with a Hierarchical Picker in which you can enter other data. For instance, if a V/Q scan is ordered, in the Edit mode, you enter Probability, and then in the Summary Hierarchical Picker, enter Low, Intermediate, or High (see the tutorial on Hierarchical Pickers earlier in this chapter).

HANDS-ON EXERCISE 5.10. NOTEKEEPER: GETTING THE MOST OUT OF DOING THE LEAST

Notes in PatientKeeper are combinations of pull-down menus and free text entry that can make quick work of admission and SOAP note writing once you've customized your data sets. All the data entered in other modules can be accessed from the NoteKeeper for your notes by using links. Your free text entry can be augmented by Qbuttons, which are customizable text buttons that allow common word entry by a simple tap of a button.

Getting There

From the mPI, access the NoteKeeper from the icon (Figure 5.76).

Editing Note Types

From the main screen in NoteKeeper, you can create and delete note types by using the Menu button on your Palm (Figures 5.77, 5.78). The program comes with the standard note types: Admit, H&P, and Progress Note. Depending on your practice, you can make detailed note types with links to data that are very specific to your work. (See the following step-by-step explanation.)

Getting back to our patient Sally "I-think-I'm-in-labor-again" Smith, let's make a note format for her admission. From the main NoteKeeper page, tap the Menu pulldown. Select "Edit Note Types" under Options. A list of current note types is shown; to add a note, choose "Add" (see Figure 5.78).

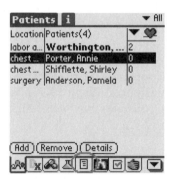

FIGURE 5.76. NoteKeeper: Access from the mPI Toolbar. (Reprinted with permission from patientKeeper, Inc.)

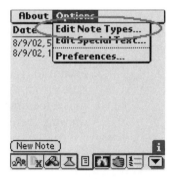

FIGURE 5.77. NoteKeeper: Access the Edit Note Types feature. (Reprinted with permission from patientKeeper, Inc.)

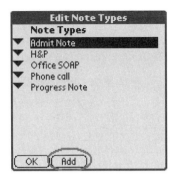

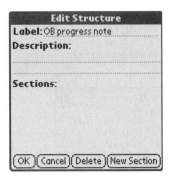

FIGURE 5.78. NoteKeeper: Select "Add" to make a new note type. (Reprinted with permission from patient-Keeper, Inc.)

FIGURE 5.79. Edit Structure: Making a new note type. (Reprinted with permission from patientKeeper, Inc.)

An "Edit Structure" screen appears, and you can choose the note type you want to make. We're making an OB progress note (Figure 5.79). For this note type, we use the basic SOAP format (Figure 5.80) but tailor it to laboring OB patients. Under Subjective, we've typed in a thumbnail of the patient (Figure 5.81). For each section, we can customize the prompts that will show up in the NoteKeeper view.

Writing Notes

Now, let's see how it looks as we use the template for Sally's admission. From the Note Type pull-down menu, select "OB progress note" (Figure 5.82). It then starts with the first section that you entered in the note you created (Figure 5.83). You can then manually insert her age and weeks of

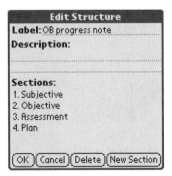

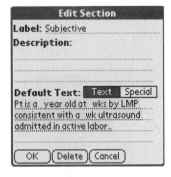

FIGURE 5.80. Edit Structure: Add new sections and customize the wording. (Reprinted with permission from patientKeeper, Inc.)

FIGURE 5.81. Edit Structure: Customize the default text. (Reprinted with permission from patientKeeper, Inc.)

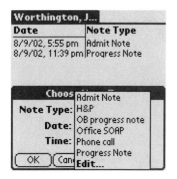

FIGURE 5.82. Writing notes: Choose the new note type from the New Note menu pulldown. (Reprinted with permission from patient-Keeper, Inc.)

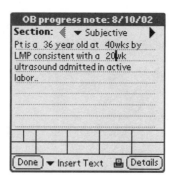

FIGURE 5.83. Writing notes: See your default text and fill in the blanks. (Reprinted with permission from patient-Keeper, Inc.)

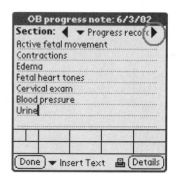

FIGURE 5.84. Writing notes: For next section, use the arrows to advance. (Reprinted with permission from patient-Keeper, Inc.)

gestation. By tapping the arrow in the upper right, corner of the screen you advance to the next section (Figure 5.84). In this screen, you can use Qbuttons to speed up the text entry. These are the fields at the bottom of the page that can be modified. For instance, you can set up your QButtons so that to say "Mrs. S is a 39 yo WF admitted in active labor" you only need to write in the name and age, and tap QButtons for the rest. If you can master the Special Text feature, you don't even need to do that!

Editing Qbuttons

Starting from the template for an Admit Note, access the Qbutton edit screen from the section page (e.g., progress record) where you want the specific information (Figure 5.85). For Sally Smith and other OB patients, your

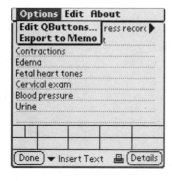

FIGURE 5.85. Edit Qbuttons. (Reprinted with permission from patientKeeper, Inc.)

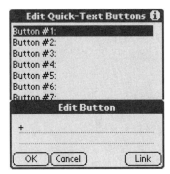

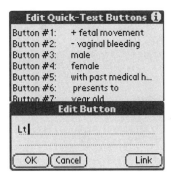

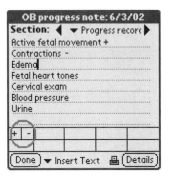

FIGURE 5.86a. Edit Qbuttons: Enter free text for Button #1. (Reprinted with permission from patientKeeper, Inc.)

FIGURE 5.86b. Edit Qbuttons: Customize your text to speed data entry. (Reprinted with permission from patient-Keeper, Inc.)

FIGURE 5.87. Edit Qbuttons: Main screen view of Qbutton text. (Reprinted with permission from patientKeeper, Inc.)

QButton set can really make short work of note writing. Up to 11 Qbuttons per page (i.e., Subjective, Objective . . .) can house short bursts of text. Select "Button #1," and an Edit Button screen (Figure 5.86a) appears. Put a "+" in, which can then be inserted into the programmed text of the section (Figures 5.86b, 5.87).

Advanced Programming

You'll note that in the Edit Qbutton screen there is an icon for inserting a Link. To access this feature, go back to the main screen of NoteKeeper and use the menu pulldown to change your preferences (Figure 5.88). Select "Advanced Mode" to insert links from other modules into your notes (Figure 5.89).

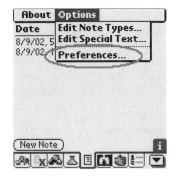

FIGURE 5.88. Preferences: Go to advanced programming to add links to other modules. (Reprinted with permission from patientKeeper, Inc.)

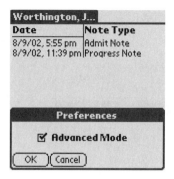

FIGURE 5.89. Preferences: Check Advanced Mode. (Reprinted with permission from patientKeeper, Inc.)

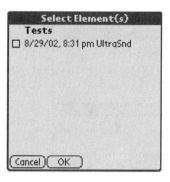

FIGURE 5.90. Qbutton link: Pick the test. (Reprinted with permission from patient-Keeper, Inc.)

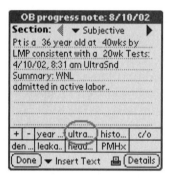

FIGURE 5.91. Qbutton link: Appearance in the text. (Reprinted with permission from patient-Keeper, Inc.)

Link to other modules now that you're in Advanced Mode so that information stored there can be easily and automatically inserted into your notes. In the Edit Qbutton mode, the link to the right of the screen allows you to select the module from which you want to link information. In our case we want to link to an ultrasound, so we select the test we want inserted into the text (Figure 5.90), and when the QButton is selected again, it inserts the summary of the test as well as when it was performed into the body of the text (Figure 5.91).

Power Users Tip

Leave a space before or after the Qbutton text to avoid having to put it in yourself as you enter data.

Inserting Text

At the bottom of the section screens, you have an opportunity to build an Hierarchical Picker. (See Hands-on Exercise 5.2 on the Hierarchical Picker, earlier in this chapter.) Click on "Insert Text," then "Edit," and use the "trees" to input information that you anticipate frequently entering.

Special Text

This is a way to link other data such as first and last name, age, gender, and billing information to Qbuttons, not just items in the modules. In the Edit Qbutton screen, select "Link" (Figure 5.92), and from the pull-down menu, choose "Edit." In the "Edit Special Text" screen, now you can enter information about fields you normally track (Figure 5.93a). In this instance, these are fields that will automatically appear in the note that you are making: age in years, gender, and reason for visit. Let's add to the preset fields a link for other diagnoses. Tap ⟨LINK⟩, which will add a link to the data (Figure 5.93b). Go to "Edit Links" in the bottom right of the screen (Figure 5.93c). Link #4 is undefined. By highlighting Link #4, you are asked to "Select Message Type" (Figure 5.93d). This gets a little complex, so hold on to your stylus! The modules contain four types of data.

1. Snippets are messages that are unchanging values for a given patient in this recorded event, such as first name, last name, age, gender. Links 1 through 3 are snippets.
2. Get Data messages come from ancillary data collected in the modules, such as tests, labs, and diagnoses.
3. Embedded modules allow you to type a new value into the note body, which will then appear in the module that you linked to, such as a new diagnosis that then ends up in DiagnosisKeeper as well.

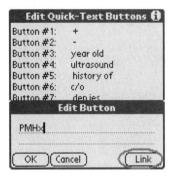

FIGURE 5.92. Edit Special Text: Get there via the link in Edit QButtons. (Reprinted with permission from patient-Keeper, Inc.)

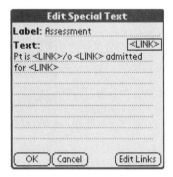

FIGURE 5.93a. Edit Special Text: Click Edit Links to customize. (Reprinted with permission from patientKeeper, Inc.)

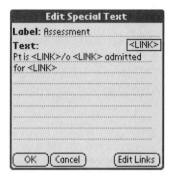

FIGURE 5.93b. Edit Special
Text: Click <LINK> to add a
link. (Reprinted with permission from patientKeeper, Inc.)

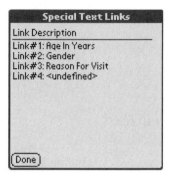

FIGURE 5.93c. Edit Special
Text: Preset fields. (Reprinted
with permission from patient-
Keeper, Inc.)

4. Summary Info is printable information that will be used by other
   programs.

For the preset fields, the messages should already be set. In the link we
are creating. Let's use a *Get Data* message that links additional diagnoses
to the patient's assessment (Figure 5.93e). This takes you to a screen where
you use the pull-down menu to access the module to which you want to
link (Figure 5.93f). Select DxKeeper, then Selected Diagnoses. After this,
you end up in the Special Text Links page again, where Link #4 shows that
it is "Select Diagnoses" (Figure 5.94).

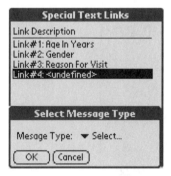

FIGURE 5.93d. Edit Special
Text: Select Message Type.
(Reprinted with permission
from patientKeeper, Inc.)

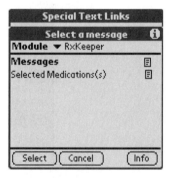

FIGURE 5.93e. Edit Special
Text: After choosing Get
Data, select module from
which to link information.
(Reprinted with permission
from patientKeeper, Inc.)

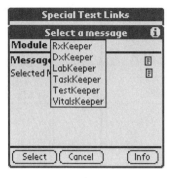

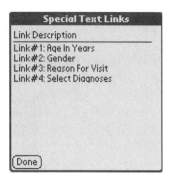

FIGURE 5.93f. Edit Special
Text: Pull-down menu for
options from which to link
information. (Reprinted with
permission from patient-
Keeper, Inc.)

FIGURE 5.94. Edit Special
Text: Link #4 is now set for
Select Diagnoses. (Reprinted
with permission from patient-
Keeper, Inc.)

HANDS-ON EXERCISE 5.11. BEAM ME UP!

Getting and giving sign-out has never been easier or more confidential
using the beaming function on your Palm! No more papers to get lost, no
more wasted time looking for the shredder. This feature allows your Palm
to "talk" to another one equipped with the current PatientKeeper program
and get its data. When you beam, you have the option of sending or receiving lists, small groups or individual patients, and then merging data to
update patient progress. With your infrared (IR) port, you can directly beam
to a printer if your institution has that capacity.

Getting There

From the mobile patient index (mPI), access the beaming feature from the
menu pulldown (circle, Figure 5.95).

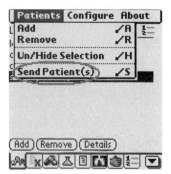

FIGURE 5.95. Send Patients: Menu pull-down.
(Reprinted with permission from patient-
Keeper, Inc.)

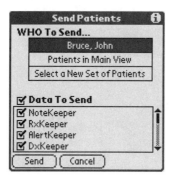

FIGURE 5.96. Send Patients:
WHO To Send. (Reprinted
with permission from patient-
Keeper, Inc.)

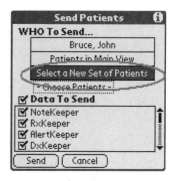

FIGURE 5.97. Send Patients:
Select a new patient to send.
(Reprinted with permission
from patientKeeper, Inc.)

Sending Patients

In sending patients, you have several options. First, make sure the recipient
is using the same version of PatientKeeper. Line up your IR ports. Access
the Send Patient(s) icon from the pull-down menu (see Figure 5.95). When
you tap this icon, you are presented with a screen giving you several options
(Figure 5.96). Send a single patient by selecting that person in the main mPI
screen before pulling down the Send Patient(s) icon. It will then be in the
top window of the selections of "WHO To Send." Alternatively, send all the
patients in your mPI screen by selecting "Patients in Main View," or select
individual patients by tapping on "Select a New Set of Patients" (Figure
5.97). Select the box to send those patients (Figure 5.98), or use a filter to
select patients based on properties that you choose (Figure 5.99).

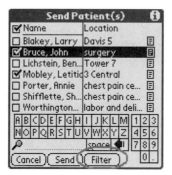

FIGURE 5.98. Send Patients:
Choose by box, or use a filter.
(Reprinted with permission
from patientKeeper, Inc.)

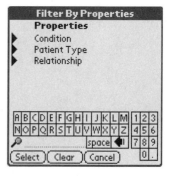

FIGURE 5.99. Filter patients:
Use the filters you designated
when you entered raw patient
data. (Reprinted with permission from patientKeeper, Inc.)

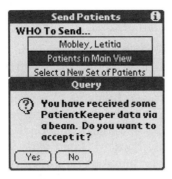

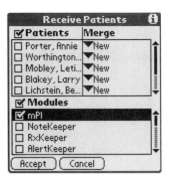

FIGURE 5.100. Receiving Patients: Accept prompt. (Reprinted with permission from patientKeeper, Inc.)

FIGURE 5.101. Receive Patients: Select information to be received. (Reprinted with permission from patient-Keeper, Inc.)

Receiving Patients

To get a patient summary from another user, line up your IR ports, and let the Palm handhelds "shake hands." It takes a few seconds to organize the data, and then your screen will "Query" you about accepting the information (Figure 5.100). Accept the patients, and you will see a screen that lets you choose which patients you want and what information regarding each one you wish to store (Figure 5.101). There are three ways of accepting data: New, Update, and Data-Only (Figure 5.102). For the New option, if you already have a patient in your list by the same name, selecting New patient will put that patient on your list twice. In Update mode, the information in the mPI screen will be changed in addition to the information from the individual modules that are selected. In Data-Only, only the information from the individual modules will be added.

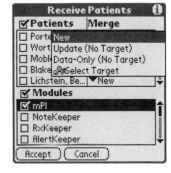

FIGURE 5.102. Receive Patients: Select mode of accepting data. (Reprinted with permission from patientKeeper, Inc.)

Pocket PC Software

The offerings for Pocket PC's, although fewer in number, are very similar. There are a few listings here with regard to patient records software. Now that you've worked your way through PatientKeeper, these other programs will be a snap. If you have a Pocket PC, many of the documents for Palm software can also be read by the Pocket PC by purchasing some additional software. Peacemaker is a program that allows you to transmit documents between a Palm OS and Pocket PC unit fairly seamlessly. Unfortunately, the programs themselves cannot be translated yet. HanDBase, one of the database template-type programs, is available on both the Palm OS and Pocket PC platforms, and other ready-made software for both platforms is increasingly available (see Table 5.1). Other software available for Pocket PC includes Quick Rounds, Noteworthy Clinical Companion 2.2, and

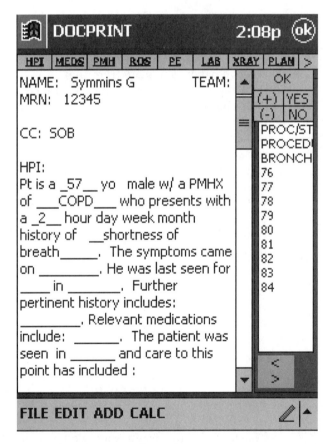

FIGURE 5.103. DOXUITE program. Quick text buttons prompt data entry. (Reprinted with permission from Cross Enterprises ON-CALL, INC.)

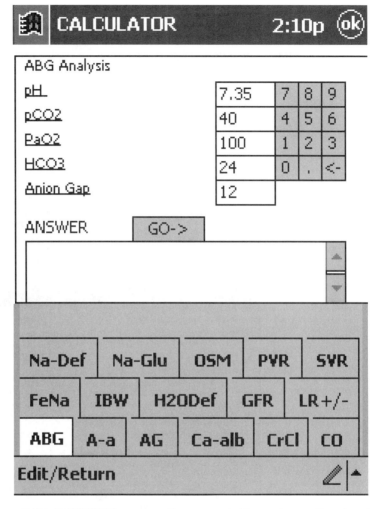

FIGURE 5.104. DOXUITE program. Data entry fields are shown. (Reprinted with permission from Cross Enterprises, ON-CALL, INC.)

DOXUITE. We'll look at a few screens of two of these programs so you can see how they function.

DOXUITE

DOXUITE is a collection of programs that links an information input program with a calculator and print-friendly module. The text is prompted by quick buttons of broad-ranging text, which you can then edit (Figure 5.103). Included are all the general components of a history, physical, labs, and notes (Figure 5.104). It has numbered fields that you can customize to the right of the screen (see Figure 5.103).

Quick Rounds

Quick Rounds completes the field as an abbreviated program that lists patient names and diagnoses (Figure 5.105), with an ICD-9 field and several

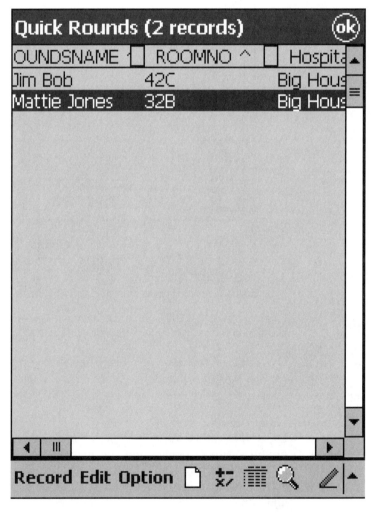

FIGURE 5.105. Quick Rounds PC program. Patient list screen with filters. (Reprinted with permission from SuiteMD)

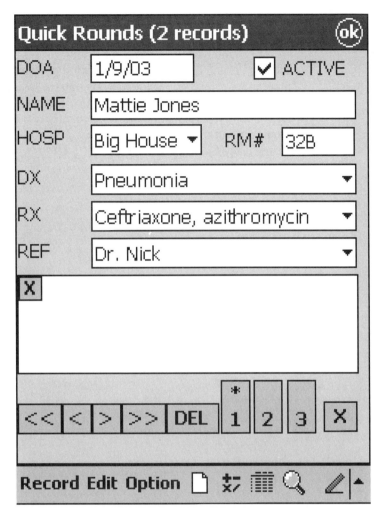

FIGURE 5.106. Quick Rounds PC program. Pull-down menus grow as you use it more. (Reprinted with permission from SuiteMD)

other fields that you can customize. It has a handy toolbar with search functions and easy new patient entry. When you enter data, the pull-down menu remembers what you've entered before, making data entry faster as you use it more (Figure 5.106).

Spend some time doing demos from these and other types of programs to see which one suits your needs, and then stop wasting all that paper and time as you begin rounding with your handheld!

Summary

Well, now you have it. . . . You can finally get rid of those pesky index cards and start doing all your patient tracking on a handheld computer. In this chapter, we talked about the various options available for patient tracking and showed you how to use one of them in great detail. Then, we showed you patient trackers available for Pocket PC's, and also an example of a simple patient tracker that could be used on both Palm and Pocket PC platforms (using HanDBase).

6

Calculator Programs for Handheld Computers: Crunching the Numbers Made Easy

Scott M. Strayer and Mark H. Ebell

Some of the more clinically useful programs developed for handheld computers include the numerous medical calculators currently available. They range in complexity from simple programs designed for calculating one type of problem (i.e., ABG Pro for blood gas analysis) to fully programmable calculators that can calculate anything from the fractional excretion of sodium for acute renal failure to pediatric weight-based dosing of commonly prescribed medications.

Although Palm Powered computers currently have an advantage in the number of programs available, many of the same programs will be available on Pocket PC units in the near future (Table 6.1). We cover ready-made calculators in this chapter and leave the programmable types for Chapter 16.

The many different programs and types of calculations are designed to appeal to a wide variety of specialists and primary care providers. Just about any medical calculation can be found between the preprogrammed and programmable calculators currently available. Of course, these calculators are not designed to replace good clinical judgment, a thorough history and physical examination, or experience solving problems using the original formulas. However, they can augment these basic principles of medicine, and may actually enhance the learning process by having the formulas available at the point of care, where questions often arise.

Single-Purpose Calculators

ABG Pro© | www.stacworks.com | free download

This is a simple, well-designed program that lets you enter blood gas analysis values including pH, pCO_2, HCO_3, Na, and Cl. It has an intuitive, clear

TABLE 6.1. Calculator programs for Palm and Pocket PC handheld computers.

Palm powered computers			
Single calculations	Multiple calculations	Programmable	Windows CE
ABG Pro	MedCalc	SynCalc	Archimedes
Stat Cardiac Clearance	HanDBase with applets	MathPad	HanDBase with applets
Stat Cholesterol	MedRules		InfoRetriever
Ranson			
PregCalc			
PregTrak			

input screen (Figure 6.1), and uses the Henderson–Hasselbach formula to calculate the expected pCO_2 values for metabolic acidosis and alkalosis and the expected HCO_3 values for respiratory alkalosis and acidosis (acute and chronic). It also uses delta–delta values to determine if there was another preexisting metabolic alkalosis or acidosis.

Ranson's Criteria | available at: www.palmgear.com | free download

This is a simple program that has checkboxes for all the criteria and then calculates the predicted mortality rate (Figure 6.2). It is helpful in identifying patients who are at risk for complications of pancreatitis and may require closer monitoring.

Stat Cardiac Clearance | www.statcoder.com | free download

This great little utility will help you take a rational, evidence-based approach to providing clearance for surgery. It lets you choose either the

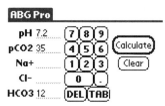

FIGURE 6.1. Inputting blood gas values into ABG Pro. (Reprinted with permission from StacWorks.)

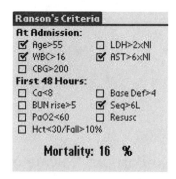

FIGURE 6.2. Ranson's criteria input screen. (Reprinted with permission from Thenar Computing.)

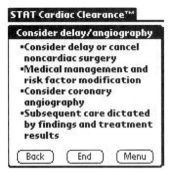

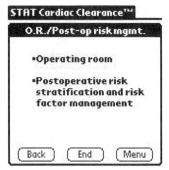

FIGURE 6.3. High-risk screen in Stat Cardiac Clearance. (Reprinted with permission from http://www.statcoder.com.)

FIGURE 6.4. Low-risk screen in Stat Cardiac Clearance. (Reprinted with permission from http://www.statcoder.com.)

American College of Cardiology/American Heart Association guidelines[1] (2002 update) or those of the American College of Physicians[2] (1997). The menus then prompt you for a series of questions that are used to determine the cardiac risk of surgery. If the patient is at high risk, the program will prompt you to consider delaying the surgery, ordering an angiogram, and modifying risk factor (Figure 6.3). If the patient is at low risk, or for emergency surgeries, the program will display a screen suggesting operative clearance and postoperative risk stratification and risk factor management (Figure 6.4). Note that the software carries a disclaimer stating that "this software is currently beta testing for demonstration purposes only." As always, good clinical judgment is paramount.

Stat Cholesterol | www.statcoder.com | free download

For clinicians still grappling with the Third Report of the National Cholesterol Education Program (NCEP),[3] otherwise known as the Adult Treatment Panel III (ATPIII) guidelines, this program may be the answer. A simple screen allows you to enter a patient's cholesterol and risk factors (Figure 6.5); the program then calculates the 10-year risk of acute myocardial infarction. It also shows you the average and low-risk values for the age and gender entered for comparison purposes. The second screen in this program lets you enter coronary heart disease equivalents including clinical coronary heart disease; symptomatic carotid artery disease; peripheral arterial disease; abdominal aortic aneurysm; diabetes; or 10-year risk greater than 20%. The third screen reviews the major risk factors including smoking, hypertension, low HDL, age, family history, and the negative risk factor of high HDL (>60). After entering this information about the patient, the program displays a risk category screen that tells users how many risk factors the patient has, what the LDL goal should be, and when to initiate treatment. Lifestyle changes are written out, including dietary recommen-

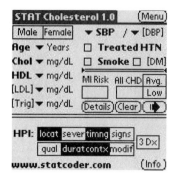

FIGURE 6.5. Main screen in Stat Cholesterol. (Reprinted with permission from http://www.statcoder.com.)

dations and the recommendation for weight management and increased physical activity. This screen also details when drug therapy should be initiated by tapping on the "drug therapy" button. The next screen identifies patients with metabolic syndrome. The final screen in the program classifies the patient's triglyceride level along with treatment recommendations. A similar program is available directly from the National Heart, Lung, and Blood Institute (http://hin.nhlbi.nih.gov/atpiii/atp3palm.htm).

PregCalc Pro | www.medicaltoolbox.com | $24.95
Pregtrak | www.stacworks.com | $15.00

Do you deliver babies? Provide prenatal care? If so, you can replace your trusty OB wheel with these programs. Not only do they calculate due dates, confirm dating by ultrasound, and let you save information about specific patients, but the time spent looking for that OB wheel when you really need it will be regained in practice! Both programs have an intuitive interface and allow for storing and beaming patients. This is ideal when checking out to colleagues or fielding late-night OB calls.

In PregCalc Pro, the opening screen prompts you to enter either the last menstrual period, estimated due date, date of conception, the ultrasound date, the given week for a certain gestational age, or the gestational age at a given time. All the buttons allow for easy calendar input when tapped (Figure 6.6), and the program shows you the gestational age, measurements, expected weight gain, relevant labs that should be ordered, and the projected next appointment date (Figure 6.7). Pregcalc Pro offers a desktop version at their website.

In PregTrak's opening screen (Figure 6.8), you are first prompted to enter either last menstrual period, estimated date of confinement, or ultrasound

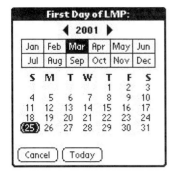

FIGURE 6.6. Last menstrual period entry in Pregcalc Pro. (Reprinted with permission from Medical Toolbox Software.)

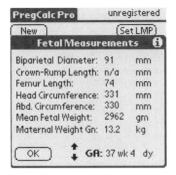

FIGURE 6.7. Measurements and Estimated Gestational Age screen in PregCalc Pro. (Reprinted with permission from Medical Toolbox Software.)

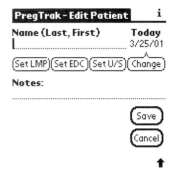

FIGURE 6.8. Opening screen for PregTrak. (Reprinted with permission from StacWorks.)

dates, along with the patient's name and the date of entry. This menu format allows you to generate a list of patients that can also be read using Preg-Trak's desktop software (Figure 6.9). The desktop software only supports the Windows operating system at this time.

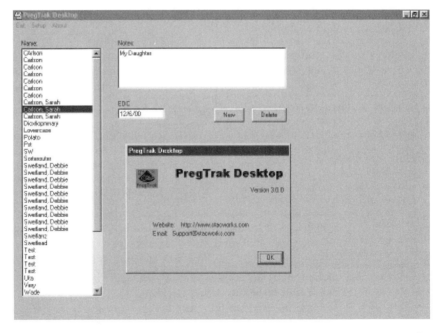

FIGURE 6.9. Desktop for PregTrak. (Reprinted with permission from StacWorks.)

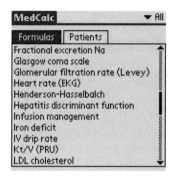

FIGURE 6.10. Menu screen for MedCalc. (Reprinted with permission from Mathias Tschopp, MD.)

Programs with Multiple Calculations

Medcalc | available at: www.palmgear.com | free download

Even if you have a penchant for memorizing medical formulas, this program has much more to offer than simple calculations. It includes dozens of formulas and uses an intuitive interface that allows you to tap on the desired formula (Figure 6.10). Once in the specific formula, you enter the data and the program calculates the answer. Values can even be saved for specific patients. This program contains calculations that will benefit nearly every specialist; see Table 6.2 for the complete list.

HanDBase | http://www.handbase.com | $29.99
HanDBase Applets | http://www.ddhsoftware.com/gallery.html | free downloads

HanDBase is a relatively powerful database application that allows you to create your own simple databases or download premade databases known as "applets" from a website gallery. Because HanDBase allows for simple calculated fields (limited to addition, subtraction, division, multiplication, averaging, and minimum/maximum values), it can be used to perform some of the simpler medical calculations such as weight-based drug dosing. Among some of the more useful applets not found elsewhere are a TPN formula calculator and an APACHE II score calculator for intensive care patients (Figures 6.11, and 6.12).

The first step is to download and install the database program HanD-Base. Then you can add or create up to 60 databases or medical calculation

TABLE 6.2. Calculations available in MedCalc.

Absolute neutrophil count
Age calculator (enter birthdate and current Date)
Alveolar-arterial O_2 gradient
Anion gap
Basal energy expenditure
Body mass index
Body surface area
Cardiac output (Fick)
Cardiac valve area (Gorlin)
Change in plasma Na
Child–Pugh score
Corrected calcium (albumin)
Corrected calcium (protein)
Corrected sodium (glucose)
Corrected sodium (lipids)
Corrected sodium (protein)
Creatinine clearance (Cockcroft)
Creatinine/urea clearance (measured)
Creatinine clearance (Schwartz)
Fractional excretion Na
Glasgow coma scale
Glomerular filtration rate (Levey)
Heart rate (EKG)
Henderson–Hasselbach
Hepatitis discriminant function
Infusion management
Iron deficit
IV drip rate
Kt/V (PRU)
LDL cholesterol
Likelihood ratios
Maintenance IV fluids (pediatric)
Mean arterial pressure
Number needed to treat (NNT)
Osmotic gap (plasma)
Osmotic gap (stool)
Oxygen index
Posttest probability (LR)
Posttest probability (sens/spec)
Predicted peak flow
Pregnancy calculator
Protein excretion
Q-Tc
Transtubular K gradient
Tubular phosphate reabsorption
Units conversion (chemistries)
Units conversion (standard)
Urinary excretion of calcium
Vascular resistances
Water deficit

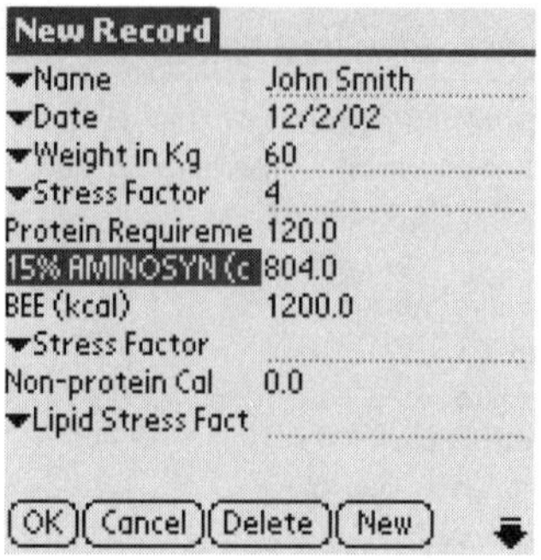

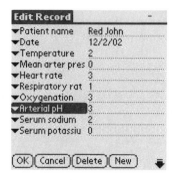

FIGURE 6.11. TPN calculator available for HanDBase. (Reprinted with permission from DDH Software.)

FIGURE 6.12. APACHE II calculator available for HanDBase (Reprinted with permission from DDH Software.).

applets. Some of the calculator programs currently available as applets are shown in Table 6.3.

MedRules | http://pbrain.hypermart.net | free download

Have you ever needed the Gail Breast Cancer Risk predictor while counseling a patient on their breast cancer risk (Figure 6.13)? How about trying

TABLE 6.3. Medical calculators available for HanDBase.

Abbreviated Mental Test score
Airway score
Apache II score
APGAR score
Body Mass Index
Cardiac drips
Cardiac Risk Factor
Creatinine Clearance
Glasgow Coma Score
Integrilin doser
LDL calculator
Mini Mental State Exam
POSSUM score
Pregnancy calculator-EDD
Pregnancy calculator-GA
Pregnancy calculator-LMP
Pregnancy wheel
Risk reduction calculation
Serum osmolality calculator
Tylenol/Motrin doser
TPN
Weight goal

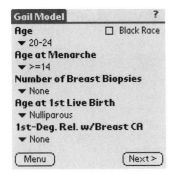

FIGURE 6.13. Gail Breast
Cancer Model in MedRules.
(Reprinted with permission
from Kent E. Wilyard, MD.)

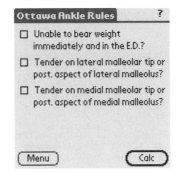

FIGURE 6.14. Ottawa Ankle
Rules in MedRules.
(Reprinted with permission
from Kent E. Wilyard, MD.)

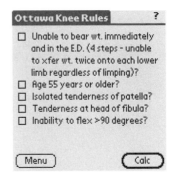

FIGURE 6.15. Ottawa Knee
Rules in MedRules.
(Reprinted with permission
from Kent E. Wilyard, MD.)

to remember the Ottawa Ankle or Knee rules when deciding whether to
order an X-ray on one of your injured amateur athletes (Figures 6.14, 6.15)?
This program has many evidence-based rules built into it and has a simple
user interface for ease of use at the point of care. Another nice feature is
that this software expires periodically, prompting users to update to the
latest version, a nice touch that shows the developer's concern for clinical
accuracy.

Using the program is simple: just select the rule that you would like to
use (Figure 6.16) and enter the values requested. The program currently
contains 40 rules (listed in Table 6.4). In addition to including rules that are
evidence based, the author includes the references used to develop the rule
in Figure 6.17.

Finally, InfoRetriever now has a Palm version of their software. It
contains more than 120 clinical decision rules. See the following for more
information.

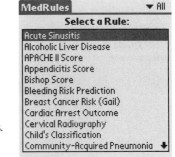

FIGURE 6.16. Rule selection screen in MedRules.
(Reprinted with permission from Kent E.
Wilyard, MD.)

TABLE 6.4. Calculations available in MedRules.

Acute Sinusitis	Mangled Extremity Score
Alcoholic Liver Disease	MI Criteria in Chest Pain w/LBBB
APACHE II Score	Ottawa Ankle Rules
Appendicitis Score	Ottawa Foot Rules
Bishop Score	Ottawa Knee Rules
Bleeding Risk Prediction	Pediatric Trauma Score
Breast Cancer Risk (Gail)	Pharyngitis Evaluation
Cardiac Arrest Outcome	Predicting Pulmonary Embolism
Cervical Radiography	Pre-Op Cardiac Risk (Detsky)
Child's Classification	Pre-Op Cardiac Risk (Goldman)
Community-Acquired Pneumonia	Pre-Op Cardiac Risk (Lee)
Coronary Disease Probability	Ranson's Criteria
Coronary Disease Risk	Renal Artery Stenosis
Croup Score	Revised Trauma Score
CT in Minor Head Injury	Romhilt–Estes Criteria for LVH
DVT Probability	Strep Pharyngitis Probability
Ectopic Pregnancy	Stroke Risk in A-Fib
Family Practice Incidence Rates	Successful VBAC
GI Bleed Mortality	Trauma Score
In-Hospital Cardiac Arrest	UTI Diagnosis

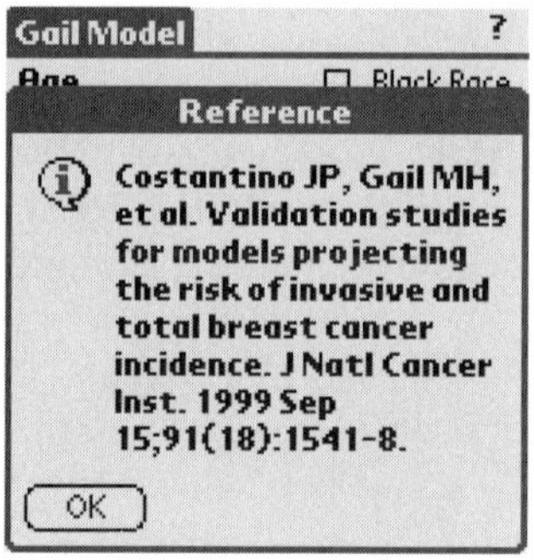

FIGURE 6.17. Reference screen in MedRules. (Reprinted with permission from Kent E. Wilyard, MD.)

Medical Calculators for the Pocket PC

One of the great things about the Pocket PC is that many of the calculators for the Palm will run just fine on the Pocket PC! That's because many are actually miniature databases or applets written for a program called HanDBase (http://www.handbase.com). We told you more about this must-have program and the various medical calculators available earlier in this section.

There are also some stand-alone programs that feature calculators. Two of the best known are Archimedes and InfoRetriever. We have to disclose that one of the authors of the book is also the author of InfoRetriever . . . it's a small world!

Archimedes | www.skyscape.com | free download

Archimedes is a collection of useful calculators and a few decision rules, organized both alphabetically and by system. The program does a great job of providing calculators that help you estimate things like a patient's A-a gradient and creatinine clearance. It doesn't have a lot of clinical decision rules, and also does not give you information on the validation or design of the rules that it does have. Using it is easy. Just select the calculation that you're interested in from the list (Figure 6.18) and enter the required values (Figure 6.19).

Due Date Calc | available at: www.pocketgear.com | $9.95
OBGynPocketPro | available at: www.pocketgear.com | $24.95

Just like the excellent due date calculators available for Palm handhelds, Pocket PC programmers have also delivered (no pun intended, honest), and Due Date Calc is one example of the type of program available for physi-

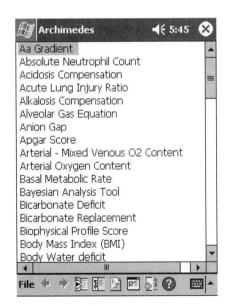

FIGURE 6.18. Calculator menu screen in Archimedes. Used with permission from Skyscape, Inc.

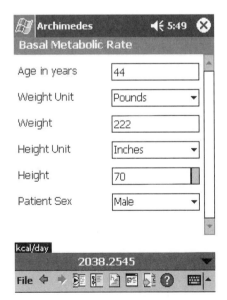

FIGURE 6.19. Basal metabolic rate in Archimedes. Used with permission from Skyscape, Inc.

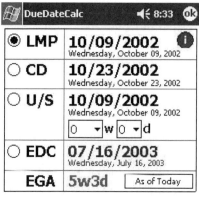
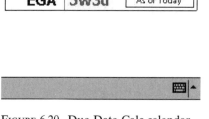

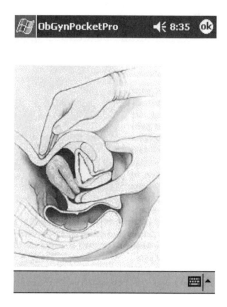

FIGURE 6.20. Due Date Calc calendar entry for calculating estimated gestational age. (Reprinted with permission from GANDM Enterprises.)

FIGURE 6.21. Counseling images in ObGynPocketPro. (Reprinted with permission from ObTech, Inc.)

cians who practice OB. Enter the last menstrual period, ultrasound date, or conception date to calculate the estimated gestational age (Figure 6.20). OBGynPocketPro has an OB wheel as well, but also offers ICD-9 and CPT codes, patient counseling images, gestational diabetes testing information, teratogen information by type and gestational age, and anomaly risk information (Figure 6.21). Unlike their Palm brethren, these two programs lack a desktop version and the ability to save individual patient records.

Inforetriever | www.infopoems.com | $249

InfoRetriever is a comprehensive collection of evidence-based medicine resources, plus Griffith's 5 Minute Clinical Consult (see Chapter 7) and a drug and formulary database. One of the most useful parts of InfoRetriever is its comprehensive collection of more than 120 clinical decision rules and calculators. Each rule is custom programmed to make the best possible use of the small screen and is accompanied by detailed information about each rule (a reference, the population to which it applies, and how it was validated).

Here is the "strep score." You quickly find it by selecting "Infectious disease" under "Clinical rules and calculators" (Figures 6.22, 6.23), and then tapping on the name of the clinical rule. Select the symptoms and age of your patient, and press "Calculate" (Figure 6.24). You not only get their probability of strep, but also the likelihood of strep after a rapid strep test. Finally, each rule has a "More info" button that tells you more about how

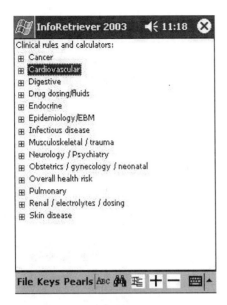

FIGURE 6.22. Clinical rules and calculators in InfoRetriever. (Reprinted with permission from InfoPOEM, Inc.)

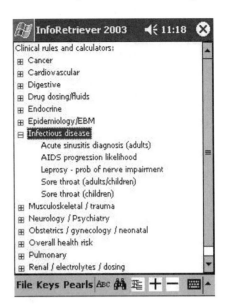

FIGURE 6.23. Selecting the "strep score" in InfoRetriever. (Reprinted with permission from InfoPOEM, Inc.)

the rule was developed and validated, so you can decide if it applies to your patient in this clinical situation.

Some of the rules also provide decision support: take a look at the National Cholesterol Education Program Adult Treatment Protocol (ATP) III guideline (Figures 6.25–6.27). Like many practice guidelines, its use has been limited by its lack of availability at the bedside; even the short version

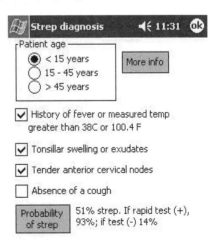

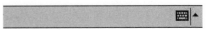

FIGURE 6.24. Information in the "strep score" in InfoRetriever. (Reprinted with permission from InfoPOEM, Inc.)

Cardiac risk (NCEP III) ◀€ 11:12 ⓞ𝐤

NCEP ATP III guidelines for treatment of hyperlipidemia

Patient's current LDL: [169]

Check all present (CHD risk equivalent)

☐ Known coronary heart disease

☐ Symptomatic carotid artery disease

☐ Abdominal aortic aneurysm

☐ Peripheral arterial disease

☐ Diabetes mellitus

[Next >]

⌨️|▲

FIGURE 6.25. Entering risk factors in the NCEPIII Clinical Calculator. (Reprinted with permission from InfoPOEM, Inc.)

Cardiac risk (NCEP III) ◀€ 11:16 ⓞ𝐤

Age (years):	[50-54 ▼]
Total cholesterol (mg/dl):	[240-279 ▼]
HDL cholesterol (mg/dl):	[40-49 ▼]
Systolic BP (mm Hg):	[130-139 ▼]

☐ Female

☑ Hypertension under treatment

☐ Smoking in past month

☐ CHD in first degree male relative < 55
years or female relative < 65 years

[< Prev]   [Estimate risk >]

⌨️|▲

FIGURE 6.26. Second screen for risk factors in NCEPIII Clinical Calculator. (Reprinted with permission from InfoPOEM, Inc.)

that they send around to clinicians is four pages long! Now, you can work through the guideline with your patient in less than a minute.

InfoRetriever focuses on rules that have been validated (tested) and shown to be accurate. Rules included in the current version are shown in Table 6.5.

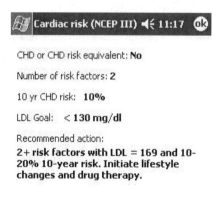

Cardiac risk (NCEP III) ◀€ 11:17 ⓞ𝐤

CHD or CHD risk equivalent: **No**

Number of risk factors: **2**

10 yr CHD risk: **10%**

LDL Goal: **< 130 mg/dl**

Recommended action:
2+ risk factors with LDL = 169 and 10-20% 10-year risk. Initiate lifestyle changes and drug therapy.

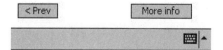

[< Prev]   [More info]

⌨️|▲

FIGURE 6.27. Patient's calculated risks using NCEPIII Clinical Calculator. (Reprinted with permission from InfoPOEM, Inc.)

TABLE 6.5. Clinical decision rules in InfoRetriever.

Cardiovascular: Acute MI
  ACI-TIPI risk score
  Probability of normal LVEF
  Risk of death in AMI
  Prognosis based on initial ECG
  Mortality in ST elevation AMI
  Prognosis in non-ST elevation AMI
  Prognosis in ST elevation AMI
Cardiovascular: Chest Pain
  Risk of AMI with normal or near-normal ECG
  Probability of significant CAD in outpatients
  Treadmill interpretation (Duke score)
  Probability of complications requiring ICU care
  Probability of left main CAD
  Acute coronary syndrome: TIMI risk score
Cardiovascular: Other
  Renal artery stenosis diagnosis
  JNC VI guideline
  DVT: clinical diagnosis
  Angioplasty: probability of complications
  AV replacement in aortic stenosis
  Aortic thoracic artery dissection diagnosis
  CPR prognosis (inpatient)
  Left atrial thrombi after commissurotomy
  Invasive vs. conservative management
  Tirofiban benefit in unstable angina/NQWMI
Cardiovascular: Pre-Op Evaluation
  Noncardiac surgery (Detsky score)
  Vascular surgery
  AAA surgery mortality
  Simple cardiac risk score (Lee)
Cardiovascular: Screening
  Cardiac risk profile (Framingham data)
  NCEP ATP III lipid guideline
Cardiovascular: Stroke
  Risk in patients with nonvalvular afib
  Acute stroke prognosis (G-score)
  Carotid endarterectomy prognosis
  Diagnosis of ischemic vs. hemorrhagic
  TIA prognosis
  30-day mortality
  5-year stroke risk
  Prediction of recovery from stroke
Drug Dosing
  Heparin dosing by weight
  Warfarin dosing in outpatients
Endocrinology
  Diabetes mellitus screening
  Basal energy requirements
  Ideal body weight calculator
  Hypercalcemia: probability of malignancy
  Body mass index calculator

TABLE 6.5. *Continued*

Epidemiology
Diagnostic test calculator (LR and PV)
Treatment calculator (NNT, RRR, ARR)
Fluids and Electrolytes
Pediatric IV fluid calculator
Anion gap
Body surface area calculator
Creatinine clearance calculator
Fractional excretion of sodium
Serum osmolality calculator
Gastroenterology
GI bleed: inpatient mortality risk
Risk of bleeding with warfarin treatment for DVT
Dyspepsia: probability of ulcer
GI bleed (upper): persistent bleeding after injection
Acute pancreatitis: prognosis (Imrie score)
Acute pancreatitis: prognosis (Ranson score)
Dyspepsia: predicting response to omeprazole
Bowel obstruction diagnosis: need for X-ray
Diarrhea: need for cultures in nosocomial diarrhea
GI bleed (upper): predicting need for intervention
GI bleed: identification of low-risk GI bleeds
Abdominal pain diagnosis (men)
Gynecology and Obstetrics
Induction of labor: Dhall score
Probability of gestational diabetes
Probability of successful VBAC
Induction of labor: Bishop score
Apgar score
Pregnancy wheel
Risk of ectopic pregnancy with pain/bleeding
Hematology/Oncology
Breast cancer: probability of CA by Gail risk model
Melanoma: 5-year prognosis
Thyroid cancer: 5-year prognosis
Infectious Disease
Acute sinusitis diagnosis in URI
Strep diagnosis in sore throat
Meningitis (bacterial) diagnosis in adults
Leprosy: predicting nerve function impairment
AIDS progression likelihood
Strep score (pediatric)
Musculoskeletal
Ankle injury: X-rays needed?
Foot injury: X-rays needed?
Knee injury: X-rays needed?
Which trauma patients need C-spine films?
Minor head injury: who needs head CT?
Minor head injury: Canadian Head CT rule
Osteoporosis screening (Dutch instrument)
Canadian C-spine rule in trauma patients
Osteoporosis screening (SCORE)
Osteoporosis screening (ORAI)
Rotator cuff diagnosis

TABLE 6.5. *Continued*

Neurology
    Syncope prognosis
    Glasgow Coma Score
    Pediatric head injury prognosis
    Mini-Mental State to screen for dementia
Overall Mortality
    Hospital d/c prognosis for elderly
    10-year mortality for various conditions
Psychiatry and Substance Abuse
    Suicidal ideation risk
    Depression screening
    CAGE score (alcoholism screening)
    Which high users are somatizers
Pulmonary Disease
    Cough: diagnosis of pneumonia
    Pneumonia: mortality in adults (Fine rule)
    Pulmonary embolism diagnosis
    ABG interpretation
    Cough/URI: diagnosis of pneumonia
    A-a gradient
    Pneumonia: diagnosis in nursing home
    Asthma relapse in adults
    Pneumonia: mortality in nursing home
    Pulmonary fibrosis survival
    Pulmonary embolism diagnosis algorithm
    Pneumonia: mortality in elderly
Renal Disease
    UTI diagnosis
    Dialysis prognosis
    Renal lithiasis diagnosis
    UTI diagnosis (Leibovici)
Skin Disease
    Braden score (pressure ulcers)
    Venous leg ulcer healing
Surgery and Trauma
    Prognosis in near drowning
    Burn injury prognosis

Summary

We hope we have shown you a few more software programs to make your life on the wards or in the office just a little bit easier. We have shown you a program to help you analyze blood gases when the situation arises instead of struggling to recall the Henderson–Hasselbach equation. In addition, several other programs were highlighted that can help you with everyday medical calculations that often come up in practice.

Regardless of whether you have a Palm or Pocket PC handheld computer, software developers around the world (including both authors) are striving to help physicians by programming useful tools such as those shown in this chapter. As we mentioned earlier, good clinical judgment is always necessary, and you should be sure to check any software for bugs or errors before relying on it too heavily.

Patients are constantly amazed when I recall their due date based on having it stored in PregTrak or Preg Calc, and I've had patients who smoke become inspired to quit by showing the dramatic decrease in risk of a heart attack by quitting using Stat Cholesterol (this can also be done using the National Cholesterol Education Program ATP III calculator in InfoRetriever). It won't be long before patients will expect this type of precise information from their doctors at the point of care, so go out and buy your handheld computer and start using some of these great programs as soon as you can. You'll be amazed by the response you get in the exam room or in the hospital!

References

1. Eagle KA, Berger PB, Calkin M, et al. ACC/AHA guideline update for perioperative cardiovascular evaluation for noncardiac surgery: a report of the American College of Cardiology/American Heart Association Taskforce on Practice Guidelines (Committee to Update the 1996 Guidelines on Perioperative Cardiovascular Evaluation for Noncardiac Surgery). 2002. American College of Cardiology website. Available at: http://www.acc.org/clinical/guidelines/perio/dirIndex.htm
2. Palda VA, Detsky AS. Clinical guideline, part II: perioperative assessment and management of risk from coronary artery disease. Annals of Internal Medicine 1997;127:313–328.
3. Third report of the National Cholesterol Education Program (NCEP) expert panel on: detection, evaluation and treatment of high blood cholesterol in adults (Adult treatment panel III). National Cholesterol Education Program. National Heart, Lung, and Blood Institute. National Institutes of Health, NIH Publication No. 01-3670. May 2001.

7

Medical References: Information at Your Fingertips

LOUIS SPIKOL

I have come to believe that medical progress can be ascertained by closely examining the contents of a medical resident's white coat pocket. Traditionally, in addition to various paraphernalia and reprinted articles, a resident's white coat has contained as much reference material and books as that particular resident was able to carry. Although maximum intracranial knowledge was encouraged, occasional perusal of reference material was tolerated at the training level. Conversely, by tradition, attending physicians could be spotted by the relative paucity of any type of onboard books or reference material. Clinical questions, whether in the hospital or the outpatient setting, are usually answered by "cranial resources," good guesses, or perhaps not at all. Clinical information is usually separated from the patient's encounter in both time and space, which presents an almost insurmountable barrier to obtaining accurate, timely, and useful critical information.

As Bob Dylan once wrote, "The times they are a-changin," and with the advent of pocket-sized PDAs and the ever-increasing capacity of memory chips it has become possible to carry multiple books and resources in a shirt or coat pocket. The purpose of this chapter is to introduce and review these resources. I will place emphasis on the World Wide Web as the ideal place to peruse, evaluate, and, in most cases, download trial and fully functional versions of reference and book software.

Also, please note that we show you alternative ways to get references on your handheld in Chapter 10 by using programs such as iSilo and AvantGo (these amazing programs allow you to put almost any Web content directly on your handheld). We also describe other references in our chapter on Evidence-Based Medicine (Chapter 14), and database references are described in Chapter 11. Finally, don't forget to mine our chapter on Web sites for your handheld (Chapter 4), where numerous treasure troves of medical references are shown.

Evaluating PDA Medical Books and Reference Material

It should come as no surprise to anyone that there is a significant difference between reading a book in paper form and reading a book formatted for a PDA. In fact, the first thing that should be considered is whether you, the reader, actually actively read medical books or use them as references. Although some PDA users are able to read lengthy sections of books on their devices without difficulties, some otherwise enthusiastic users consider this task an exercise in patience and eyestrain. My advice for those wishing to read long sections of medical textbooks is to consider either regular books or electronic books for full-size computers/laptops. The PDA platform really shines for medical books used as references and evidence-based sources.

The functionality of medical references for PDAs is dependent on both hardware and software factors. Hardware considerations with both the Pocket PC and Palm platform relating to the viewing of books and other references include the following:

- Screen size does vary somewhat across and within both platforms. A larger screen size provides for easier reading, with a trade-off being a larger device size.
- Two devices having the same screen size can differ in their resolution and total number of pixels produced, with the higher-resolution device being easier to read.
- Color versus black and white: color screens are generally easier to read at the expense of shorter battery life, and devices using black and white can vary in shades of gray produced.
- Various software tricks and processes can be used to make print on a small screen appear sharper and easier to read, such as the Microsoft process called ClearType.
- The hardware and the operating system should be able to accommodate different font sizes and appearances that can be adjusted by the user.
- Finally, and perhaps most important, the hardware and operating system should allow expansion cards to hold the large amount of data contained in books and other references. The Palm platform has lagged in this area until recently, with newer models having adequate expansion capability. The software itself should be able to be installed and run from the expansion card.

Software considerations for individual medical books and references are also critically important. Considering the small size of the screen, medical books and other resources ported to the PDA platform must have increased functionality to be useful. Some attributes to look for in PDA books and other medical references include the following:

- The ability to search for topics in multiple ways, such as the table of contents, the index, and ability to search for specific words and other topics.
- The ability to fit words on the screen in a fashion that is convenient and readable. Many but not all programs have the ability to resize fonts.
- The ability to scroll both vertically and horizontally if needed. The text should be constructed so that scrolling horizontally is minimized. It is also useful to be able to rapidly go between pages as well as go to a specific page.
- The program ideally should allow the user to set multiple bookmarks and return to those bookmarks at a later time as needed.
- Determine if the reference is updated often and, if so, does it cost extra? Many references provide free updates for a year.

A Survey of PDA Medical Book Resources

Skyscape: www.skyscape.com

Products

Skyscape is the "800-pound gorilla" of the PDA medical book field. They have been releasing and perfecting medical references for the PDA platform since the Apple Newton. They carry well over 100 reference books and drug guides (see their website for a listing of all titles) for both the Palm and Pocket PC platform. They have a sophisticated interface that is carried throughout their titles.

Cost

Cost of Skyscape resources depends on the reference; it is comparable to hard copy, with some specials.

Highlights

The typical well laid out format is shown by their Primary Care Medical References (Figure 7.1). The software can show figures, graphs, and charts, as in The Harriet Lane Handbook (Figure 7.2). Search by index (Figure 7.3) or table of contents (Figure 7.4), and choose different text sizes (Figure 7.5). A unique feature of Skyscape references is the ability to link to other Skyscape titles installed on your PDA (Figure 7.6). Demo versions of books are provided. Updates are free for 1 year. The company discounts certain multiple book packages and runs various specials throughout the year.

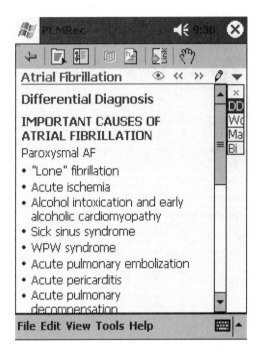

FIGURE 7.1. A typical Skyscape medical book. Used with permission from Skyscape, Inc.

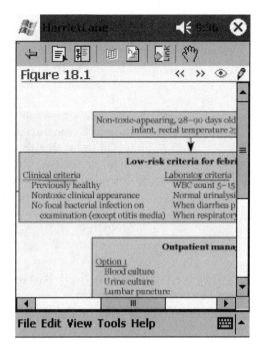

FIGURE 7.2. Harriet Lane table. Used with permission from Skyscape, Inc.

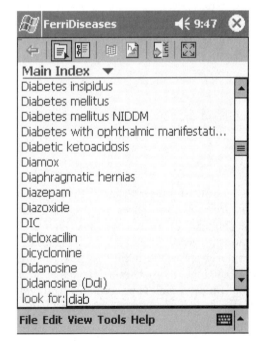

FIGURE 7.3. Index search. Used with permission from Skyscape, Inc.

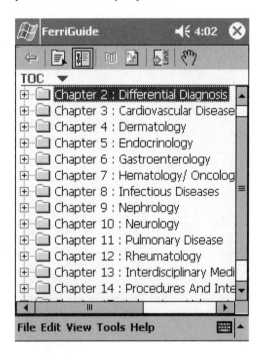

FIGURE 7.4. Table of contents search. Used with permission from Skyscape, Inc.

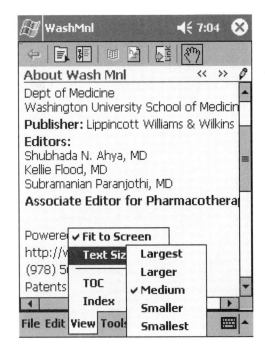

FIGURE 7.5. Different text size. Used with permission from Skyscape, Inc.

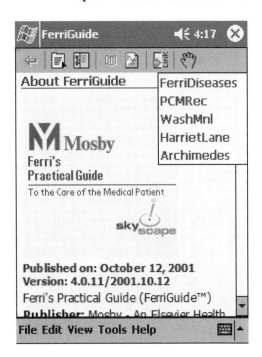

FIGURE 7.6. Links to other titles. Used with permission from Skyscape, Inc.

Handheld Med: www.handheldmed.com

Products

About 30 different medical books including the Merck manual (see their Web site for full listing).

Cost

Cost depends on the book; comparable to hard copy.

Highlights

About 30 different books including the Merck manual. Palm and Pocket PC platform. EZReader software (Figure 7.7) provides one reading platform. Multiple ways to search including chapters (Figure 7.8) and index (Figure 7.9).

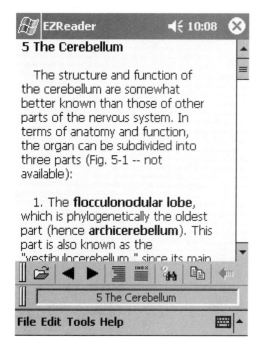

FIGURE 7.7. EZReader software. (Reprinted with permission from Handheldmed, Inc.)

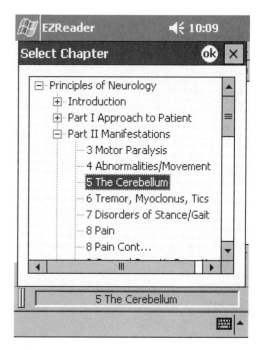

FIGURE 7.8. Chapter search. (Reprinted with permission from Handheldmed, Inc.)

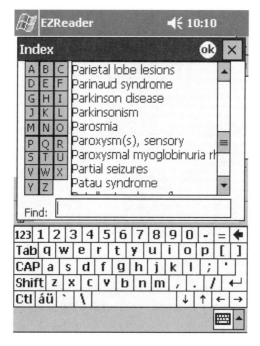

FIGURE 7.9. Index search. (Reprinted with permission from Handheldmed, Inc.)

Unbound Medicine: www.unboundmedicine.com

Products

> Unbound Medicine offers a number of electronic books and CogniQ, "a knowledge management platform integrating handheld devices and the web." They also have Harrison's and Ovid online with PDA components, for both Palm and Pocket PC.

Cost

> *British Medical Journal* content is offered through CogniQ as a free trial. It is uncertain what the future price will be. Harrison's is $250/year, and Ovid online is sold through resellers.

Highlights

> Medical books and journal reference. Routine updates available. CogniQ represents a unique approach to books and journals. The CogniQ main interface (Figure 7.10) shows active subscriptions that are updated via the Internet when the PDA is synched to the computer. Tapping on subscriptions expands into the appropriate submenus (Figures 7.11, 7.12) and appropriate further information (Figures 7.13–7.15). Also notice that the program gives the user the opportunity to either ask more clinical questions or request the full topic. During the next Hotsync, the user is taken to his or her personal information retrieval desktop on the Web (Figure 7.16). Information can then be managed with the online interface as well as the handheld computer.

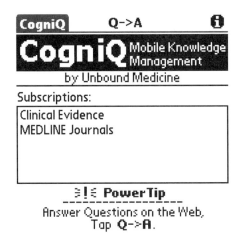

FIGURE 7.10. CogniQ main menu. (Reprinted with permission from Unbound Medicine.)

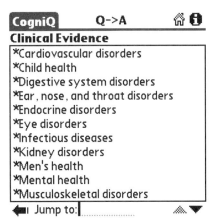

FIGURE 7.11. CogniQ clinical evidence. (Reprinted with permission from Unbound Medicine.)

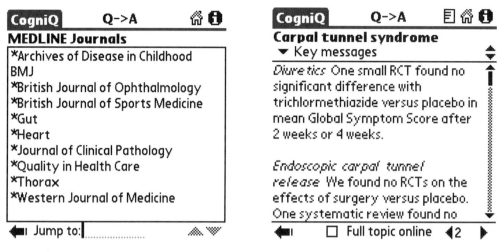

FIGURE 7.12. CogniQ journals. (Reprinted with permission from Unbound Medicine.)

FIGURE 7.13. CogniQ citation. (Reprinted with permission from Unbound Medicine.)

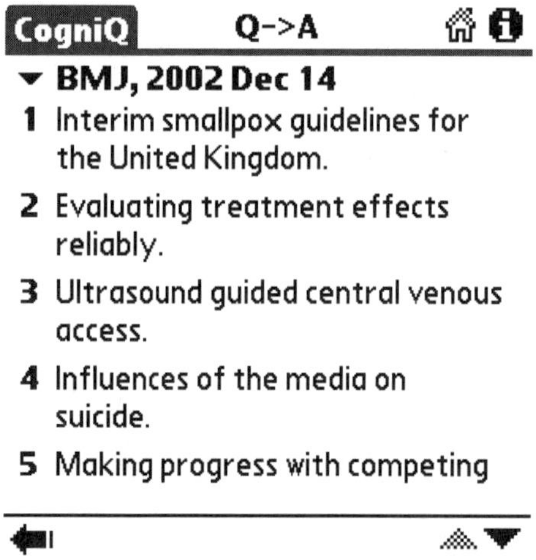

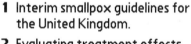

FIGURE 7.14. CogniQ journal. (Reprinted with permission from Unbound Medicine.)

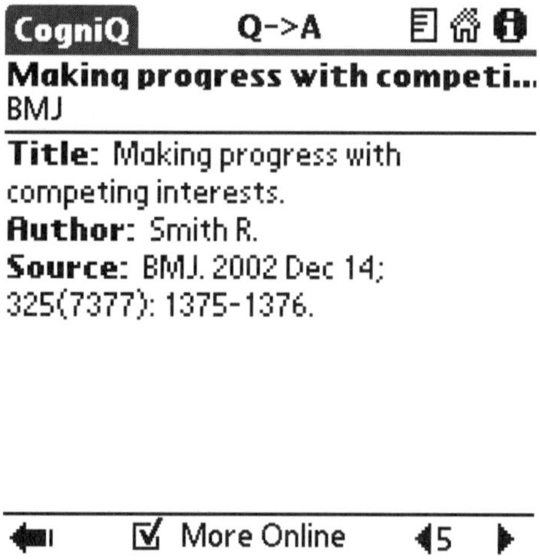

FIGURE 7.15. CogniQ more information. (Reprinted with permission from Unbound Medicine.)

Electronic Drug References

By far the most popular use of PDA's among healthcare professionals has been electronic drug references. In my opinion, all of them are easy to use and provide a wealth of features. Special features to be noted include drug interaction checking, updates via the Web, and state-specific formulary checking.

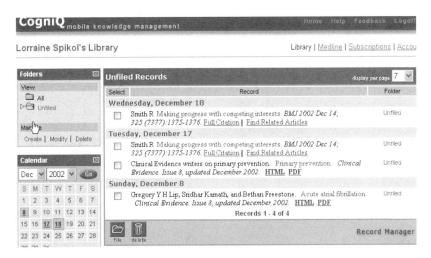

FIGURE 7.16. CogniQ Web interface. (Reprinted with permission from Unbound Medicine.)

Epocrates: www.epocrates.com

Products

Epocrates Rx (Palm Platform only) and Rx Pro (Palm and Pocket PC).

Cost

Epocrates Rx, free; Epocrates Rx Pro, $50/year.

Highlights

Both versions have interaction checking, formularies, and auto-updates. The Pro version has infectious disease information, alternative medicine, clinical tables, and med math. The Pocket PC version doesn't offer infectious disease information, Doc Alert Messages, or MedMath at the time of this printing. They are scheduled to be added.

Highlights

Epocrates is the most popular medication PDA reference. It has a very nice clean interface (Figures 7.17, 7.18), with sections for pediatric dosing (Figure 7.19) and pregnancy and lactation (Figure 7.20). A particularly useful aspect of the program provides specific insurance formulary information with drug alternatives (Figure 7.21). Other parts of the professional edition include doctor alerts (sent to your handheld each time you synchronize over the Internet), infectious disease information, and tables (Figures 7.22–7.25).

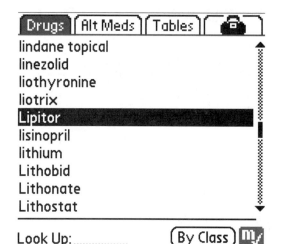

FIGURE 7.17. Epocrates lookup. (Reprinted with permission from Epocrates.)

FIGURE 7.18. Epocrates drug information. (Reprinted with permission from Epocrates.)

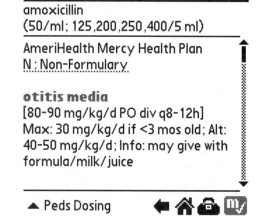

FIGURE 7.19. Epocrates pediatric dosing. (Reprinted with permission from Epocrates.)

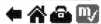

FIGURE 7.20. Epocrates pregnancy information. (Reprinted with permission from Epocrates.)

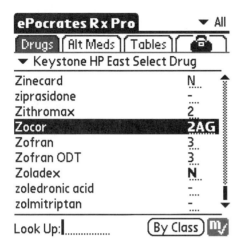

FIGURE 7.21. Epocrates formulary information. (Reprinted with permission from Epocrates.)

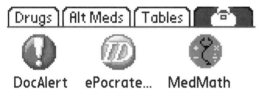

FIGURE 7.22. Epocrates extras. (Reprinted with permission from Epocrates.)

Bone/Joint
CNS
ENT
Eye
Genital
GI
Heart
Lung
Other
Skin/Soft Tissue
Systemic

Look Up:

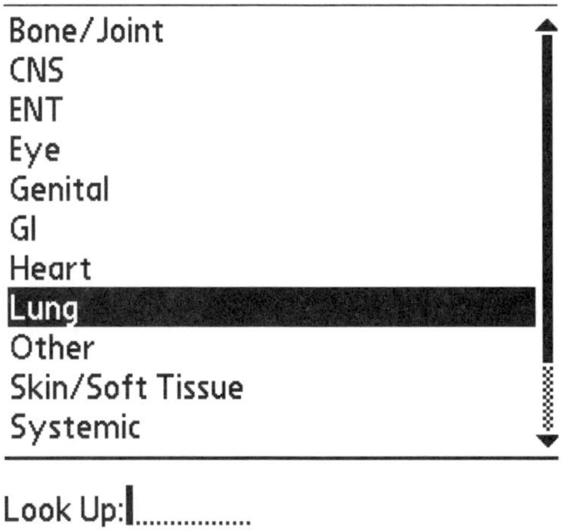

FIGURE 7.23. Epocrates infectious disease. (Reprinted with permission from Epocrates.)

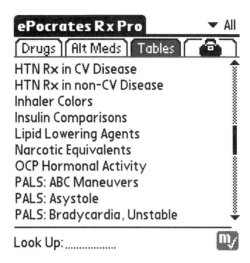

FIGURE 7.24. Epocrates tables. (Reprinted with permission from Epocrates.)

DocAlert

You have new DocAlert(s):

1) ePocrates tips for formulary users
2) Melatonin may exacerbate asthma symptoms

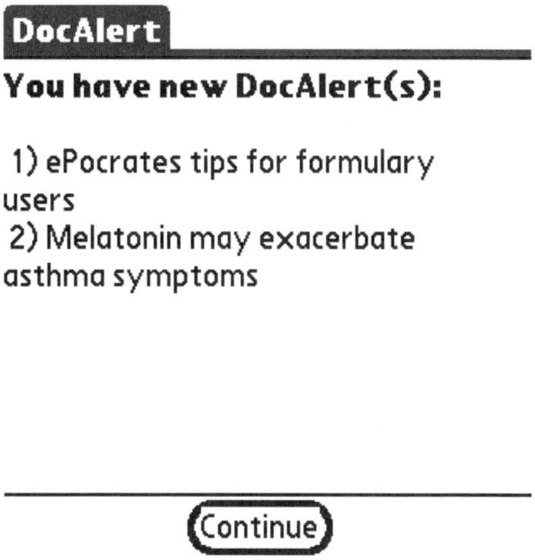

FIGURE 7.25. Epocrates doctor alerts. (Reprinted with permission from Epocrates.)

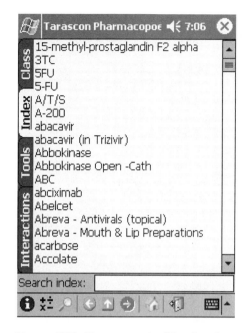

FIGURE 7.26. Tarascon main. (Reprinted with permission from Tarascon publishing and USBMIS, Inc.)

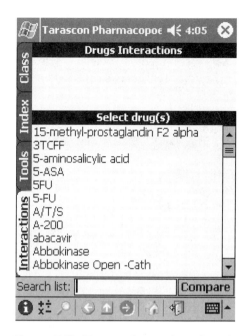

FIGURE 7.27. Tarascon interactions. (Reprinted with permission from Tarascon publishing and USBMIS, Inc.)

Tarascon Pharmacopoeia: www.tarascon.com

Products

Tarascon Pharmacopoeia is the electronic version of the well-known pocket drug reference (Palm and Pocket PC platform).

Cost

Approximately $30 annually.

Highlights

Drug search by index or class (Figure 7.26). The program has drug interaction checking (Figure 7.27).

Mobile PDR: www.mobilepdr.com

Products

Mobile PDR (Palm and Pocket PC platforms).

Cost

Free.

Highlights

Drug search by index (Figure 7.28). Well laid out information (including "black box" warnings) with the ability to add notes (Figure 7.29). The program provides interaction checking (Figure 7.30) and medication alerts that are updated when you synchronize (Figure 7.31).

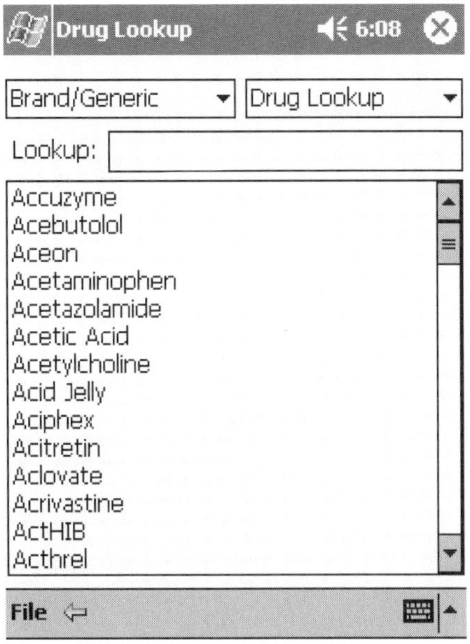

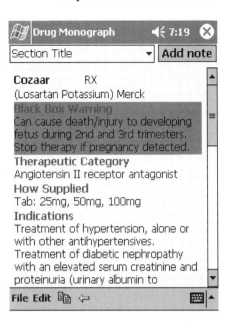

FIGURE 7.28. Mobile PDR index. (Reprinted with permission from The Thomson Corporation.)

FIGURE 7.29. Mobile PDR drug information. (Reprinted with permission from The Thomson Corporation.)

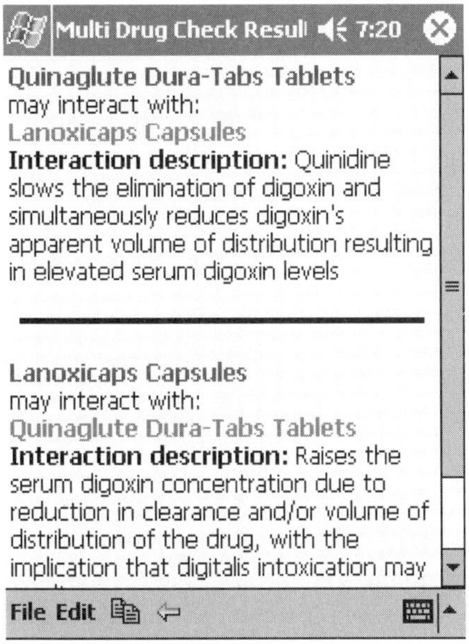

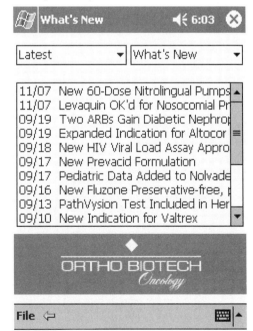

FIGURE 7.30. Mobile PDR interactions. (Reprinted with permission from The Thomson Corporation.)

FIGURE 7.31. Mobile PDR alerts. (Reprinted with permission from The Thomson Corporation.)

Medication Program (Platform)	Cost	Web Updates	Interactions	Formulary Information	Extras
Epocrates (Palm)	**Rx-free Rx Pro-50$\Yr**	**Yes**	**Yes**	**Yes**	**Rx-Doctor alerts Rx Pro:Infectious disease,clinical tables, medmath, alternative medications**
Mobile PDR (Palm and Pocket PC)	**Free**	**Yes**	**Yes**	**No**	**Doctor Alerts**
Tarascon Pharmacopeia (Palm and Pocket PC)	**Free (During beta test)**	**Yes**	**Yes**	**No**	**Medical calculator Drugs by class Tables**

FIGURE 7.32. Drug reference comparison table.

Shown in Figure 7.32 is a table comparing the salient features of the drug database programs. Please check the Web sites for the individual products because features and cost tend to change over time.

HANDS-ON EXERCISE 7.1. DOWNLOADING AND INSTALLING A MEDICAL REFERENCE

In this tutorial, we download and install the trial version of 5 Minute Clinical Consult from Skyscape to our Palm and Pocket PC, respectively. First, go to the Skyscape Web site (www.skyscape.com), click on "Products," and navigate to your desired book.

1. Click on "Download the trial version" (Figure 7.33) and then choose your platform (PC or Macintosh, Palm or Pocket PC; Figure 7.34).
2. When the download dialog box appears, click on "Save" (Figure 7.35). Remember to note where on your computer the book file is being saved and what it is called (Figure 7.36). The download will then proceed (Figure 7.37).

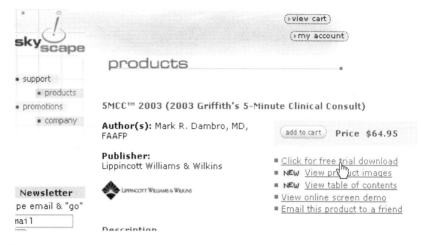

FIGURE 7.33. Skyscape download. Used with permission from Skyscape, Inc.

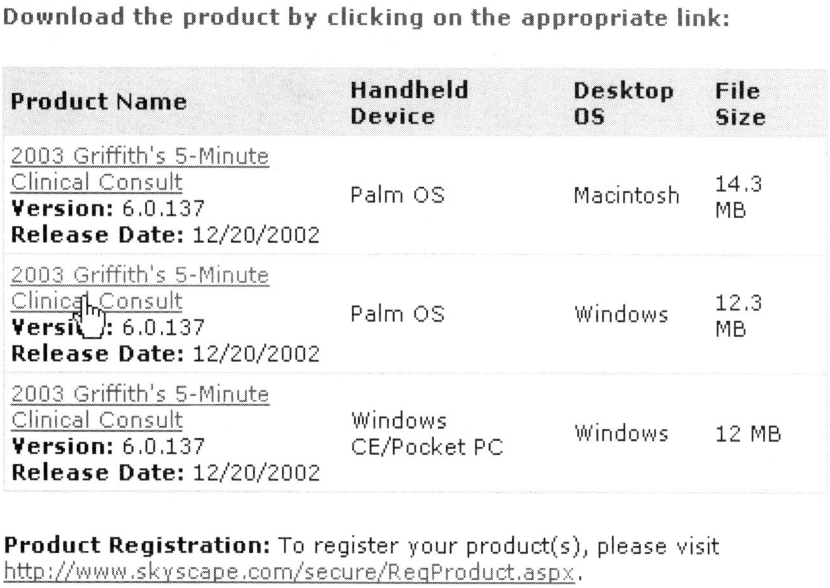

Download the product by clicking on the appropriate link:

Product Name	Handheld Device	Desktop OS	File Size
2003 Griffith's 5-Minute Clinical Consult **Version:** 6.0.137 **Release Date:** 12/20/2002	Palm OS	Macintosh	14.3 MB
2003 Griffith's 5-Minute Clinical Consult **Version:** 6.0.137 **Release Date:** 12/20/2002	Palm OS	Windows	12.3 MB
2003 Griffith's 5-Minute Clinical Consult **Version:** 6.0.137 **Release Date:** 12/20/2002	Windows CE/Pocket PC	Windows	12 MB

Product Registration: To register your product(s), please visit
http://www.skyscape.com/secure/ReqProduct.aspx.

FIGURE 7.34. Skyscape choose product. Used with permission from Skyscape, Inc.

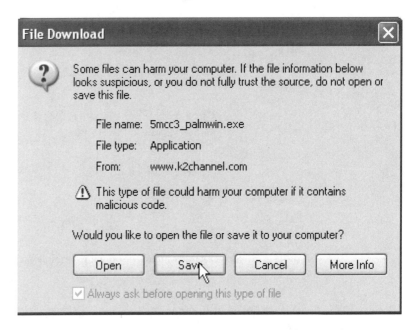

FIGURE 7.35. Skyscape save. Used with permission from Skyscape, Inc.

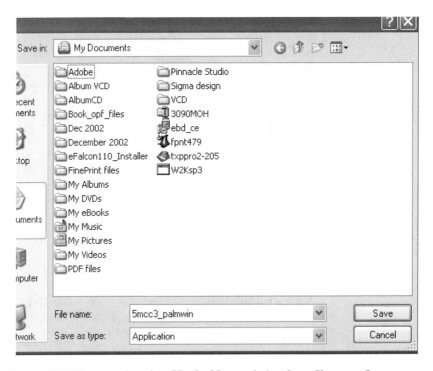

FIGURE 7.36. Skyscape location. Used with permission from Skyscape, Inc.

3. For the Palm: after the file has transferred to your computer, find it and click on it. Click on the type of installation you prefer (Figure 7.38) and which device you prefer (with one device, it will just say "Next sync operation"; Figure 7.39).

4. The next dialog box (Figure 7.40) gives you a choice between putting the book in main memory or a storage card. Most of the time, you will choose a storage card. The program will then be installed on the next Hotsync.

For the Pocket PC, go through a similar routine of downloading the appropriate file. Make sure your Pocket PC is connected and ActiveSync is running.

1. Clicking on the program will produce similar screens as the Palm version, with a different screen detecting the Pocket PC and offering to proceed with the installation (Figure 7.41).

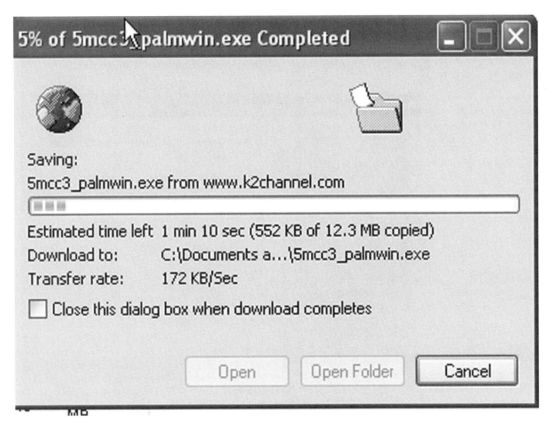

FIGURE 7.37. Skyscape downloading. Used with permission from Skyscape, Inc.

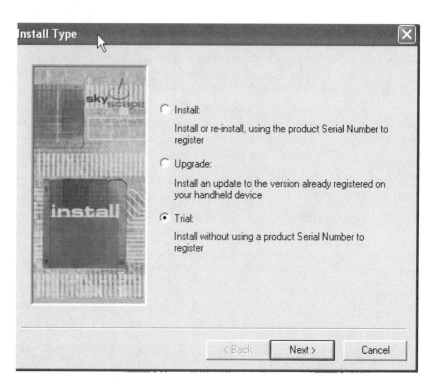

FIGURE 7.38. Skyscape trial. Used with permission from Skyscape, Inc.

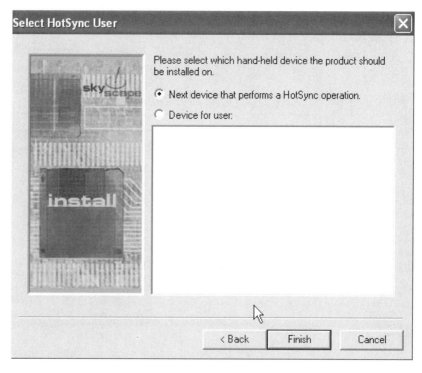

FIGURE 7.39. Skyscape user. Used with permission from Skyscape, Inc.

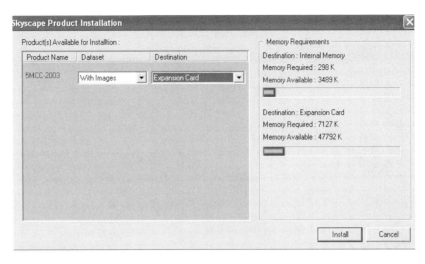

FIGURE 7.40. Skyscape Palm install. Used with permission from Skyscape, Inc.

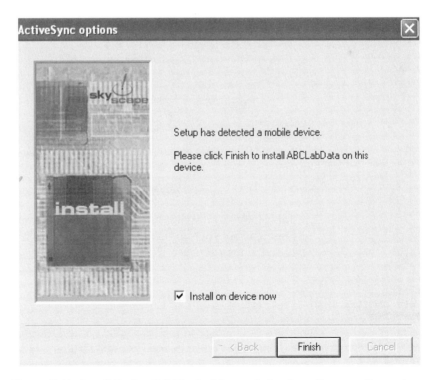

FIGURE 7.41. Install Pocket PC. Used with permission from Skyscape, Inc. and Microsoft Corporation.

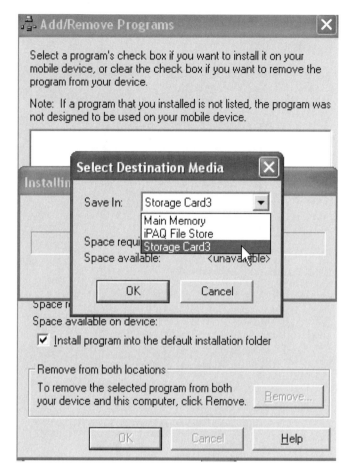

FIGURE 7.42. Install card. Used with permission from Skyscape, Inc. and Microsoft Corporation.

2. Choosing not to install in the default installation directory will bring up a screen where you can specify the location for installation (Figure 7.42), which will then proceed (Figure 7.43).

Final Words and Hot Tips

There is an old adage in medicine that clinical questions remain the same but the answers change every 5 years. I strongly believe that medical references in electronic format should take advantage of the strengths of this format. These main strengths include the ability to be easily updated and easily searched and the potential to provide personalized information.

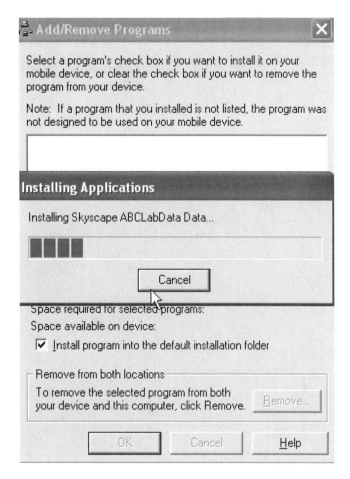

FIGURE 7.43. Install Pocket PC finish. Used with permission from Skyscape, Inc. and Microsoft Corporation.

Certainly some of these references (drug references and CogniQ from Unbound Medicine, in particular) have taken advantages of the strengths of the electronic format. Most of the other references can be easily updated, but continue to be connected to the printed version, in my opinion. So, I leave you with a few quick tips regarding electronic references on PDAs:

- Many companies offer trial downloadable versions from the Web. Take advantage of this to try out the products and see how often you need to use them. Also, pay attention to the book's functionality and ease of use.
- Carefully match the particular drug database to your needs.
- Strongly consider products that have frequent updates.
- Backup your electronic medical books in case of a computer crash.

- Make sure the books or drug database are compatible with your particular PDA and can be run from expansion cards if you desire.
- Finally, carry your PDA with you during rounds and in the office. Patients will certainly be impressed that you are consulting up-to-date information to better care for them with such information at your fingertips!

8

Getting Paid for What You Do: Avoid Losing Your Shirt by Using a Handheld Computer for Billing

SCOTT M. STRAYER

Moving Beyond Scraps of Paper for Billing: Handheld Charge Capture

This book is devoted to the many clever uses for handheld computers we have found in our years of combined experience. What about billing, or charge capture as it is now called? The idea of using my handheld for billing struck me like a lightning bolt out of the sky, the first week I owned my new Palm III back in 1999.

At the time I wasn't aware of any programs for billing using a handheld computer, and I knew of the many inefficiencies of using index cards, scraps of paper, gum wrappers, yellow stickies, and the many other innovative ways devised to capture those late-night ER admissions, ICU trips for crashing patients, and nursing home visits. These scraps of paper sometimes made it back to the billing office, but on many occasions they ended up as illegible balls of paper after going through the wash, or were discovered in the trunk of my car a year or so after they were recorded. God forbid you own a convertible! Not only would you lose your billing revenue, but also with the Health Insurance Portability and Accountability Act (HIPAA) security and privacy regulations, you might even have to sell the convertible to pay the fine.

So I set out to create the ultimate billing program for handheld computers, and have a patent pending on the process. Well, they say when you have a great idea, at least 40 or so more people have the same idea. It wasn't long before the simple idea of a "billing program" became known as "charge capture," and now there are several companies who have been financed to the tune of millions of dollars by venture capitalists looking to make a quick buck in this market.

Most doctors and health professionals who do patient billing (especially in mobile locations such as the hospital, ER, nursing homes, and home visits) probably have a sense that using index cards is not perfect for this function and that some charges get lost this way. Most were probably shocked to learn the costs of lost charges when it was actually quantified in a market analysis piece by W.R. Hambrecht.[1] The report quoted numerous industry studies and Health Care Financing Administration (HCFA) data showing that practicing physicians were actually losing in excess of $25 billion per year in denied or reduced fee-for-service claims because of improper documentation and failing to bill for services outside the office setting, for example. Another study by Synergy Medical Informatics estimated that lost billings totaled $60,000 per year for each actively practicing physician in the United States.

Several industry studies also show rather generous returns on investment or ROIs for using handheld charge capture products. That is, for every dollar spent on the software and transaction fees to process claims using a handheld computer, the average return is from $5 to $10 in billed charges.[2,3] An abstract presented at the American Medical Informatics Association Meeting in October 2001 (by "yours truly") showed that physicians easily adopt handheld charge capture and that this leads to increased capture of patient encounters.[4]

Despite this admittedly rosy picture that I'm painting for handheld charge capture, a recent report from Fulcrum Analytics and Deloitte Research showed that only about 6% of physicians using a handheld computer used it for charge capture in 2001.[2] I would speculate that the reasons for this are many, including

- Lack of time to learn new technology
- High cost of the software from some companies
- Belief that they aren't losing charges

Read on if you want to join the early adopters, and become a member of this elite group using handheld computers to recoup lost billing charges. It's really not that difficult, and the range of options is quite wide, allowing you to start with a simple program such as PocketBilling (the one I developed) for under $50 (www.pocketmed.org), all the way to a fully implemented system that interfaces with your scheduling, practice management, and EMR system from companies like Allscripts (www.allscripts.com), Patientkeeper (www.patientkeeper.com), and MDeverywhere (www.mdeverywhere.com).

Designing the Ideal Solution: Telepathic Billing

Of course we all dream of the day when we are rounding on our complicated patient, Hallie (whom you will learn more about in our next chapter on electronic prescribing), who has the too-numerous-to-count-diagnoses syndrome (TNTCDS), and the billing gets submitted to your office staff based on your thoughts while seeing the patient (an implant captures neural impulses and wirelessly transmits them to the office). Until that day, we are going to have to settle for what we have. But, believe it or not, a lot of things can be automated and only entered once using a handheld computer.

First of all, having the patient's name and demographic data already entered can easily be done by synchronizing with your hospital or office computer system. Many companies are already doing this (although the cost is pretty significant). You can also easily enter the most basic information and then have office staff fill in the blanks later. The date of service can be automatically entered as you enter the charge, or you can have the program provide a calendar "date-picker" if you enter the charges later.

Entering the diagnoses can be done by synchronizing with the hospital system (again, this can be costly, but may be worth it), or you can select diagnoses from well-organized pick lists without having to write anything in the handheld. Then, CPT codes for Evaluation and Management or Procedures can also be selected from pick lists. Some of the software automatically provides guidelines for the levels of service, and there are also separate programs that can help you with this if it's not built into your software.

Finally, getting this information back to the billing staff can be accomplished either wirelessly, by synchronizing over a network, or by simply printing out the data on a daily or weekly basis or when your schedule allows. Although this isn't as elegant as the telepathic billing we would all love to have, it's a heck of a lot better than the current system of index cards and paper scraps. You are almost certain to more accurately and completely capture your billing charges, and your office staff will love you for it—trust me.

Creating Your Own Program

It's easy to create your own program for billing. You can use one of the many database programs described later in Chapter 11, and use our "how-to" section on programming databases (Chapter 17) to create your own unique billing program designed specifically for your needs. Let's just say you want to capture patient names, date of service, and the level of charge. Let your office staff fill in the diagnoses from hospital discharge information, and let them get the demographic information and enter it into your office billing software. All you want to do is show them whom you saw, when, and your level of service, right? Figure 8.1 is just what you ordered, or created, as the case might be. This simple program was created using HanDBase, as described in further detail in Chapter 17.

Simply write in the patient's name in the "name" field, and then tap on the "date of service" field to get a pop-up calendar for entering the date (Figure 8.2). Finally, you can select from a few simple preentered CPT codes in the "level of service" field (Figure 8.3). You could certainly add more

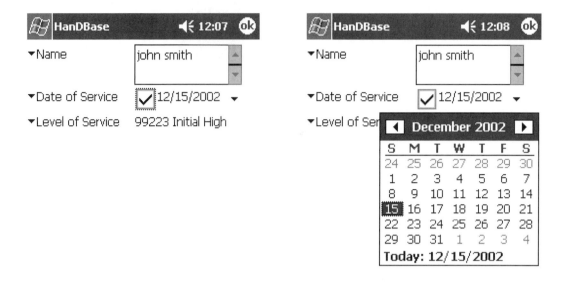

FIGURE 8.1. A simple charge capture program created using HanDBase. (Reprinted with permission from DDH Software.)

FIGURE 8.2. Pop-up calendar for entering date of service in our simple charge capture program. (Reprinted with permission from DDH Software.)

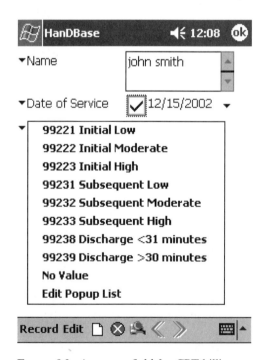

FIGURE 8.3. A pop-up field for CPT billing codes. (Reprinted with permission from DDH Software.)

fields than this, but this might do as a basic billing sheet. The advantages over index cards and other paper-based forms of billing are numerous:

- You are much less likely to lose your $500 iPaq than your stack of index cards.
- Data are now in digital form, and in addition to being readable, can be printed out, exported to other database formats, e-mailed, and so on.
- You can also beam a list of patients to your colleagues for weekend coverage.

This is the simplest and least expensive way to do billing on your handheld computer. Chapters 11 and 17 go into great detail on how to create your own databases, and you can easily use that information to create your own solution. If you would rather let someone else do the work of creating your program, however, read on.

Stand-Alone Solutions for Handheld Charge Capture

In looking at the various options for capturing charges on your handheld computer, it quickly becomes clear that there are two basic options: the stand-alone solutions, which basically reside on your handheld and synchronize with your desktop computer, and "extra strength" solutions that integrate with practice management software or hospital legacy computer systems (Table 8.1).

TABLE 8.1. Stand-alone versus "extra strength" solutions for charge capture.

	Stand-alone solutions	Extra strength solutions
Practice type	Smaller groups or solo practitioners	Larger or hospital-based groups
Cost	$30 (create your own using a database program) to $50–$200 for ready-made solutions	Monthly service fee of $50–$100 (varies) Implementation fee (up to several thousand dollars depending on company and difficulty of implementation)
Advantages	Easy to learn Minimal implementation time	Integrate with practice management systems Submit charges with minimal office support Built-in error checking
Disadvantages	Still need to process claims Lack of integration	High cost Steeper learning curve
Solutions	PocketBilling ZapBill	ChargeKeeper EveryCharge Allscripts

Stand-alone solutions are more likely to be used by individual practitioners, or health professionals in a small group practice without a lot of information technology support or budgetary resources. They are also useful for health professionals who don't have a lot of time to implement a major overhaul of their computer system and interfaces between the handheld and their office or hospital systems. Two examples of these simple, stand-alone solutions are PocketBilling by PocketMed (www.pocketmed.org) and ZapBill by ZapMed (http://www.zapmed.com/).

These solutions are all similar in that they are database programs that enable mobile charge capture by having fields to capture patient names, dates of service, ICD-9 codes, and CPT codes. The interfaces vary in their design and have different features.

PocketBilling

Web site: (www.pocketmed.org)
Cost: $49.99
Platform: Palm OS and Pocket PC

This was one of the first handheld charge capture programs, and we happen to like it because it was designed by one of the authors, Dr. Scott Strayer. It features a simple interface that is intuitive and enables entry of patient name, date of service, visit codes, and a minihistory, as well as a field for note-taking (Figures 8.4–8.6). The software synchronizes with a full-featured desktop program (Figure 8.7) that can export into various database formats (including csv, xls, html, xml, and doc). The software is downloadable from the Web or can be shipped in CD-ROM format.

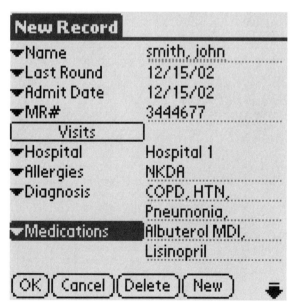

FIGURE 8.4. Main patient entry screen in PocketBilling. (Reprinted with permission from PocketMed.)

FIGURE 8.5. Initial visit CPT codes in PocketBilling. (Reprinted with permission from PocketMed.)

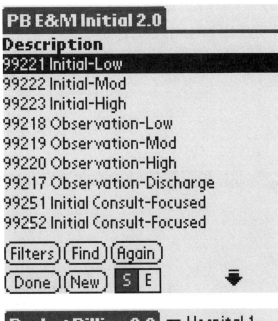

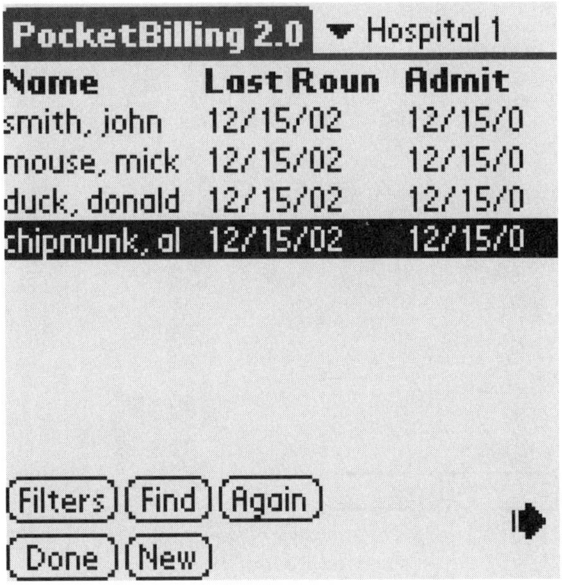

FIGURE 8.6. Rounding screen in PocketBilling. (Reprinted with permission from PocketMed.)

ZapBill

Web site: (www.zapmed.com)
Cost: $89
Platform: Palm OS

Another intuitive, simple, and easy-to-use handheld charge capture program created by a practicing physician, Dr. Mark Spohr (Figures 8.8,

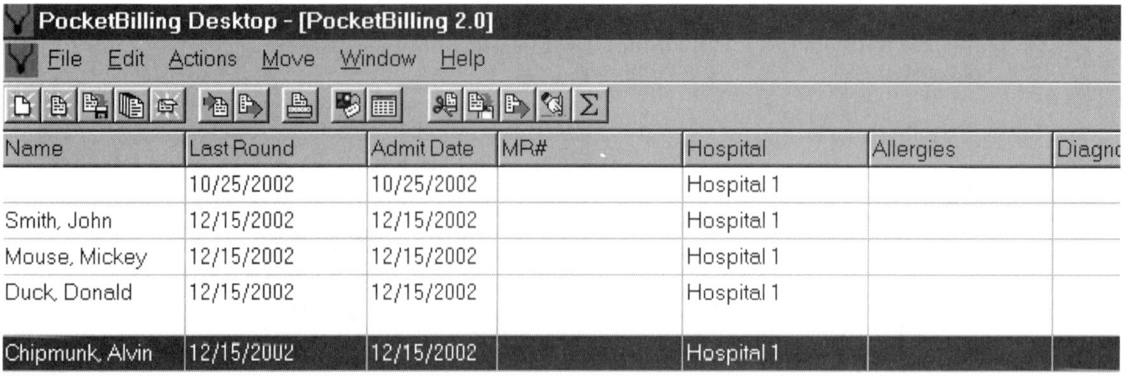

FIGURE 8.7. PocketBilling Desktop. (Reprinted with permission from PocketMed.)

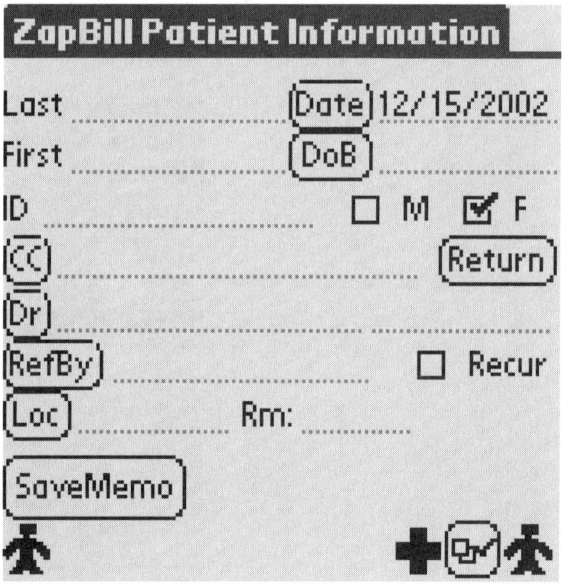

FIGURE 8.8. ZapBill Patient Information Screen. (Reprinted with permission from ZapMed.)

8.9), this one allows you to download and customize lists of ICD-9 codes and CPT codes from the Web site. For an extra $69 you can add on ZapCode, which checks your coding using either the 1995 or 1997 HCFA rules. This program enables patient entry using popular scheduling programs such as Microsoft Outlook or the Palm Desktop scheduling application.

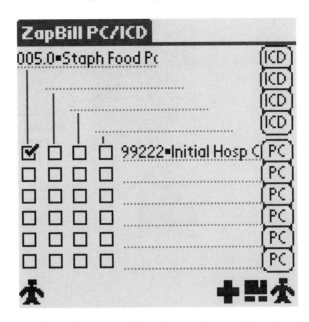

FIGURE 8.9. ZapBill coding screen. (Reprinted with permission from ZapMed.)

Extra Strength Charge Capture Solutions

These solutions are the "big kahunas" of charge capture. The software will integrate with most office or hospital practice management systems and submit claims to be processed after your handheld is synchronized (some of them automatically). Although many doctors and healthcare professionals dream about this type of automation, others are terrified by the prospect. Advantages include a high degree of automation, which can lead to fewer errors and increased charge capture. It also may decrease the need for certain office staff or clerical help. On the other hand, the cost can be significant, and a much steeper learning curve is involved in learning these systems (see Table 8.1).

Practices need to decide if they desire this level of automation and also evaluate the many offerings before proceeding with implementation of these systems. Budgets need to be carefully considered, and information technology support is obviously highly desirable. These types of systems tend to be favored by larger group practices or hospital systems due to the costs and support associated with them. When properly implemented, they come close to the ideal of "telepathic billing" described in our introduction.

Solutions that fall in to the extra strength category include TouchWorks Charge by Allscripts, Inc., EveryCharge from MDEveryWhere, and Charge-Keeper by PatientKeeper.

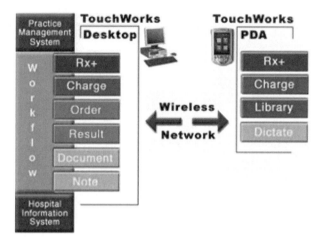

FIGURE 8.10. Modular implementation of TouchWorks. (Reprinted with permission from Allscripts, Inc.)

TouchWorks Charge

Web site: (www.allscripts.com)
Cost: Implementation and monthly subscription, varies by practice
Platform: Pocket PC

Allscripts is one of the few publicly traded companies in the handheld market and has been around since the 1980s. This is an important consideration when investing significant capital in a solution for charge capture (or any medical information technology investment for that matter). Their solution allows for modular implementation (i.e., charge capture, EMR, e-prescribing) and integration between desktop computers and handhelds (Figure 8.10). Basically, TouchWorks Charge digitally routes the paper encounter form, and has built-in Evaluation & Management coding assistance, medical necessity checking, and subsequent Advance Beneficiary Notification collection. The software has an intuitive interface and is easy to use (Figures 8.11–8.17). Basically, patients are selected from the main patient screen after synchronizing your daily schedule, and then the date of service, diagnosis, E/M codes, and Procedure Codes are selected from customizable pick lists. Once the encounter is finished, simply select "Submit," and the charges are entered in the main system. All these features will lighten the load on your office staff, and may even make coding and billing fun—is that possible?

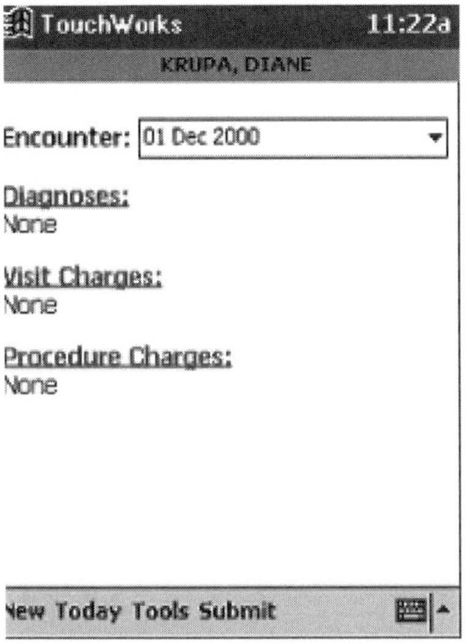

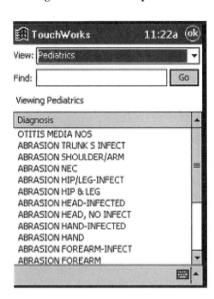

FIGURE 8.11. Main charge screen in TouchWorks Charge. (Reprinted with permission from Allscripts, Inc.)

FIGURE 8.12. Diagnosis pick list in TouchWorks Charge. (Reprinted with permission from Allscripts, Inc.)

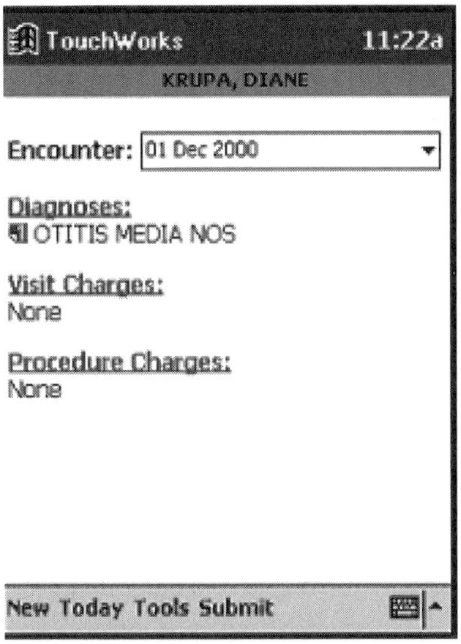

FIGURE 8.13. Diagnosis entered in TouchWorks Charge. (Reprinted with permission from Allscripts, Inc.)

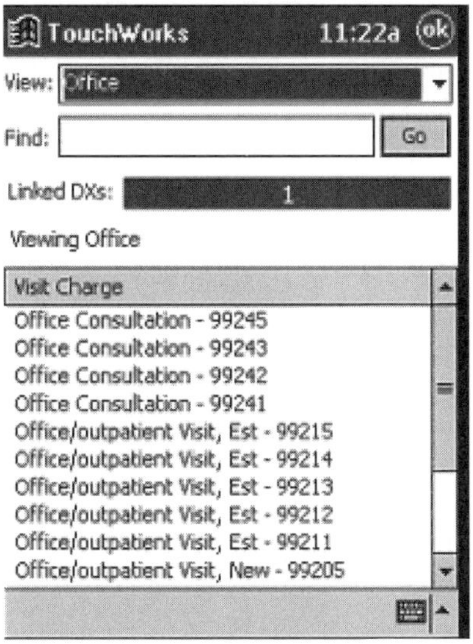

FIGURE 8.14. Office Evaluation and Management (E/M) Codes in TouchWorks Charge. (Reprinted with permission from Allscripts, Inc.)

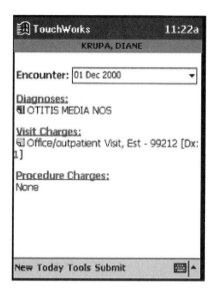

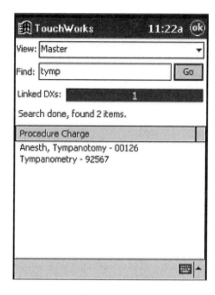

FIGURE 8.15. Diagnosis and E/M code entered in TouchWorks Charge. (Reprinted with permission from Allscripts, Inc.)

FIGURE 8.16. Procedures pick list in TouchWorks Charge. (Reprinted with permission from Allscripts, Inc.)

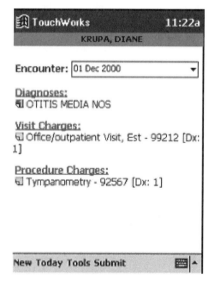

FIGURE 8.17. Finished encounter in TouchWorks Charge. (Reprinted with permission from Allscripts, Inc.)

EveryCharge

Web site: www.mdeverywhere.com
Cost: Implementation and monthly subscription, varies by practice
Platform: Palm OS and Pocket PC

MDeverywhere's EveryCharge is also part of a suite of solutions for physicians using handheld computers. Although not offering the full set of solutions available from Allscripts, MDeverywhere features their charge capture solution as well as voice dictation, order entry, and reference tools. EveryCharge synchronizes with existing practice management systems to upload your daily schedule, and professional services, diagnoses, and procedures can then be entered at the point of care. The software does come with a rules engine to assist with coding, and batched, error-checked charges are sent from MDeverywhere's data center to your billing system for forwarding to payers. This software also features a simple, intuitive interface (Figure 8.18a–c).

ChargeKeeper

Web site: www.patientkeeper.com
Cost: Contact company
Platform: Palm OS

PatientKeeper was actually first programmed as a patient tracker by a medical student. It subsequently grew to become a patient tracker with an open architecture capable of communicating with hospital and office computer systems. This tracking system with its communicating software mobilizes patient indexes, lab data, alerts, memos, and now charge capture with ChargeKeeper. The software has built-in error and validity checking and is quite robust. We review the patient-tracking program in Chapter 5, if you would like to see screen shots of this program.

Coding Guidelines for Your Handheld

So, after all these years, you have a clear concept of the 1995 and 1997 HCFA E/M guidelines, right? You know exactly how many HPI and ROS items are needed for all the levels of visits. If you do, you might be spending too much time memorizing useless information, instead of using some of the great coding tools available for handheld computers. And now, there's talk that they might actually change or be replaced. What is one supposed to do? We highly recommend keeping an updated coding tool on your handheld to help you when there are any doubts. After all, this is another way to lose the convertible—getting fined for miscoding patient visits. Why take a chance? These are also great tools to help residents learn coding, if you happen to be in a training program.

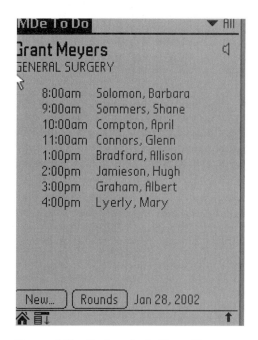

FIGURE 8.18a. Patient list in EveryCharge. (Reprinted with permission from MDEverywhere, Inc.)

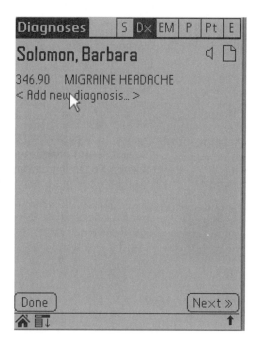

FIGURE 8.18b. Patient diagnoses are displayed when patient is selected. (Reprinted with permission from MDEverywhere, Inc.)

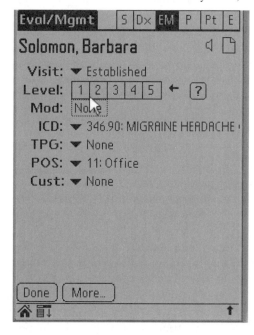

FIGURE 8.18c. Coding screen in EveryCharge. (Reprinted with permission from MDEverywhere, Inc.)

For the stand-alone billing solutions we have covered, you will need an add-on tool such as those described in this section. Otherwise, most of the extra strength solutions come with built-in coding wizards and guidelines.

Stat E&M Coder

Web site: www.statcoder.com
Cost: $75 for 2-year license
Platform: Palm OS

This little gem was created by a practicing physician with an MBA—go figure. The program is very intuitive and easy to use. It walks you thorough

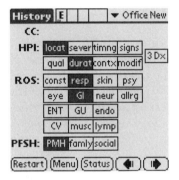

FIGURE 8.19. Initial screen for Stat E&M Coder. Users simply tap completed components of the HPI, ROS, and PFSH, and they are automatically considered in the coding. (Reprinted with permission from StatCoder.com.)

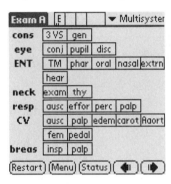

FIGURE 8.20. First exam screen for Stat E&M Coder. Tap completed exam items and they are automatically entered into the coding algorithm. (Reprinted with permission from StatCoder.com.)

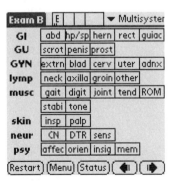

FIGURE 8.21. Second exam screen for Stat E&M Coder. (Reprinted with permission from StatCoder.com.)

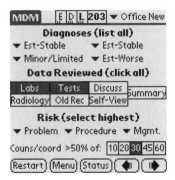

FIGURE 8.22. After selecting the appropriate components in this final screen, the code is shown on the top of the screen (in this case it is a level 203 for a new patient office visit). (Reprinted with permission from StatCoder.com.)

the components for E&M coding with simple pick and tap menus and then spits out a suggested code at the end. Users can either select the 1995 or 1997 HCFA guidelines (Figures 8.19–8.22). In addition to the E&M Coder, there are two other programs available to help you with your coding: STAT ICD-9 Coder and STAT CPT Coder. These two programs can be used for looking up ICD-9 codes and CPT codes, respectively.

InfoRetriever E/M Wizard

Web site: www.infopoems.com
Cost: See Web site
Platform: Palm OS and Pocket PC

Truly one of the best coding tools I have seen to date, this was created by one of our authors, Dr. Mark Ebell. It has one of the simplest interfaces, and is remarkable for the fact that it all fits on one screen. Users can choose the 1995 or 1997 HCFA guidelines, and all entries are "pick and tap." It comes with your annual subscription to InfoRetriever, which is an awesome Evidence-Based Medicine resource (see Chapter 14). This program also has an ICD-9 lookup list to further assist you with your coding (Figures 8.23, 8.24).

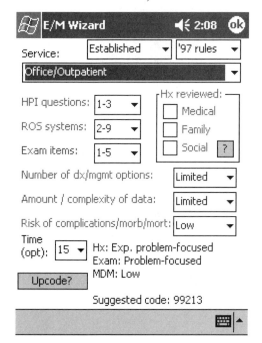

FIGURE 8.23. InfoRetriever E/M Wizard. (Reprinted with permission from InfoPOEM.)

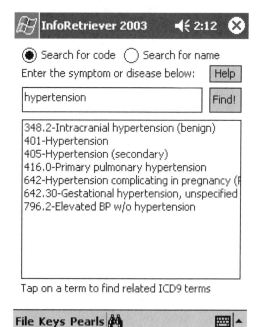

FIGURE 8.24. InfoRetriever ICD-9 Lookup Tool. (Reprinted with permission from InfoPOEM.)

Summary

We've covered quite a bit of ground in this chapter, and we hope you're feeling it might be worth it to venture out and try charge capture on your handheld computer, instead of your hand (or index cards as the case may be). These programs have pretty good evidence that they are worthwhile and will increase your billing accuracy and revenue.

A small investment in time and money is likely to yield significant returns and may lessen the drudgery of billing for all the hard work you do. We recommend trying one of the many stand-alone solutions for solo and small group practitioners; the extra strength solutions are more likely to apply in larger groups and hospital settings. Even if you're not ready to take the plunge into charge capture, at least try one of the coding assistants we described, as they are sure to assist you in billing accurately.

References

1. Fisher J, Wang R. The Cure is in the Hand: Bringing Information Technology to Patient Care. WR Hambrecht, San Francisco, CA, 2000.
2. Walpert B. Software to Help Your Billing—and Your Bottom Line. ACP-ASIM Observer. Retrieved from the World Wide Web at http://www.acponline.org/journals/handhelds/nov02/billing.htm, December 15, 2002.
3. MDEveryWhere case studies. Retrieved from the World Wide Web at http://www.mdeverywhere.com/ProvenValue/CaseStudies/index.aspx, December 15, 2002.
4. Strayer SM. Study evaluating handheld computer software to increase inpatient billing charge capture. J Am Med Inform Assoc 2001; Suppl. 5:837.

9

Electronic Prescribing: Drug Dealing Twenty-First Century Style

Gary N. Fox

Three billion prescriptions are filled each year in the United States (and remember that's only the ones patients choose to fill). That's 3 billion-plus chances for error—AND for callbacks from the pharmacy about illegibility, drug interactions, and formulary issues. According to estimates, medication errors kill thousands of Americans each year—7,000 by the Institute of Medicine's estimate. Incredibly, this exceeds the number of deaths from workplace injuries. There are other reasons (besides error reduction) to consider electronic prescribing, including speed, patient "wow," too many drugs and formulations to remember, and reducing those dreaded pharmacy callbacks.

Let's take a little trip to the future and design the perfect electronic prescribing solution. Then, we'll explore in detail one option that requires little investment and is a "safe" starting option for someone who wants to test things by gingerly putting a toenail edge into the water.

OK, fast forward your DUD player (a generation up from those old DVD players) past Orwell's *1984* and past *2001*: HAL, the talking computer in *Space Odyssey*, to sometime in the 2000-teens. You have been selected by your specialty organization, the AARP (American Academy of Remarkable Physicians—after all, you *are* reading this), to be on the committee to design the ultimate prescribing solution. With the plethora of new sound-alike, look-alike drugs, handwritten solutions are no longer acceptable. Really now, how many docs could read their OWN handwriting to distinguish reliably between Zaditor, Zagam, Zantac, Zebeta, Zerit, Zestril, Zemplar, Zarontin, Zaroxolyn, Zemuron, Zenapax, zanamivir, zafirlukast, Ziagen, zaleplon, Zinacef, Zinecard, Z-max (who's got time to write it out?), Ziac, Zocor, Zofran, Z-pak, Zonegran, Zonalon, Zostrix, Zosyn, Zovia, and Zovirax. Oops (sorry), I forgot Zyflo, Zyloprim, Zyprexa, Zyrtec, Zydone, and Zyban.

In addition, "regular" computer systems are now out of the question. The worldwide ban on nuclear power brought about by the Kyoto Treaty of 2009 and the precipitous decline in hydroelectric power from the unprecedented drought conditions from global warming have made electricity to run such systems unavailable and unaffordable. Plus, with President Hillary's imposition of strict cost controls and the socialization of medicine, there simply isn't the budget for widespread computerization or the extravagant use of electricity. (Gee, I miss air conditioning.) So, the committee has decided to go the handheld computer prescribing route.

What Elements Should Handheld Electronic Software Ideally Possess?

Basic Information, Patient Demographics, and Physician Identifiers

Now let's start with intuitive design, something that "looks and feels" a lot like a prescription pad, including speed and ease of use. The handheld will "know" the date and "automagically" transfer that to the prescription, as well as the physician's DEA number (entered once) *when needed*. Patient names will be transferred from the practice management system (yes, most practices can still finagle one such machine). But names can also be entered on the fly ("Mrs. Jones wants to know if you can also look in Johnnie's ears even though he's not been seen here before . . .) *or*, actually, to skip the name altogether ("Mrs. Jones' grandma is here visiting from Moosebreath and thinks she may have acute prescriptophilia—she will never be seen here again") and just print the prescription without entering a name.

Drug Information Entry

There should be an expansive drug list. For each drug, available forms (e.g., drops, tablets) should be listed and, for each form, available dosages (e.g., 125 mg/5 mL, 250 mg/5 mL) should also be listed. There should be default instructions ("sig"), specifically the "usual and customary" labeling, but it should be easily customized *and* stored for future use if desired. (President Hillary's quality initiatives still haven't forced us all to prescribe the same way.) We need to include refills, "dispense as written," and multiple options for prescription transmittal (e.g., beaming, printing, faxing). There should be an option to produce a paper copy of the prescription for documentation. Additionally, the prescription needs to be saved electronically for reference and future renewal.

New drugs should appear on the handheld's drug prescribing screen at the same time they are hitting pharmacy shelves—and vice versa for the all-too-common drug withdrawals. So, the drug list should be reasonably complete and up-to-date.

There should be a mechanism to enter prescriptions without printing or transmitting them. So that you have a record in the handheld for drug interactions checking or future reference, you might wish to enter a prescription called in for a patient, drugs prescribed by consultants, or drugs taken by a new patient who doesn't yet need renewals.

The prescription "writing" process on the handheld should follow a logical sequence, similar to what physicians are used to, maintaining traditional office systems, functions, and work flow. The technology should be unobtrusive and not interfere or adversely impact patient–physician interactions.

The Big Drug Fix

The prescription *generating* technology should be more than just "prescription *writing*." More like prescription *righting*. Specifically, we are going to design in all the error-checking capability that we can into our ideal system. The handheld could even guesstimate appropriateness of the prescription if other key information were entered—diagnosis code, age (calculated from one-time, stored entry of patient's birth date), renal and hepatic function, drug allergies, and adverse reactions. For example, a flag may appear if the physician enters a diagnosis code of 462 (pharyngitis, acute) or 034.0 (streptococcal sore throat) and, in a non-penicillin-allergic patient, chooses something *other than* penicillin in an adult or other than penicillin or amoxicillin in a child (so the gizmo's protocol uses birth date information). It would also flag the choice of these first-line antibiotics if they *were* selected in a penicillin-allergic individual.

And, just to make life interesting, should the physician choose Avelox (moxifloxacin) or Cipro for one of these diagnoses (OK, you could argue that maybe the patient has gonorrhea, but let's not go there), the handheld could start its alarm, could vibrate, maybe remotely set off all the car alarms in the parking lot, and could squirt one of those bank robbery dye packs onto the physician's white coat. (Wouldn't that make for fun lunches in the physicians' dining room?) Appropriateness criteria could also include drug–age warnings, such as quinolones (Cipro and cousins) in children and metformin (Glucophage) in patients age 80 and older. Of course, these would be warnings, because there are circumstances where these prescriptions would be appropriate (no dye packs for these).

Other error checks should include drug interactions checking and drug allergy checking. Have you ever looked at the allergy list, seen "sulfa," and 5 to 10 minutes later starting writing for Bactrim/Septra, only to have the patient say "This doesn't contain sulfa, does it doc?" Even if that's never happened to you, now there are complex relationships among drug structures that create theoretical cross-allergenicity, such as between sulfonamides and thiazide diuretics, furosemide (Lasix), celecoxib (Celebrex), sulfonylureas (Amaryl, Diabeta, Glucotrol), and zonisamide (Zonegran), for example.

Do we really need to say anything about drug–drug interactions testing? Everybody knows some drugs that interact with everything including water, air, ozone, and comets passing too close by. But now patients are seeing multiple physicians and may end up on a dizzying array of less familiar drugs (don't forget the herbs!)—and less familiar interactions. That's one reason efficient (so it's not an annoyance) "automagic" drug interactions is a good idea as part of electronic prescribing.

Drug–disease interactions can also be checked, particularly drug dosage adjustments in renal failure, cautions with hepatic insufficiency, and, if age qualifies, quinolones in youth and metformin (Glucophage) in the over-80 crowd. Certainly the algorithm should flag metformin in anyone with a creatinine or creatinine clearance above prescribing thresholds (at least, the prescriber should be vibrated if the device is capable—REALLY!!).

Of course, to make all this happen, multiple things need to be entered (Do YOU drink grapefruit juice?) in addition to chart numbers, pharmacy numbers, etc. These error-checking processes, after initial entry (*once*), should be transparent, rapid, and require *no* active effort on the part of the prescriber, except if an error is detected.

The Output

One patient may wish a prescription sent directly to the pharmacy (and doesn't care whether it gets there by e-mail, cellular technology, or horse-n-buggy, so long as it gets there before he or she does). Another may wish a paper prescription to hang onto (a "backup prescription") or to comparison shop. Most physicians will want printed local documentation.

How does a TV, radio, or cell phone work? Who cares? It just does. A signal is generated somewhere and is deciphered somewhere else. Using such magic, our gizmo could deliver a prescription to the pharmacy before the ink is dry on the encounter form. Needless to say, there are multiple other methods. Briefly, with "docking" methods, that is likely to be the rate-limiting step in the prescription production process. For "printer" methods, it is worth the investment in a fast and reliable printer to avoid this as a bottleneck that could sabotage an otherwise workable electronic prescribing solution.

Data Security, Connectivity (Data Sharing), and Backup

Somehow, all these data need to be secured in case the handheld device is lost, misplaced, or stolen—or just falls prey to some rug rats who want to see what games are installed. The handheld device should require a login password and have a time-out feature. The data need to be backed up. If information is stored solely on the handheld and the handheld is lost or damaged (or the battery runs completely out), the data may be lost. Ouch.

There needs to be a mechanism for the practice's handhelds to communicate with each other. If you and a partner each see 25 patients who average 2.5 prescriptions each, that's 125 prescriptions. Each handheld can send its data to a central source, then redownload the mother-of-all-data from the central source. This could be accomplished in "real time" via a continuous exchange between the handhelds and a wireless network or at the end of sessions via docking with hardwired connections.

Bells and Whistles

Renewals of medications should be a snap. Remember Hallie? She's the 62-year-old with obesity, COPD, DM type 2, hypertension, dyslipidemia, osteoarthritis, hypothyroidism, and irritable bowel, bladder, and brain. In short, she's got the TNTCD (too numerous to count drugs) syndrome. It takes a whole week just to write out her scrips. Time for renewal of Hallie's prescriptions? Simple. Select each drug for renewal from her list on the handheld, modify any (maybe the ACE or antihyperlipidemic needs increasing) that need adjustment (a simple process from drop-down lists of available dosages), hit "transmit" or "print" and—voila—we've done a week's work in a few stylus taps.

Ideally, data should be accessible from anywhere. A handheld that downloads fresh data daily or periodically from a central computer is one solution. That central computer could be in the office, or on the Web. If Web based, that would allow password-protected access from other locations, such as when on call, at home, or in the hospital, without even having to carry the prescribing handheld. That would be helpful for prescription renewal calls, or other prescription- or medication-related calls, during these times. And by office staff when the office is open but *you're* not. How would that work? You or another authorized individual will go to the secure site, renew or generate the appropriate prescription, and have it transmitted to the pharmacy (with in-office documentation).

Other bells and whistles: some form of authentication so the pharmacy knows it's you and not one of the other neighborhood drug pushers; and, when printing locally, a software-printed, digitized, tendon-sparing signature.

And, I'm sorry to say, in the 2000-teens, we still have "formulary" issues. So, despite a large chunk of the populace being victims of HillariCare, there are dozens of companies dividing up the remaining pieces of the pie. So, except for the docs who use the various formulary charts as wallpaper in the exam rooms, the incessant phone calls about which ACEs, HMGs, NSAIDs, antibiotics, and PPIs are and are not covered continue. So, our handheld should allow us to enter the patient's insurance plan and should allow us to determine *in advance* whether the drug is a preferred one, an acceptable formulary preparation, or a-phone-call-waiting-to-happen.

Class II controlled substances—the methylphenidates (Ritalin, Concerta, others), the amphetamines (Adderall, others), oxycodone (Oxycontin, OxyIR, others)—still need monthly prescriptions. Wouldn't it be nice to be able to "tag" prescriptions that need refill the first of every month? Like Hattie (Hallie's cousin) with cancer who needs oxycodone monthly. And meds for those 50 kids with attention-getting disorder (the new name for you-guessed-it) that need to be generated each month. Note that, for some states, laws may not allow e-prescribing of Class II's.

OK, we're doing a good job so far. Let's keep designing a little more. During the winter, how many new reactive airways with cough, possible pertussoid syndrome, I-better-use-my-favorite-macrolide-plus-reactive-airways-multi-med-regimen-plus-some-symptomatic-therapy patients are there? And what about multimodal treatment for sinusitis, including a prescription in-your-nose spray, antibiotic, decongestant-plus-loosification agent? Wouldn't it be nice if we could just pull up Hammie's (yes, you guessed right) patient entry, and click "Winter-rot-with-cough-regimen" or "Super Sinus Blaster Special #1" (or both when needed) rather than having to select a half-dozen individual drugs? (Sort of like ordering electrolytes rather than sodium, potassium, bicarb, chloride. . . .)

Remember Hallie? She needed refills on *everything*. HillariCare doesn't include BRAIN monitoring (Bloodless Real Accurate Instantaneous Numbers—the transcutaneous monitoring stuff for glucose). So we have to refill Hallie's old-fashioned diabetes monitoring strips and, while we're at it, her meter dates from the 1990s (can you imagine!) and she needs a new one. Be nice if the same gizmo printed those things, too. And, because we are the ones designing it, it will. (That probably means our Unique Physician Identification Number (UPIN) number will need to be added somewhere into gizmo's memory but that's probably required on everything by now, anyway.)

So, can we get rid of that paper prescription pad yet? What about physical therapy prescriptions and work excuses? Yep, let's add those, too. That way, when Hackie (Hammie and Hallie's kid) comes in, you select his name from the patient list, tap "Winter-rot-with-cough-regimen" and "Work excuse," tap a couple entries from drop-down lists, hit "print," and you have the whole pile of scrips and a completed work excuse (maybe even transmitted direct to the employer!) with Hackie's name, visit date, and so on.

All variable fields would have drop-down lists (options represented here by <brackets>), and the text would be user entered once and saved for the future: "Please excuse me for writing this note, but I can't figure out why this guy hasn't been to work for the last <1, 2, 3, 4, infinity> <hours, days, weeks, months, years, millennia>." These free-form prescriptions should also allow users to enter those special mixes (like dilute nitroglycerin ointment for anal fissures), dermatologic formulations, and so on, that just aren't going to be in any formulary.

Now, with all this printing, faxing, e-mail, beaming, and digitized signatures, we won't need drug company pens any more.

OK, a new drug, Liverrotatoxacin, is recalled. Wouldn't it be nice to be able to retrieve a list of all patients on it? Because extensive searching on a handheld device tends to be slow at this juncture (the future may be different), it makes more sense to perform such a search on the PC or server-based backup file. It would also be nice to be able to cross reference whatever data are in the software. For example, assuming health maintenance information is entered, "Which patients on estrogen age 40 or older have not had a mammogram in the last year?" Or, "List the patients on insulin who are not on an ACE inhibitor." It would also be nice to be able to retrieve drugs for prescription by classification during attacks of "Acute Brain Spongiosis" ("What is the name of that drug for . . .").

Also, the software should allow drugs to be deleted from the patient's history list (e.g., erroneous entry or malaria prophylaxis for a prehistoric trip). Users may consider *retaining* but *inactivating* old episodic medications on the patient's drug history to save a lot of thumbing through the chart to find "that stuff that worked so well before." Furthermore, annotating inactive medications for future reference ("ACE-induced cough") is highly desirable. For drugs that have a finite quantity prescribed (10 days of Amoxil® prescribed 3 months ago) the software should "automagically" flag them for inactivation.

One of the most important aspects is that the whole process be *fast*, at least as fast as generating a handwritten prescription. The gizmo must be portable, light, instant-on, reliable, legal (state laws vary), and sufficiently affordable so as not to present an obstacle to experimentation.

OK, we're back off the starship *Enterprise* and down to reality. Many of the features we've discussed—and even more—for example, some voice recognition technology and the software "automagically learning" each user's preferred prescriptions—are already available. But some aren't (like "Fox's Sinus Blaster #1"). Since we've done all the work of listing ideal features, I compiled them in Table 9.1 for convenience.

Handheld Prescription Writing as an Incremental Technology

As typewriters have given way to word processors, and as the power of "average" computers has increased, the features of word processors have increased. Also, users have learned to use slews of new features built into word processors. Earlier, we talked about including all the "error checking" that we could in our prescription writer, even to the point of including health maintenance and disease data. As speed and memory on palmtops increases and, as users begin to use more features of prescription writers,

TABLE 9.1. Considerations in selecting a handheld prescribing system.

Practice considerations
What are the motivations for starting handheld prescribing? How likely is handheld
 prescribing to fulfill these expectations?
How many providers are involved? Is there adequate "buy in"?
Is there adequate room for hardware and consensus on where it will be located?
Is the system going to be used at multiple locations? If so, how is that going to be
 managed?
How will the technology influence patient–physician interaction?
What are the start-up costs, including data transfer, and ongoing costs, including
 subscription fees and prescription paper (if applicable)?
What changes in workflow will occur? For example, will management of telephone
 prescription renewals change?
In the future, might there be a desire to add other modules that integrate and, if so, does
 this system allow (vendor have) such modular additions?

Hardware considerations
What types of specific hardware (operating system and brand, amount of memory) and
 software will be required, including detailed specifications?
Is the hardware sufficiently durable to withstand clinical use?
Is the battery life sufficient for office needs? Rechargeable (if a concern)?
Warranties?

Software and product considerations
General and administrative:
Can patient demographic data be transferred from existing systems?
Would the information be transferrable to another system if the vendor goes out of
 business or you decide to take your business elsewhere?
How are prescription data going to be shared among providers' handheld units?
What is the minimum amount of patient information that needs to be entered to write a
 prescription? Can a prescription be written *without* entry of any patient information?
Is there a mechanism for offsite production of prescriptions, or remote access to data,
 such as through the Internet?
How user friendly is the software?
If prescriptions are transmitted directly to pharmacies, how will that fit into workflow?
How is physician name and practice identification information handled?
How is the DEA number handled?
Prescription generation:
  How fast is the process? If it will slow you down, will you *really* use it?
  How complete is the drug listing for your specialty?
  Can the default prescription instructions, quantities, and so on, be modified and saved
   for future use? If so, how rapidly and easily can this be accomplished? (One product
   actually "memorizes" each user's most common prescriptions, including Sig, by
   diagnosis, e.g., for sinusitis.)
  How "good" are the default prescriptions (especially the "sig")?
  How quickly are newly available drugs put into the drug list and how quickly are
   withdrawn drugs removed?
  How are prescriptions for compounded preparations, medical devices, physical therapy,
   radiographic tests, work excuses, and other things for which physicians use their
   prescription pads handled with the software?
  Is there formulary coverage in the software? Does it include the major formularies for
   your practice? Does it suggest formulary alternatives?

TABLE 9.1. *Continued*

Do printed prescriptions have to be signed manually, or is there a digitized signature capability?

Is the software approved by your state for generating prescriptions for Class II controlled substances?

How are transmitted prescriptions authenticated?

If prescriptions are printed, can they be queued for printing?

What options for producing and transmitting prescriptions are there?

What mechanisms are there for producing documentation for the chart?

How does the software handle prescription renewals?

Are there unnecessary screens or keystrokes in the prescription generation process?

Prescription database and database functions:

Can notes be attached to patient listings?

Can patient listings be deleted?

Can individual drugs in patients' drug histories be deleted?

Can drugs in drug histories be inactivated? Can notes be attached to inactivated drugs for allergy or intolerance notations?

What are the report and search capabilities of the product? Could you find all patients who have been prescribed a recalled drug?

Is there a mechanism for recalling and producing "monthly" (Class II controlled substance) prescriptions?

Error checking:

Is there capability for drug–drug interactions error checking? If so, are such things as alcohol use included?

Is there capability for drug–allergy checking?

Can diagnoses be entered?

If so, is there drug–disease interaction checking? If so, can renal and hepatic function be entered?

Can error checking (if present) be turned off? Can the error checking sensitivity be adjusted?

Security, data backup, and recovery:

Are there adequate security measures for patient-specific data on the handheld? During backup and transmissions?

Are the data reliably and securely backed up to ensure against data loss or corruption?

Vendor considerations

How long have the hardware and software vendors been in business? Are they likely to be in business for the duration you plan to use the products? What is their track record on support? What are the warranties?

Is there corporate sponsorship that might bias drug lists or other features?

an evolution of prescription software, similar to that seen with word processing software, may occur.

Specifically, let's look at a few features that could be added by the time the planets next align in the Western sky. Wouldn't it be convenient to "jot" down the monitoring protocol in the handheld for a drug we don't use often? What about reminders or notes of *any* sort, for that matter? Notes could be date-tagged, and could be the first thing that comes when the handheld is activated on or after the note's date stamp. Adding health maintenance protocols is not much of a stretch. As voice-to-text voice recognition software improves, the handheld's "basic prescription writer" of the early 2000s—plus add-ons—could become the electronic medical record platform of the foreseeable future.

Handhelds Do Not Eliminate Human Prescription Errors

Types of prescribing error include choosing the wrong medication, the wrong route, a suboptimal dosage (too high or too low), or an incorrect frequency of administration. Default sigs ("apply Sloppy Goo FIVE times a day") help, but things such as weight-based dosing and dosage recommendations based on diagnosis (e.g., different antibiotic dosages for UTI and otitis media) are beyond *current* capabilities of most of the handheld prescribing software products.

Errors can occur with handheld prescribing. It can be difficult to tell which "John Jones" is which from the patient list. (Hint: Pull up the correct patient before going in the exam room.) Also, it is easily to tap the stylus one line high or low, especially if talking or distracted. So, one can generate a perfect prescription—for the wrong patient. A slight misapplication of the stylus can also occur in the drug list; sustained-release preparations are listed right under their nonsustained counterparts. The default "sig" may not be *your* default. For nortriptyline (Pamelor), the default sig in *iScribe* is "tid," whereas I prescribe it as a single nightly dose.

All prescriptions, *e-* or traditional, in my opinion, should be double- and triple-checked for (in)accuracy. On the flip side, sometimes when I'm going for 250 mg tid and see the tempting 400 mg bid dosage listed, I switch to shoot for better compliance (at the expense of increasing cost). So, for us in the "geriheimer's club," the "pick lists" offer alternatives to our last millennium's automatisms. The things that handheld prescribing unquestionably cure are legibility *and spelling*—they are gifts for physicians who couldn't pass the spell checker's test at the M&M factory. They also make it pretty hard to prescribe a dosage or form that isn't available.

Key Points

- Prescribing is the most visible, integral, and potentially error-prone (even fatal) endeavor in routine outpatient clinical practice.
- Electronic prescribing via handheld devices is a technology that can be introduced in a manner "minimally invasive" to the typical office routine and culture.
- Handheld prescribing promises to reduce some types of prescribing error, most especially those from mistaken drug names and dosages resulting from misspelled and illegible prescriptions.
- Formulary compliance can be easily checked before a prescription is produced.

- Only available formulations and dosages are listed to be prescribed, so the physician cannot write for a nonexistent 20-mg pill (although a prescription for 40 mg ½ po qd is no problem).
- One possible scenario is that electronic prescribing software will continue to add more advanced features and, as more and more bells and whistles are added, this technology could form the nucleus of a handheld mini-electronic medical record.

Handheld Prescription Writers in Action

We'll graphically review two programs, one for the Palm OS (iScribe, used by the author) and one for Pocket PC devices (Touchworks Rx+ from Allscripts). These are by no means the only options available. Table 9.2 lists some vendors, complete with propaganda from their websites (because,

TABLE 9.2. Selected vendors of handheld prescribing solutions.

Product: Allscripts
Platform: Pocket PC
Cost: Monthly subscription and one-time hardware and installation fees (practice dependent).
Web site: http://www.allscripts.com/
Clips from Web site (material deleted):
TouchWorks Rx+
The TouchWorks Rx+ module is an ambulatory medication management and prescription communication tool featuring drug and allergy interaction checking and plan-specific formularies. With the Rx+ PDA companion, physicians can prescribe and route prescriptions directly from the exam room. The entire process is faster than using a script pad and reduces the need for pharmacy callback, saving time for physicians and their patients.
The Rx+ advantage:

- Streamlined office efficiency
  Medication questions and prescription renewals are managed online, eliminating paper chart pulls to answer questions, improving turnaround time for renewal requests, and facilitating communication with pharmacies and pharmacy benefit management (PBM) companies.
- Enhanced health care decision making
  Drug utilization review and smart links to appropriate knowledge sources provide staff with valuable on-the-spot information.
- Improved quality of care
  Using Rx+, medication errors arising from illegible handwriting (misinterpretation of the drug name or dosage) are reduced. Physicians are proactively notified of prescription expirations and can check on patient compliance with medication fulfillment to ensure that patients are receiving the maximum health benefits with the recommended course of treatment.

Product: Pocketscript
Platform: Pocket PC
Cost: Variable—practice dependent; estimate about $150 per physician per month. Vendor may have methods of offsetting charges (e.g., electronic drug detailing agreements).

TABLE 9.2. *Continued*

Web site: http://www.pocketscript.com/
Clips from Web site (material deleted and edited for brevity):
PocketScript, Inc. has created a highly efficient way to write electronic prescriptions with voice commands or only a few touches of the screen. . . . the system wirelessly communicates with a server in the physician's office and interfaces with existing medical records. . . . doctors can obtain patient information, insurance coverage information, formulary listings and potential drug interactions, and then use the technology to send prescriptions via fax or the Internet.
PocketScript was designed with a physician's natural workflow in mind.

- . . . enables physicians to transmit electronic prescriptions directly from the examining room to the pharmacy. . . . Before the prescription is transmitted, PocketScript flags possible drug interactions and supplies provider-specific approved formulary drug listings . . . Sends prescriptions via the Internet through a 128-bit encrypted, secure application directly to the pharmacy.
- Physicians can access more than 60,000 patient records in a single second. . . . the PDA is a thin client that wirelessly connects to the server (that is, the PDA is a remote screen viewing data that "lives" on the central computer) to obtain all current patient . . . information. . . . Assures patient confidentiality because most information resides on the physician's office server.
- The PocketScript PDA has a 10-hour battery life. . . . allows physicians to write up to 350 prescriptions a day, without recharging the battery.
- PocketScript meets state pharmacy board compliance standards in more than 30 states and complies with all DEA regulations regarding electronic prescription of Schedule III, IV, V drugs.
- PocketScript Releases World's First Speech-Driven Prescription Writer (BUSINESS WIRE)—Feb. 5, 2001—New Next Generation e-Prescribing Tool lets Doctors simply say names of Patients and Prescriptions to Dramatically Improve Use of PDAs at Point of Care.

Product: iScribe
Platform: Palm OS
Cost: Vendor has not yet released cost information. WAG (wild-ass guesstimate) is $20 per month per physician.
Web site: http://www.iscribe.com/
Clips from Web site (material deleted and edited for bevity):
iScribe Electronic Prescribing
Write prescriptions, access formulary information, and print legible prescriptions—all at the point of care.
The iScribe System:

- helps decrease the chance of medication errors.
- reduces the need for pharmacy callbacks with legible, printed prescriptions that are prechecked for formulary coverage.

Features include:

- Access approximately 8000 drug formulations and medical supplies.
- Easily customize and save a list of your preferred Sigs to quickly generate prescriptions.
- Build your database of patient medication histories on the handheld for easy reference and simplified renewals.
- Easily generate a second prescription for your patients to send to their mail-order facility.
- Interface to your practice management, billing, or scheduling system. An easy interface loads your patient demographics from your practice management system onto your handheld.

after all, this book is *so* captivating you wouldn't want to have to put it down just to go to their Web sites now).

Allscripts Touchworks Rx+

Remember the "incremental technology" thesis? Well, a company called Allscripts also believes it is a possibility. So rather than be forced to take the giant leap to an electronic record, the physician can start with any one of Allscripts' modular products, such as charge capture or dictation—or Rx+, the electronic prescribing module for Pocket PCs. (It's sort of like Microsoft making "Office," one component of which is Word, another Excel, etc.) If a user chooses all the modules, the result approaches that of an electronic record.

Let's briefly walk through Rx+ with Dr. Chip Ahoy, who has plenty of money to spend on technology having made a fortune in the cookie business. (As you know, those are the things online services put on your hard drive.) Dr. Ahoy starts his office session by logging into Rx+ on his Pocket PC handheld. Although he can search for any patient registered with the practice, he pulls up his daily schedule, which naturally, has his patient list (Figure 9.1).

It is now time to see Diane Krupa. Her demographic information is in the registration system—including formulary benefits, pharmacy, date of birth, and so on. This info can then be viewed immediately on the handheld because the handheld is simply a "window" that allows access to the data on the main office computer.

Ms. Krupa has sinusitis. To begin the prescribing process, Chip taps Ms. Krupa's name. After the patient is selected, the next step in Rx+ is to choose the diagnosis, as illustrated in Figure 9.2. Sinusitis is on Chip's list of most frequent diagnoses. For other diagnoses, he can "search" for the diagnosis.

TouchWorks		6:03a
Name △	DOB	
BAILEY, MARY	1/31/1943	
BARRETT, NORIENE	10/15/1916	
CALDWELL, MARY	10/7/1927	
FAFARD, TENA	10/10/1926	
GADDINI, JEAN	12/12/1977	
GALASKE, TRACY	6/21/1973	
KRUPA, DIANE	5/15/1952	
KRUPAN, JIMMY	1/30/1952	
ROSS, HENRY	1/1/1953	
SMITH, DAVID	10/5/1950	
SMITH, MONA	12/12/1978	
WEIN, DEBORAH	9/20/1999	

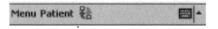

FIGURE 9.1. Daily schedule for Dr. Chip Ahoy. (Reprinted with permission from Allscripts, Inc.)

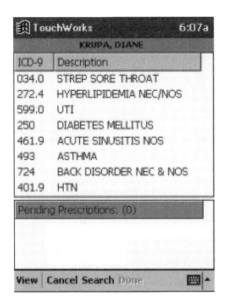

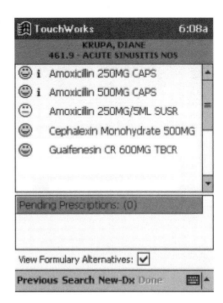

FIGURE 9.2. Rx+'s "diagnosis" step. (Reprinted with permission from Allscripts, Inc.)

FIGURE 9.3. Dr. Ahoy's personal most frequently used drugs for diagnosis 461.9, acute sinusitis, as illustrated at the top of the figure. Note the colored smiley-face "emoticons," which indicate each drug's formulary status for Diane's pharmacy benefit plan. (Reprinted with permission from Allscripts, Inc.)

Rx+ "remembers" Chip's drug choices for each diagnosis, thus the logic of forcing a choice of diagnosis first. Now that sinusitis has been chosen as a diagnosis, the drugs Chip most frequently individually prescribes for that particular diagnosis are displayed (Figure 9.3).

Chip chooses amoxicillin 500mg for Diane. Once Chip taps this drug, a default sig is displayed, which Chip can either choose or he can choose to write a new instruction to replace the default (Figure 9.4). After choosing the default sig by a stylus tap, Chip is immediately taken to the next screen, which shows that the prescription for amoxicillin is "pending" (Figure 9.5).

At this point, Chip can either decide he's "done" or continue adding more drugs to send all at once. Once done, Chip taps "destination" and the scrip wings its way to its final resting place via wireless magic (Figure 9.6).

Note the formulary status of each drug is shown in the drug screens (e.g., Figure 9.3) via colored "smiley face" emoticons, green being preferred formulary alternatives, yellow being allowable options, and red being nonformulary products. If Chip chooses a nonformulary drug, Rx+ will suggest formulary alternatives. Note that all error checking—drug–drug, drug–allergy/intolerance, drug–disease—occurs in the background, and the user is notified only if an interaction is detected.

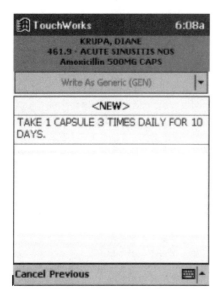

FIGURE 9.4. Chip can select the default "sig" or choose to write a new one. (Reprinted with permission from Allscripts, Inc.)

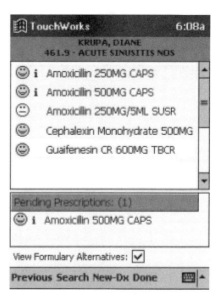

FIGURE 9.5. Prescription pending: Amoxicillin 500 mg, a green, smiley-faced drug, is on the list to be sent. (Reprinted with permission from Allscripts, Inc.)

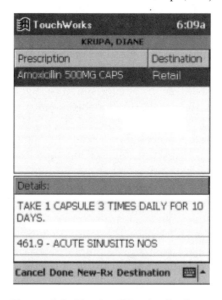

FIGURE 9.6. Tapping "Destination" sends the prescription via wireless magic to its destination, the retail pharmacy. (Reprinted with permission from Allscripts, Inc.)

One User's Experience: iScribe

Figures 9.7 through 9.53 illustrate how prescribing works with *iScribe*, an easy-to-use Palm OS electronic prescribing product. Because I work in a system where it would have been complicated to have data transferred into *iScribe* from the registration/billing system, I manually enter new patients just before the start of office hours. I use the Palm's Graffiti entry method, but the Palm's built-in, tappable keyboard or one of the external keyboard units for the Palm could be used.

It generally takes no longer than a couple of minutes to add patients. I use one printer that is situated right outside my suite of examination rooms. Each prescription is printed on one sheet of paper. Each contains the prescription on the top half of the sheet and an address label-sized "sticky" on the bottom half. The "sticky" contains all the prescription information for charting, serving as a duplicate prescription for documentation. In a multiphysician practice, each handheld unit needs to be synchronized via the Internet with iScribe to back up the data and share the practice's patient information. Each synchronization also downloads the latest drug list and formulary information. Note that iScribe does not do any error checking (drug–drug, drug–allergy, drug–disease) and does not automatically link to any "drug of choice" or drug comparison sources.

When laid out step by step, the prescribing process may look slow and cumbersome, but selections can be made quite rapidly from the drop-down lists or via Graffiti entries. On my Palm IIIC, iScribe's latest version is notably slower than the pre-7/1/02 version (which was quite rapid), particularly when entering multiple prescriptions ("+Rx" in the figures) and is also slower in printing. As for me, I have a hard time envisioning living without ePocrates, electronic Tarascon, and iScribe. Follow the figures for a walk-through of the prescribing process in the Hands-On Exercises. Go to https://physician. advancepcs.com/advpcs_phyres/index.html for software updates.

HANDS-ON EXERCISE 9.1. ENTERING A PATIENT AND PRODUCING PRESCRIPTIONS IN ISCRIBE

The user taps the iScribe icon on the handheld to arrive at the password screen (Figure 9.7). Physical possession of the unit constitutes the first level of security; the password requirement further protects patient data (Figure 9.8). Once the password is entered, the patient list appears (Figure 9.9). The patient list scrolls as the user types in letters of the patient's name (Figure 9.10). We are looking to see whether Gary N. Fox has been entered and, if not, we are going to enter him. After entering two letters (f, o), we can see that only Caroline Fox is in the patient list (Figure 9.11). We next tap "New" to enter our new patient.

We have entered our patient's first name, last name, date of birth, sex, SSN, and patient number (Figure 9.12). We need actually enter *none* of this

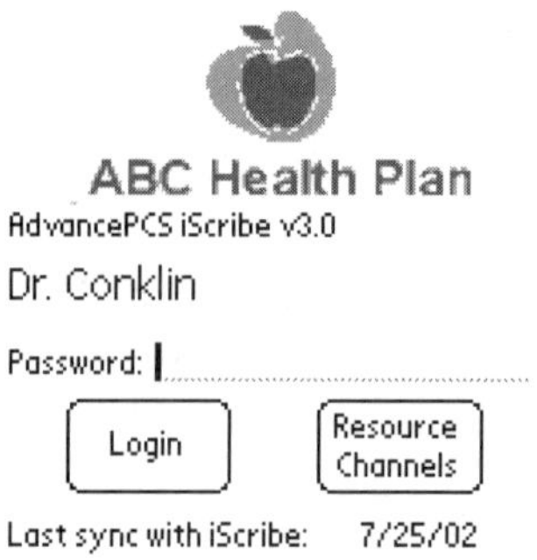

ABC Health Plan
AdvancePCS iScribe v3.0

Dr. Conklin

Password: |

[Login]   [Resource Channels]

Last sync with iScribe: 7/25/02

FIGURE 9.7. Tapping on the iScribe icon on the handheld opens the password screen. (Reprinted with permission from Caremark, Inc.)

ABC Health Plan
AdvancePCS iScribe v3.0

Dr. Conklin

Password: 123|

[Login]   [Resource Channels]

Last sync with iScribe: 7/25/02

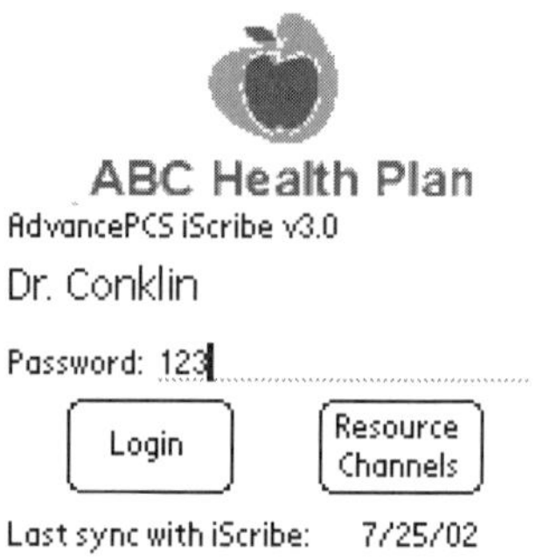

FIGURE 9.8. The user enters the password. Physical possession of the unit constitutes the first level of security; the password requirement further protects patient data. (Reprinted with permission from Caremark, Inc.)

information if we choose; we can tap the "Skip" option at the bottom of Figure 9.9, 9.10, or 9.11 and begin prescribing (but the information would then not be saved because there is no associated name to save it with). The name can then be handwritten onto the prescription.

Alternatively, we could have just entered the patient's name. For our example, next we tap on "Baseline Formulary," also an optional entry. The list of formulary options appears (Figure 9.13). The user selects these on the basis of his or her practice's insurance plans. The choices that appear on the handheld are selections made by the user on iScribe's Web site and downloaded onto the user's handheld during synchronization with the Web site.

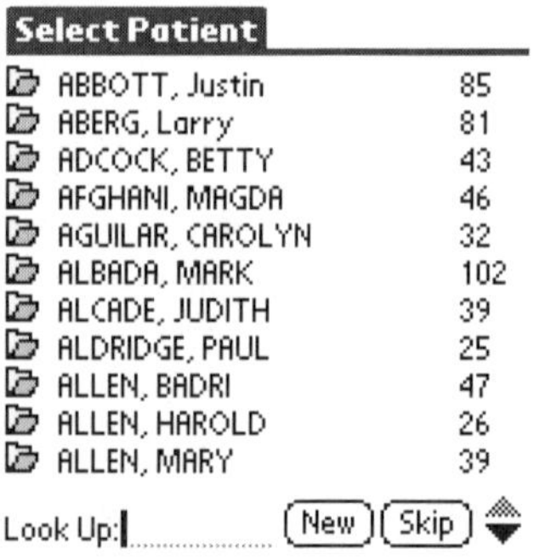

Select Patient	
ABBOTT, Justin	85
ABERG, Larry	81
ADCOCK, BETTY	43
AFGHANI, MAGDA	46
AGUILAR, CAROLYN	32
ALBADA, MARK	102
ALCADE, JUDITH	39
ALDRIDGE, PAUL	25
ALLEN, BADRI	47
ALLEN, HAROLD	26
ALLEN, MARY	39

Look Up: | [New] [Skip]

FIGURE 9.9. Once the password is entered, the patient list appears. (Reprinted with permission from Caremark, Inc.)

Select Patient	
FACAS, MELISA	42
FARAVELLI, ANTHONY	42
FEDERWITZ, RAED	93
FELDE, HERBERT	39
FELLOWS, LAURA	102
FERREIRA, JANET	32
FERREIRA, JOHN	57
FILIPELLI, MARYL	37
FINATO, SCOTT	19
FINNEGAN, EMILY	54
FINNEGAN, JOHN	46

Look Up: f   [New] [Skip]

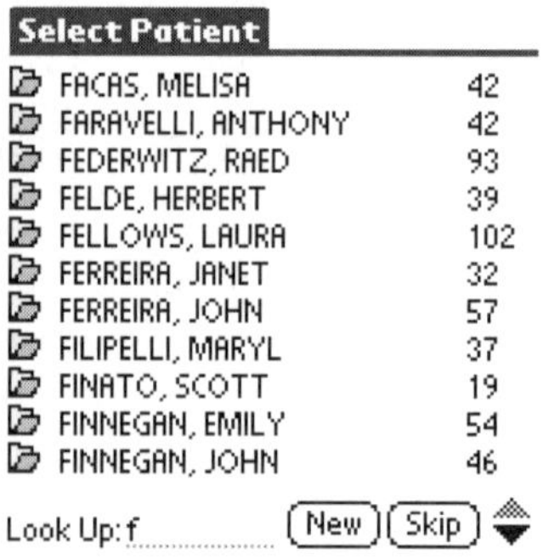

FIGURE 9.10. The patient list scrolls as the user types in letters of the patient's name. We are looking to see whether Gary N. Fox has been entered and, if not, we are going to enter him. (Reprinted with permission from Caremark, Inc.)

Select Patient	
FOILES, PAMELA MICHELLE	75
FOLLOSCO, MARILYN	45
FORREST, JANICE	72
FORREST, KELLY	76
FOX, CAROLINE	60

Look Up: fo   [New] [Skip]

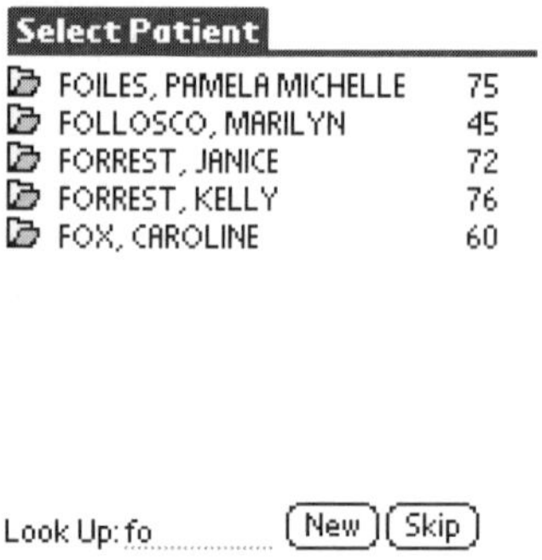

FIGURE 9.11. After entering two letters (f, o), we can see that only Caroline Fox is in the patient list. We next tap "New" to enter our new patient. (Reprinted with permission from Caremark, Inc.)

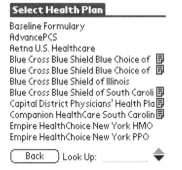

Patient Info   ▼ Demographics
First Name: Gary N.
Last Name: Fox
DOB: 01/01/1950 Sex: M F ?
SSN: 123 - 45 - 6789
Pt. #: FoxGN0001
Health Plan:
Baseline Formulary

(Back) (New Rx) (Save)

FIGURE 9.12. We have entered our patients first name, last name, date of birth, sex, SSN, and patient number. We need actually enter *none* of this information if we choose; we can tap the "Skip" option at the bottom of Figure 9.5 and begin prescribing. The name can then be handwritten onto the prescription. Alternatively, we could have just entered the patient's name. For our example, next we tap on "Baseline Formulary," also an optional entry. (Reprinted with permission from Caremark, Inc.)

Select Health Plan
Baseline Formulary
AdvancePCS
Aetna U.S. Healthcare
Blue Cross Blue Shield Blue Choice of 🗐
Blue Cross Blue Shield Blue Choice of 🗐
Blue Cross Blue Shield of Illinois
Blue Cross Blue Shield of South Caroli 🗐
Capital District Physicians' Health Pla 🗐
Companion HealthCare South Carolin 🗐
Empire HealthChoice New York HMO
Empire HealthChoice New York PPO

(Back) Look Up: _____ ◈ ▼

FIGURE 9.13. The list of formulary options appears. These are selected by the user based on his or her practice's insurance plans. The selections are actually made on iScribe's Web site and downloaded onto the user's handheld during synchronization with the Web site. (Reprinted with permission from Caremark, Inc.)

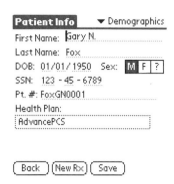

Patient Info   ▼ Demographics
First Name: Gary N.
Last Name: Fox
DOB: 01/01/1950 Sex: M F ?
SSN: 123 - 45 - 6789
Pt. #: FoxGN0001
Health Plan:
AdvancePCS

(Back) (New Rx) (Save)

FIGURE 9.14. For illustration, we have selected the "AdvancePCS" formulary. Once we have entered this information, we can tap "Save," which would save this entry and bring us back to the entry patient list. In this case, we are going to write a prescription for this patient, so we tap "New Rx" instead. (Reprinted with permission from Caremark, Inc.)

For illustration, we have selected the "AdvancePCS" formulary (Figure 9.14). Once we have entered this information, we can tap "Save," which would save this entry and bring us back to the entry patient list. In this case, we are going to write a prescription for this patient, so we tap "New Rx" instead to bring up the prescription list (Figure 9.15). The user has a choice in setting up the preferences to have a preselected "Quick List" ("QL") or "All" available products shown as the default. I have selected the "Quick List" as the default here.

To change to the full list, the user taps the drop-down list at "QL" (arrow in Figure 9.16). Tapping "All" brings up a more extensive list of drugs. However, switching to "All" is *not* necessary. As soon as the user enters the first letter of a drug "look up," the software automatically begins searching in the "All" list. "TC" is "therapeutic class," which allows searching by drug class. In iScribe, the "Quick List" is best reserved for drugs with customized instructions, such as your standard prednisone taper. Users must scroll to these drugs because beginning a "Look Up" automatically switches to the "All" list.

We have now switched to "All" (Figure 9.17). Note the abbreviations in front of the drug names; these are formulary status indicators (e.g., F = Formulary; NF = Not Formulary). Users can tap on the abbreviation to obtain an explanation of the code.

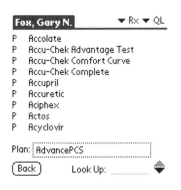

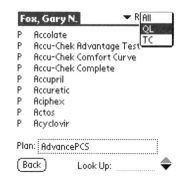

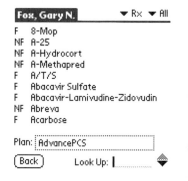

FIGURE 9.15. Tapping "New Rx" brings up the prescription list. The user can choose the preselected "Quick List" ("QL") or "All" available products as the default. I have selected the "Quick List" as the default here. To change to the full list, the user taps the drop-down list at "QL" (*arrow*). (Reprinted with permission from Caremark, Inc.)

FIGURE 9.16. Tapping "All" brings up a more extensive list of drugs. However, switching to "All" is *not* necessary. As soon as the user enters the first letter of a drug "Look Up," the software automatically begins searching in the "All" list. "TC" is "therapeutic class," which allows searching by drug class. In iScribe, the "Quick List" is best reserved for drugs with customized instructions, such as a standardized prednisone taper. Users must scroll to these drugs because beginning a "Look Up" automatically switches to the "All" list. (Reprinted with permission from Caremark, Inc.)

FIGURE 9.17. We have now switched to "All." Note the abbreviations in front of the drug names: these are formulary status indicators (e.g., F = Formulary; NF = Not Formulary). Users can tap on the abbreviation to obtain an explanation of the code. (Reprinted with permission from Caremark, Inc.)

Gary's blood pressure could use some more lisinopril. We begin entering the appropriate letters. Had we been in the "Quick List," using the "Look Up" feature would have taken us to the "All" (complete list), even if we had a customized prescription for lisinopril in the "Quick List" (Figure 9.18). For many drugs, the drug name will appear on the handheld's screen after entry of the first three or four letters. The software finds only two entries beginning with "lis" (Figure 9.19). Tapping the drug name then selects it.

Now that we have selected lisinopril (Figure 9.20), completing the prescription is much like producing a written one (Figure 9.21). The drop-down box by "Tablet" is grayed, indicating there is no selection here (no capsule, syrup, drops). However, we have choices of dosage, quantity, instructions, and refills. Additionally, we can select (tap) "DAW" (dispense as written) and "MO," which produces not only the prescription we see but also an additional one for a 3-month "*Mail Order*" supply. We've now chosen "30 mg" and honored the patient's request for a 1-month supply to fill

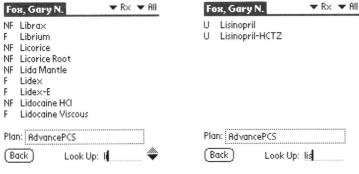

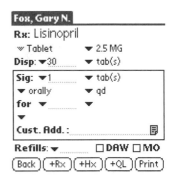

FIGURE 9.18. Gary's blood pressure could use some more lisinopril. We begin entering the appropriate letters. Had we been in the "Quick List," using the "Look Up" feature would have taken us to the "All" (complete list), even if we had a customized prescription for lisinopril in the "Quick List." (Reprinted with permission from Caremark, Inc.)

FIGURE 9.19. For many drugs, the drug name will appear on the handheld's screen after entry of the first three or four letters. The software finds only two entries beginning with "lis." Tapping the drug name then selects it. (Reprinted with permission from Caremark, Inc.)

FIGURE 9.20. We have now selected lisinopril. Completing the prescription is now much like producing a written one. The drop-down box by "Tablet" is grayed, indicating there is no selection here (no capsule, syrup, drops, etc.). However, we have choices of dosage, quantity, instructions, and refills. Additionally, we can select (tap) "DAW" (dispense as written) and "MO," which produces not only the prescription we see but an additional one for a 3-month "Mail Order" supply. (Reprinted with permission from Caremark, Inc.)

locally and a 3-month mail-order prescription (Figure 9.22). Our patient needs more prescriptions, so we'll next tap "+Rx" to add to the list. We'll "Print" after queuing all the prescriptions for the patient.

Our new patient also takes hydrochlorothiazide, so we enter letters of that drug name until the drug appears on our screen (Figure 9.23). Then we tap the drug name. Unlike lisinopril, hydrochlorothiazide comes in several formulations, so we have the option to choose the solution, capsule, or tablet (Figure 9.24). We've chosen tablets, and selected 25-mg tablets from among the choices of 25-; 50-; or 100-mg tabs (Figure 9.25). We're now going to change the quantity from 30 to 100 (Figure 9.26). We can also enter this manually from the Graffiti writing area or "keyboard" on the handheld; the figure illustrates choosing from the drop-down list.

Next, we choose how many pills to take for each dose from the drop-down list (Figure 9.27). This can also be entered manually if desired. We are going to choose $\frac{1}{2}$ per day (note 0.5 is another option), then tap the drop-down area that is circled to provide further instructions, a method for making the prescribing instructions more explicit (Figure 9.28), such

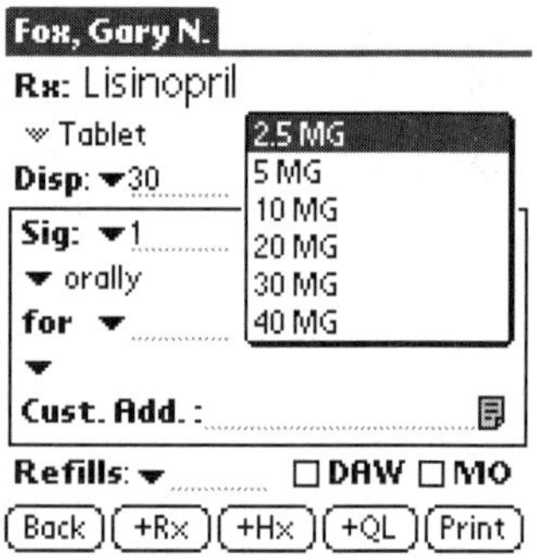

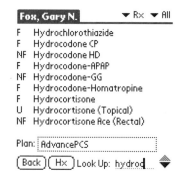

FIGURE 9.21. Example of a writter prescuption. (Reprinted with permission from Caremark, Inc.)

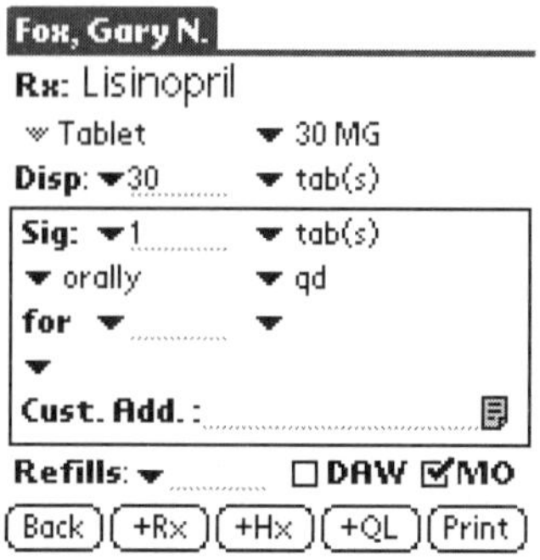

FIGURE 9.22. We've now chosen 30 mg (*1*) and honored the patient's request for a 1-month supply to fill locally and a 3-month mail-order prescription (*2*). Our patient needs more prescriptions, so we'll next tap "+Rx" (*3*) to add to the list. We'll "Print" after queuing all the prescriptions for the patient. (Reprinted with permission from Caremark, Inc.)

FIGURE 9.23. Our new patient also takes hydrochlorothiazide, so we enter letters of that drug name until the drug appears on our screen. Then we tap the drug name. (Reprinted with permission from Caremark, Inc.)

as giving the diuretic in the morning. The completed prescription is for hydrochlorothiazide, 25 mg, #100, ½ po qd in the AM (Figure 9.29). We have a 200-day supply here, so have not checked "refills." We could also choose a spelled-out "zero" for the printed prescription.

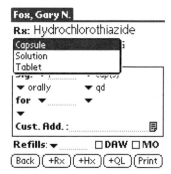

FIGURE 9.24. Unlike lisinopril, hydrochlorothiazide comes in several formulations, so we have the option to choose the solution, capsule, or tablet. (Reprinted with permission from Caremark, Inc.)

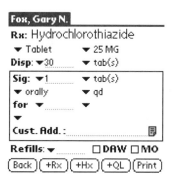

FIGURE 9.25. We've chosen tablets, and selected 25-mg tablets from among the choices of 25-, 50-, or 100-mg tabs. (Reprinted with permission from Caremark, Inc.)

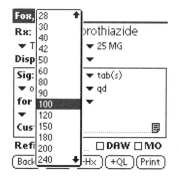

FIGURE 9.26. We're now going to change the quantity from 30 to 100. We can also enter this manually from the Graffiti writing area of the handheld; the figure illustrates choosing from the drop-down list. (Reprinted with permission from Caremark, Inc.)

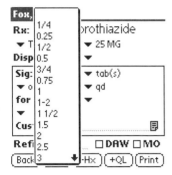

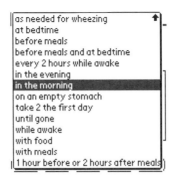

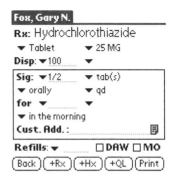

FIGURE 9.27. Next, we choose how many pills to take for each dose from the drop-down list. This can also be entered manually if desired. We are going to choose ½ per day (note 0.5 is another option), then tap the drop-down area that is circled to provide further instructions. (Reprinted with permission from Caremark, Inc.)

FIGURE 9.28. Additional options for making the prescribing instructions more explicit. We want to give the diuretic in the morning. (Reprinted with permission from Caremark, Inc.)

FIGURE 9.29. The completed prescription for hydrochlorothiazide, 25 mg, #100, ½ po qd in the A.M. We have a 200-day supply here, so have not checked "refills." We could also choose a spelled-out "zero" for the printed prescription. To produce another prescription, we would again tap "+Rx." (Reprinted with permission from Caremark, Inc.)

To produce another prescription, we would again tap "+Rx." To add atenolol, we type successive letters (Figure 9.30). Formulary status "NP" means "Non-Preferred," which can be discerned by tapping on the abbreviation; "P" means "Preferred" formulary status. We have now completed an atenolol prescription and tapped on the drop-down arrow selector by "Refills" (Figure 9.31). We have choices from "zero" to 1 year. We can also put a number in manually. After making our refill selection, we bring our handheld to the printer, align the infrared ports, and then tap "Print." Printing takes a few seconds. During that time, I'm usually coding the encounter form, gathering patient education materials, completing lab slips, or, if none of that is still pending, doing documentation.

Once we have completed Gary's visit, we can look at his prescription history (Figure 9.32). We see that he had four prescriptions issued (the two for lisinopril reflect the 1-month supply plus the 3-month mail order one). Details of each prescription can be viewed by clicking on the corresponding page icon (circled). To renew the prescription for lisinopril next year, all we have to do is tap on the former prescription, and up it pops, ready to print (or to add another rx via "+Rx") (Figure 9.33).

Let's say Gary has lost his mail-order insurance and only wants monthly prescriptions. We can "delete" the 3-month prescription. We check it (via a tap in the box), and then tap "Delete" (Figure 9.34). The software asks for confirmation of the deletion (Figure 9.35).

Gary also now reports a cough that started very shortly after the lisinopril. We have an option to "Deactivate" the prescription. We again check it,

Fox, Gary N. ▼ Rx ▼ All

```
NP  Atacand
NP  Atacand HCT
F   Atamet
F   Atarax
P   Atenolol
F   Atenolol-Chlorthalidone
F   Ativan
P   Atorvastatin Calcium
NF  Atovaquone
```

Plan: `AdvancePCS`

(Back) (Hx) Look Up: at| ◆

FIGURE 9.30. To add atenolol, we type successive letters. Formulary status "NP" means "Non-Preferred," which can be discerned by tapping on the abbreviation; "P" means "Preferred" formulary status. (Reprinted with permission from Caremark, Inc.)

Fox, Gary N.

Rx: Atenolol

~ Tablet   ▼ 100 MG
Disp: ▼ 100   ▼ tab(s)
Sig: ▼ | tab(s)
  ▼ oral| zero | qd
  for ▼ 1
       ▼ 2
         3
Cust. | 4
       5
Refills PRN   □ DAW □ MO
(Back)(×1yr   ) (+QL)(Print)

FIGURE 9.31. We have now completed an atenolol prescription and tapped on the drop-down arrow selector by "Refills." We have choices from "zero" to 1 year. We can also put a number in manually. After making our refill selection, we bring our handheld to the printer, align the infrared ports, and then tap "Print." Printing takes a few seconds. During that time, I'm usually coding the encounter form, gathering patient education materials, completing lab slips, or, if none of that is still pending, doing documentation. (Reprinted with permission from Caremark, Inc.)

Fox, Gary N. ▼ Rx History

```
□ Atenolol            7/25/02  ▤
□ Hydrochlorothiazide 7/25/02  ▤
□ Lisinopril          7/25/02  ▤
□ Lisinopril          7/25/02  ▤
```

□ Check All   (Deactivate)
(Back)(New Rx)(Delete)

FIGURE 9.32. Once we have completed Gary's visit, we can look at his prescription history. We see that he had four prescriptions issued (the two for lisinopril reflect the 1-month supply plus the mail-order one). Details of each prescription can be viewed by clicking on the corresponding page icon (*circled*). (Reprinted with permission from Caremark, Inc.)

Fox, Gary N.

Rx: Lisinopril

~ Tablet   ▼ 30 MG
Disp: ▼ 3   ▼ months supply
Sig: ▼ 1   ▼ tab(s)
  ▼ orally   ▼ qd
  for ▼   ▼
  ▼
Cust. Add. :   ▤
Refills: ▼ 3   □ DAW □ MO
(Back)(+Rx)(+Hx)(+QL)(Print)

FIGURE 9.33. To renew the prescription for lisinopril next year, all we have to do is tap on the former prescription, and up it pops, ready to print (or to add another rx via "+Rx"). (Reprinted with permission from Caremark, Inc.)

Fox, Gary N. ▼ Rx History

```
□ Atenolol            7/25/02  ▤
□ Hydrochlorothiazide 7/25/02  ▤
☑ Lisinopril          7/25/02  ▤
□ Lisinopril          7/25/02  ▤
```

☑ UnCheck All   (Deactivate)
(Back)(New Rx)(Delete)

FIGURE 9.34. Let's say Gary has lost his mail-order insurance and only wants monthly prescriptions. We can "delete" the 3-month prescription. We check it (via a tap in the box), then tap "Delete." (Reprinted with permission from Caremark, Inc.)

Fox, Gary N. ▼ Rx History

```
□ Atenolol            7/25/02  ▤
□ Hydrochlorothiazide 7/25/02  ▤
☑ Lisinopril          7/25/02  ▤
□ Lisinopril          7/25/02  ▤
```

Delete Prescription(s)

(?) **Are you sure you want to delete the selected prescription(s)?**

(Yes) (No)

FIGURE 9.35. The software asks for confirmation of the deletion. (Reprinted with permission from Caremark, Inc.)

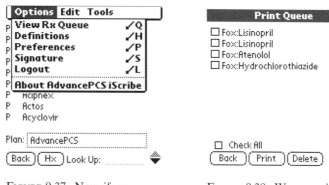

FIGURE 9.36. Gary also now reports a cough that started very shortly after the lisinopril. We have an option to "Deactivate" the prescription. We again check it, then tap "Deactivate." Subsequently it appears grayed on the screen. Unfortunately, there is no facility to attach an annotation about Gary's ACE-induced cough. (Reprinted with permission from Caremark, Inc.)

FIGURE 9.37. Now, if we hadn't printed Gary's prescriptions, they'd still be waiting in the "Rx Queue." We can view the Queue from the Options menu. (Reprinted with permission from Caremark, Inc.)

FIGURE 9.38. We can print the waiting prescriptions or select individual ones for deletion. If the lisinopril prescriptions were duplicate entries, or perhaps one was an erroneous dosage, we can determine which is which by tapping on the page icon to see the details of each prescription. Any can be deleted from the queue. We'll tap the page icon by hydrochlorothiazide for illustration. (Reprinted with permission from Caremark, Inc.)

and then tap "Deactivate" (Figure 9.36). Subsequently it appears grayed on the screen. Unfortunately, there is no facility to attach an annotation about Gary's ACE-induced cough. Now, if we hadn't printed Gary's prescriptions, they'd still be waiting in the "Rx Queue" (Figure 9.37).

We can view the Queue from the Options menu. We can print the waiting prescriptions or select individual ones for deletion (Figure 9.38). If the lisinopril prescriptions were duplicate entries, or perhaps one was an erroneous dosage, we can determine which is which by tapping on the page icon to see the details of each prescription. Any can be deleted from the queue. We'll tap the page icon by hydrochlorothiazide for illustration (Figure 9.39). Here's our HCTZ prescription, exactly as written, 200-day supply, take $\frac{1}{2}$ tablet in the morning, with no refills.

HANDS-ON EXERCISE 9.2. SETTING USER-MODIFIABLE PREFERENCES IN ISCRIBE

Completely switching gears, here are the user-definable preferences (Figure 9.40). If the prescription paper and handheld printing format do not exactly match, "fine tuning" can be done with X and Y offsets. When the iScribe

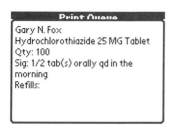

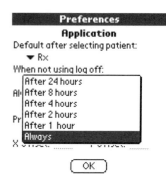

FIGURE 9.39. Here's our HCTZ prescription, exactly as written, 200-day supply, take ½ tablet in the morning, with no refills. (Reprinted with permission from Caremark, Inc.)

FIGURE 9.40. Completely switching gears, here are the user-definable preferences. If the prescription paper and handheld printing format do not exactly match, "fine tuning" can be done with X and Y offsets. (Reprinted with permission from Caremark, Inc.)

FIGURE 9.41. When the iScribe software has not been accessed for a specific length of time, the application automatically logs off. I have mine set to log out after 2 hours of inactivity. (Reprinted with permission from Caremark, Inc.)

software has not been accessed for a specific length of time, the application automatically logs off (Figure 9.41). I have mine set to log off after 2 hours of inactivity. I prefer to have my DEA print only on prescriptions for controlled substances (Figure 9.42). Other options include printing the DEA on all prescriptions or no prescriptions. Users can also enter their signatures, which will then be digitized and print on the prescriptions (Figure 9.43). I have chosen to sign manually because it gives me another second to verify that I have produced the exact prescription I wish, and I feel this step adds another layer of security.

HANDS-ON EXERCISE 9.3. FORMULARY FEATURES OF ISCRIBE

Formulary definitions and abbreviations in iScribe are shown in Figure 9.44. I will explain how to use formulary designators and choice of formulary alternatives in iScribe with the following scenario (Figure 9.45). Gloria comes in with a cough and I wish to use Humibid-DM. However, Gloria's insurance does not cover it ("NF"). When I click on the "NF," the software tells me what NF stands for, but also presents a list of suggested formulary alternatives. A scrollable list of formulary alternatives is presented but, interestingly, none of them is a guaifenesin-dextromethorphan combination (Figure 9.46). When dextromethorphan-guaifenesin is specifically sought, it appears that its formulary status is "U," Unknown (Figure 9.47). Therefore, it was not retrieved among the suggested formulary options. This example illustrates that although the system is powerful when used to its full advantage, there are still gaps.

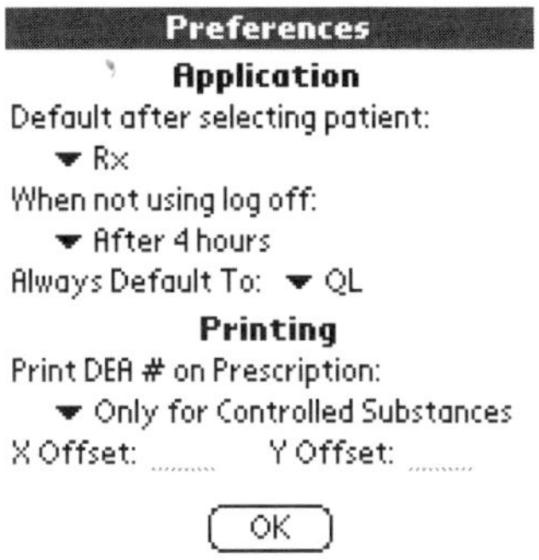

Preferences

Application

Default after selecting patient:
▼ Rx
When not using log off:
▼ After 4 hours
Always Default To: ▼ QL

Printing

Print DEA # on Prescription:
▼ Only for Controlled Substances
X Offset: .... Y Offset: ....

(OK)

FIGURE 9.42. I prefer to have my DEA print only on prescriptions for controlled substances. Other options include printing it on all prescriptions or no prescriptions. (Reprinted with permission from Caremark, Inc.)

Signature

Please Sign in the Box Below

(Back) (Clear) (Save)

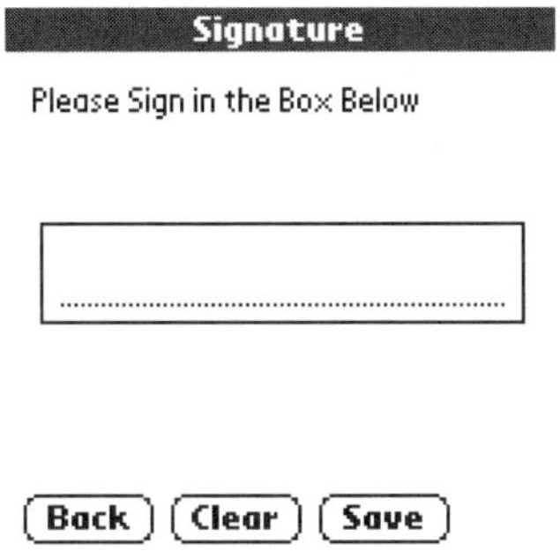

FIGURE 9.43. Users can also enter their signatures, which will then print on the prescriptions. I have chosen to sign manually because it gives me another second to verify that I have produced the exact prescription I wish, and I feel this step adds another layer of security. (Reprinted with permission from Caremark, Inc.)

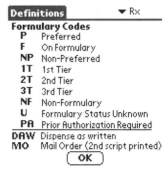

Definitions   ▼ Rx

Formulary Codes
P   Preferred
F   On Formulary
NP   Non-Preferred
1T   1st Tier
2T   2nd Tier
3T   3rd Tier
NF   Non-Formulary
U   Formulary Status Unknown
PA   Prior Authorization Required
DAW   Dispense as written
MO   Mail Order (2nd script printed)

(OK)

FIGURE 9.44. Formulary definitions and abbreviations in iScribe. (Reprinted with permission from Caremark, Inc.)

REED, GLORIA   ▼ Rx ▼ All

F   Humibid LA
NF   Humibid Pediatric
NF   Humibid-DM
U   Humidifiers

Plan: AdvancePCS
(Back) (Hx) Look Up: humi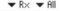

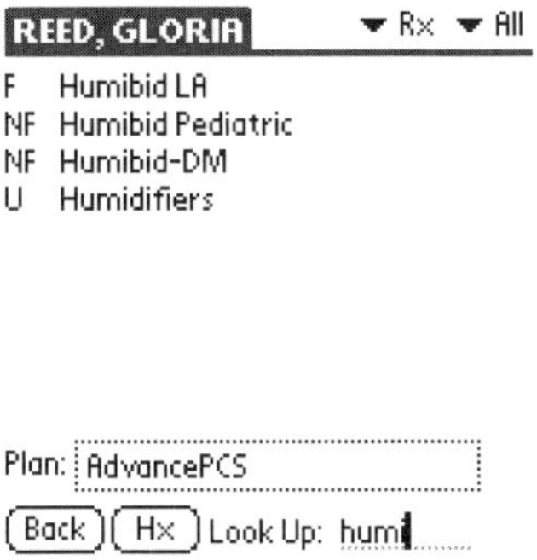

FIGURE 9.45. Use of formulary designators and choice of formulary alternatives. Gloria comes in with a cough and I wish to use Humibid-DM. However, Gloria's insurance does not cover it ("NF"). When I click on the "NF," the software tells me what NF stands for, but also presents a list of suggested formulary alternatives. (Reprinted with permission from Caremark, Inc.)

Formulary Alternatives

Humibid-DM is Non Formulary.
Select an alternative:

F   Codeine-GG
F   Diabetic Tussin C
F   Entex PSE
F   Guaifen PSE

or to continue:
▼ <select reason code>

(Back)

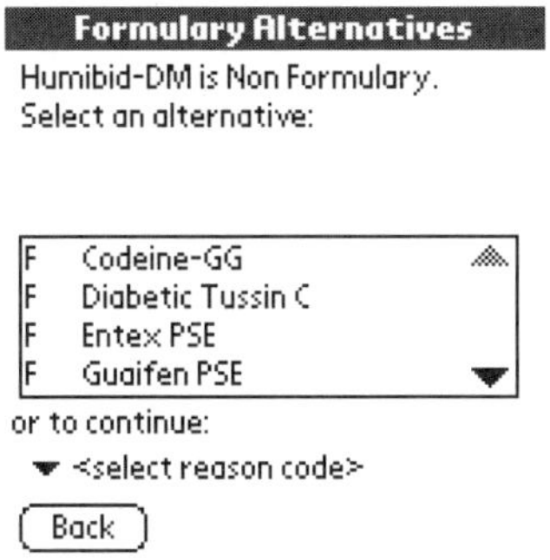

FIGURE 9.46. A scrollable list of formulary alternatives is presented but, interestingly, none of them is a guaifenesin-dextromethorphan combination. (Reprinted with permission from Caremark, Inc.)

REED, GLORIA   ▼ Rx ▼ All

F   Dextroamphetamine Sulfate
F   Dextroamphetamine Sulfate CR
U   Dextromethorphan-GG
F   DextroStat

Plan: AdvancePCS
(Back) (Hx) Look Up: dextr

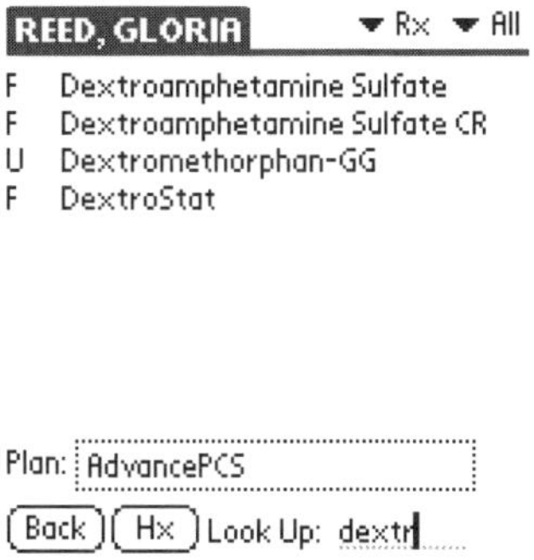

FIGURE 9.47. When dextromethorphan-guaifenesin is specifically sought, it appears that its formulary status is Unknown ("U"). Therefore, it was not retrieved among the suggested formulary options. This example illustrates that although the system is powerful when used to its full advantage, there are still gaps. (Reprinted with permission from Caremark, Inc.)

Select Patient	
ABBOTT, Justin	85
ABERG, Larry	81
ADCOCK, BETTY	43
AFGHANI, MAGDA	46
AGUILAR, CAROLYN	32
ALBADA, MARK	102
ALCADE, JUDITH	39
ALDRIDGE, PAUL	25
ALLEN, BADRI	47
ALLEN, HAROLD	26
ALLEN, MARY	39

Look Up: .... (New)(Skip) ▲▼

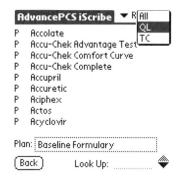

Plan: Baseline Formulary

(Back)   Look Up: .... ▲▼

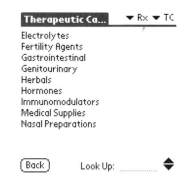

(Back)   Look Up: .... ◆

FIGURE 9.48. Let's say a newly diagnosed diabetic comes in and the two of you want to check the formulary status of glucose meters, but do not wish to enter the patient's name now. Tap "Skip" from the main patient menu. (Reprinted with permission from Caremark, Inc.)

FIGURE 9.49. From the "List" choices (All, Quick, Therapeutic Categories), choose Therapeutic Categories (TC). (Reprinted with permission from Caremark, Inc.)

FIGURE 9.50. In Therapeutic Categories, "Look Up" or scroll down to "Medical Supplies." (Reprinted with permission from Caremark, Inc.)

Let's say a newly diagnosed diabetic comes in and the two of you want to check the formulary status of glucose meters, but do not wish to enter the patient's name now. Tap "Skip" from the main patient menu (Figure 9.48). From the "List" choices (All, Quick, Therapeutic Categories), choose Therapeutic Categories (TC) (Figure 9.49). In Therapeutic Categories, "Look Up" or scroll down to "Medical Supplies" (Figure 9.50). Under "Medical Supplies," one choice is "Diabetic Supplies" (Figure 9.51). These next two screen pages on the software show the Accu-Chek and One Touch systems are Preferred (P) formulary options for the selected insurance plan (Figures 9.52, 9.53). Note that the physician can print these items or any other prescription *without* the patient name having been entered by simply "skipping" the name. The name can then be handwritten on the prescription after it is printed, just as would be on any traditional paper prescription (but will not be saved in the system). In other words, we can choose a product, such as the One Touch Ultra System Kit, and print directly from this screen.

Summary

The most overwhelming reason for considering e-prescribing is error reduction, which, if it already isn't a huge issue, is destined only to become more so. At absolute minimum, e-prescribing solves the problem of legibility and dosage selection (e.g., not writing for 10 mg when the smallest size is 20 mg). And let's get real—nobody can keep up with all the incompatibilities from all those P-450 interactions and from prolonged cutie (QT) intervals.

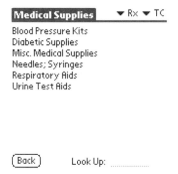

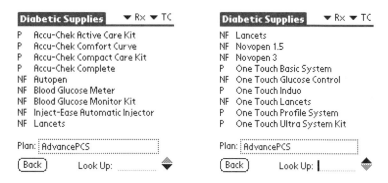

FIGURE 9.51. Under "Medical Supplies," one choice is "Diabetic Supplies." (Reprinted with permission from Caremark, Inc.)

FIGURES 9.52 and 9.53. These two screen pages on the software show the Accu-Che and One Touch systems are Preferred (P) formulary options for the selected insurance plan. Note that the physician can print these items or any other prescription *without* the patient name having been entered by simply "skipping" the name. The name can then be handwritten on the prescription after it is printed, just as it would be on any traditional paper prescription. In other words, we can choose a product, for example, the One Touch Ultra System Kit, and print directly from this screen. (Reprinted with permission from Caremark, Inc.)

Another good reason is patient "wow." As one smart airline executive once noted, the airline's passengers judge the quality of the airline's maintenance based on the cleanliness of the flip-down trays. Likewise, prescribing is one very visible aspect of one's medical practice. Hammie, Hallie, Hattie, and Hackie may have no idea whether you gave them the correct medication, dosage, duration, and instructions, but they can judge the "quality" of what you've flipped 'em—and of the pharmacist's reaction to it. And, e-prescribing is fun.

e-Prescribing can be fairly simple and inexpensive—a handheld, an infrared printer, and a software subscription. Or, systems can be more complex, including wireless office networks and internet or cell phone-type "magic" connections to pharmacy fax machines and messaging systems (Figure 9.54). Regardless of the chosen system and infrastructure, producing e-prescriptions via handheld devices certainly requires no more time than old-fangled, illegible p-p-prescribing (paper-pen). Almost any basic prescription consisting of a drug, dosage, quantity, "usual" sig, and refill instructions can be produced in a couple of seconds with a few rapid taps of the stylus selecting from scrolling and drop-down lists. And, prescribers can be confident of the drug's formulary status at the time of prescribing. By the time prescription renewals are needed (which means demographics and the initial scripts have to be in the system)—certainly when refilling Hallie's walk-in drug cabinet—these e-systems save time up front and later by reducing pharmacy callbacks.

What are you waiting for? . . . YOU CAN DO THIS!!

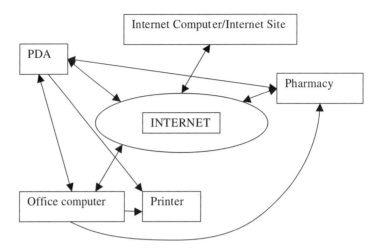

FIGURE 9.54 Possible mechanisms of "producing" prescriptions. Most of the connections diagrammed can be wireless. Examples include wireless transmission from the PDA to the printer or from the PDA directly to the pharmacy. The PDA may connect wireless to the office computer, which might transmit the prescriptions via wired connections either to the pharmacy directly or through the Internet to the pharmacy. Alternatively, the PDA may connect to an office computer, which in turn may connect to the Internet, which connects to the vendor's Internet site, which in turn connects via Internet to the pharmacy. Prescriptions need not originate from the PDA. They may originate from the office computer or from a secure logon the vendor's Internet site (for renewals, for example). Note that virtually everything can be connected through the Internet bidirectionally. That way, formulary information, drug list updates, synchronization of patient information (from backup of multiple physician users in one office), and so on, can be accomplished *from* a vendor's site, in addition to routing prescriptions *to/through* the site.

Key Points

- Handheld prescribing solutions are available for practices ranging from a single physician to an ARMY (aggregation of real multispecialty yahoos).
- Some require more infrastructure and expense (wireless network) and others less (one handheld, one printer).
- If you've figured out how to use a pocket calculator and how to graduate from medical school, you can do this!

Reference

1. Kohn LT, Corrigan JM, Donaldson MS, eds. To Err is Human: Building a Safer Health System. Committee on Quality of Healthcare in America. Institute of Medicine, National Academy Press, Washington, D.C., 2000.

10

Medical Documents in Your Pocket

PETER L. REYNOLDS

As health professionals, we would quickly lose our way without the medical texts we reference daily. There's just too much critical information these days for one person to memorize. What's more, the things we do know change at a breakneck pace. Fortunately, the day of the electronic medical book has truly arrived with handheld computing. Many medical textbooks, journals, and other media are now available in an electronic form that is portable on handheld computers. All types of references have been adapted to handheld formats, with new ones popping up weekly. And most interesting, more and more Internet content is accessible using a handheld, either in real time or in novel ways we'll discuss in this chapter.

In 1994, Slawson, Shaughnessy, and Bennett published a paper in the *Journal of Family Practice* that sparked the evidence-based medicine revolution.[1] Their landmark work defined the usefulness of any piece of medical information to the practicing medical professional. USEFULNESS, they said, equals the product of VALIDITY and RELEVANCE divided by the TIME it takes, from the point of care, to obtain the information. Validity and relevance are complicated topics and require more explanation elsewhere. On the other hand, everyone understands the time component, and handheld computers offer unmatched time efficiency when it comes to bringing excellent quality medical evidence to the bedside. Less time translates into greater usefulness. Your bookshelf in the palm of your hand . . . it's no longer too good to be true!

What's a Document Reader?

For our purposes, we'll consider a document reader to be any program whose primary aim is to present information rather than create, modify or transform it. In their simplest form, these programs allow you to move existing digital media from a desktop computer to your pocket device. Early document readers focused on text only, because first-generation handhelds lacked sufficient memory or screen resolution for graphic intensive applications. The latest handhelds, with color screens and expandable memory, promise desktop-like multimedia capabilities, and document reader software has advanced accordingly. Just about any desktop computer format can be reproduced on a handheld device, including some digital movies.

Beware . . . despite oodles of hype, more graphics doesn't always mean better quality. Many of the medical documents you'd like on your handheld just don't need graphics. Patient data, coding information, facts and formulas, and pharmacopoeia are well represented with text-only documents. Other documents are just too big to be well represented on a handheld screen. For example, I have yet to see a clinically useful facsimile of a radiograph or a 12-lead ECG displayed on a handheld device (although I'm sure that it's only a matter of time).

More advanced document readers seek to present information, both text and graphical, in special formats designed from the ground up for handheld devices. Although the mechanics are usually transparent to the user, the results can be impressive. Take AvantGo, a Web page viewing program that we discuss in detail here, and compare how a standard Web page looks compared to one customized for handhelds. You'll undoubtedly prefer the customized version.

Other types of programs besides document readers suit themselves to document management. For example, a list of medical facts and formulae might be better represented using a database program than one of the document readers discussed in this chapter. Also, outliner software, such as Bonsai Outliner ($24.95 at www.natara.com), works well for organizing information into categories. You just have to jump in, give this and that a try, and you'll quickly figure out what you like best.

Eliminating 2-by-2 Scraps of Paper: Using Palm OS MemoPad or Pocket PC PocketWord

If you do anything relating to medical documents on your handheld, please, please, PLEASE do something with those little notes you've been jotting down all these years. Many of us entrust the most amazing pearls of wisdom to 2-by-2 scraps of paper with sticky on the back. The perfect steroid taper, the favorite insulin-drip protocol, a tried-and-true lab workup for anemia, your top-secret country remedy for smelly feet: they're all priceless. Sometimes, you find them when needed. Sometimes, they're lost forever.

Consider a digital transfer! It's as easy as using any desktop word processor. Pocket PC devices can read Microsoft Word documents right out of the box. With Palm OS, you can just as easily cut and paste from any word processor program into Palm Memopad entries using the Palm Desktop software. If you prefer, you can enter these notes into Palm OS Memos or Pocket PC Word documents right on the handheld. It's not quite as fast,

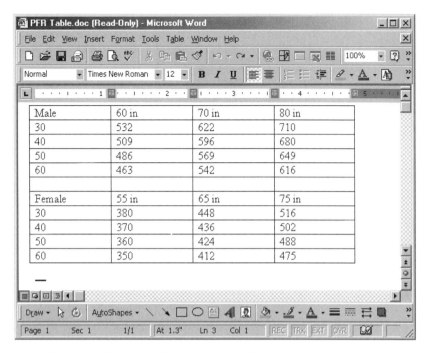

FIGURE 10.1. Peak flow rate table on Microsoft Word.

but it's just as easy. Once on your handheld, you can categorize entries by subject and search through entries using the Find feature on your handheld. If you want to share a pearl, your entries can be beamed to other handheld users. You'll stun your colleagues with your tech savvy (and generosity).

In Chapter 2, you saw several examples of medical-related, Palm OS Memopad entries. One, a peak flow rate table, was cut from the Microsoft Word table in Figure 10.1 and then pasted to a new Palm Memopad entry created on the Palm Desktop software. After a bit of formatting on the desktop—a few tabs here and a few tabs there—synchronization brought the table to the handheld as shown in Figure 10.2. Memopad entries look exactly the same on the Palm Desktop as they do on the handheld.

Transfer of Word documents to Pocket PC devices is even easier. Just drag and drop the Word document to your Pocket PC "synchronization folder" on your Windows Desktop. Once you synchronize your device, you'll see the peak flow rate table (Figure 10.3). No cutting and pasting or additional formatting is required other than a few tab strokes to make the columns line up.

The point is you can and should take advantage of the document reader capability that comes installed on your handheld. Palm Memopad entries are limited to 4 KB or approximately 800 words. (The Palm Desktop soft-

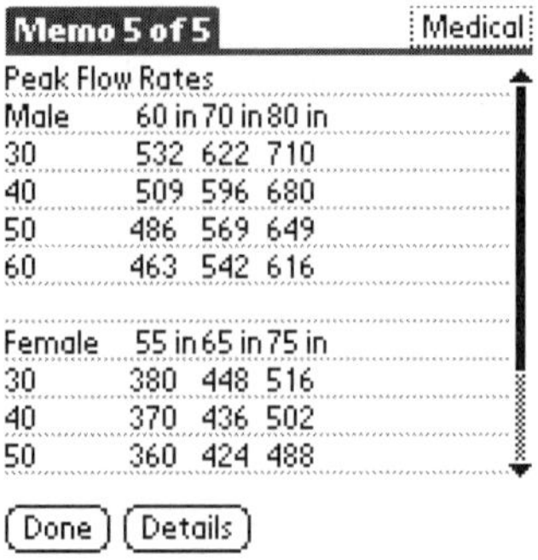

FIGURE 10.2. Peak flow rate table with Palm OS.

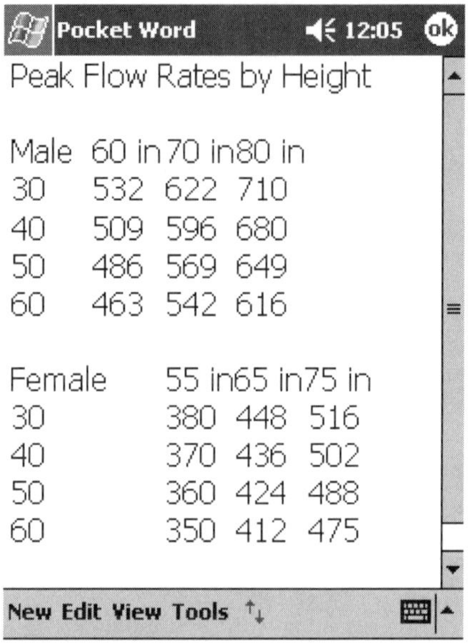

FIGURE 10.3. Peak flow rate table with Pocket PC.

ware automatically segments larger files into sequential Memopad entries.) Apart from that limitation (which isn't present in Pocket Word), you can move just about any text document to Palm Memos or Pocket PC Word documents. It's fast and efficient and requires no additional software.

As a final note, some folks find they'd like to organize Palm OS Memopad entries further into subfolders. Although you can't do this with the included software, several third-party solutions work well, such as QuickMemo from QuickTap Software ($14.95 at www.quicktap.com).

Third-Party Document Readers

So what about third-party document readers you can purchase for your handheld? They cost extra money and take up space, but are they worth it? Every new program you purchase takes time to learn and master. It's also something else that can break or crash, and yet another program to update. As a busy professional, you should think hard before investing time and resources in new software. In this case, the document reader included with your handheld might just meet your needs. If so, then great! You're set and don't need more software.

On the other hand, several benefits of add-on document readers stand out. Popular programs used as document readers are summarized in

Table 10.1. Some readers offer greater data compression and, therefore, smaller file sizes. Most include some kind of bookmark function, which allows you to mark commonly referenced sections of a document for easy retrieval later. Both the Palm Memopad and Pocket PC reader include a search function, but it's not as fast as bookmarking.

To preserve the original formatting of a document, third-party document readers can be a necessity. That is to say, you can copy and paste text from a Microsoft Word or Adobe PDF document to a Palm Memopad document (using the Palm Desktop software), but it won't look the same. Rather, you need Documents-to-Go or Quick-Word to view Word documents and Adobe Acrobat to view PDF files. Programs like these preserve the original structure of documents, even on the handheld device. A word of warning, however; a 2-inch-square screen is a 2-inch-square screen is a 2-inch-square screen. I remember my first trial of Adobe Acrobat on my old Palm III—I was disappointed! The document was there on the screen, but to my eye, it was fuzzy and hard to read. The new Adobe Acrobat has improved, however, especially when viewed on the latest high-resolution color screens.

TABLE 10.1. Document management software.

Document reader	Web site	Supported formats	Approximate cost[a]	Platform
Aportis Doc	www.aportis.com	DOC	$30 (+ $20 converter)	Palm/PPC
Teal Doc	www.tealpoint.com	DOC	$17	Palm
Documents To Go (DataViz)	www.dataviz.com	DOC MS Word MS Excel	$50–$70	Palm[b]
Quick Word	www.cesinc.com	MS Word	$20–$40	Palm[b]
iSilo	www.isilo.com	DOC iSilo	$17.50	Palm/PPC
LIT "Reader" files	www.microsoft.com/reader/ default.asp	[c]	Free	PPC
Adobe Acrobat	www.adobe.com/products/ acrobat/readerforpalm.html	PDF	Free (+ $249 converter)	Palm
FireViewer by Firepad	www.firepad.com	[d]	$30	Palm
Bdicty	www.beiks.com	[c]	Free–$10	Palm
InfoDB	www.handtop.com	[c]	$50	Palm
HanDBase	www.ddhsoftware.com	[c]	$30	Palm/PPC
J File	www.land-j.com	[c]	$25	Palm
MobileDB	www.handmark.com	[c]	$20–$30	Palm/PPC
TomeRaider	www.tomeraider.com	[c]	$20–$25	Palm/PPC

[a] Prices quoted from product Web sites or www.palmgear.com November 2002.
[b] Pocket Word and Pocket Excel included with all Pocket PC (PPC) handhelds.
[c] Proprietary only.
[d] JPEG, GIF, TIFF, BMP, RLE, PNG, AVI, MOV, and HTML.

In point of fact, convenience is the most common reason medical users buy third-party document readers. Many available documents are formatted for specific document readers and are not readable using software included on your handheld. Consider the example of a Palm-toting, Brazilian physician looking for the International Code of Diseases in Portuguese. He hops on the Internet and goes to www.memoware.com, a popular online PDA library. Sure enough, they have the ICD-10 International Code of Diseases in Portuguese (no joke, they do!). Unfortunately, it's only in the J File format, and he doesn't have J File on his handheld. What does he do? Option #1: install Palm OS Emulator on his desktop (hard!), install a trial version of J File on the Emulator and run Portuguese International Code of Diseases, cut and paste each field from the Emulator to a Palm Memopad entry on his Palm Desktop software, synchronize his handheld, and presto, he's done. Option #2: buy J File for $25. (Option 1 is crazy and probably illegal in all 50 states. I don't recommend it!)

Web sites such as www.memoware.com include thousands of documents of all kinds and hundreds of medical-specific ones. These documents include full textbooks, medical dictionaries, various "peripheral brains," lists of diagnostic and billing codes, drug databases, and everything else but the kitchen sink. If you find just the document you're looking for, take the step and purchase the document reader that goes with it. Although you pay for the reader, the documents themselves are usually free. Still, try to keep document reader creep to a minimum.

Clearly some document readers are more popular than others. Authors and other contributors (plagiarists, pilferers, thieves, etc.) tend to go with tried-and-true document formats. Most recently, Memoware offered close to 400 medical document titles with all formats combined. Of these, the formats of the 50 most popular titles are summarized in Table 10.2. (Note

TABLE 10.2. Popular document viewers in medicine.	
Document format[a]	Popularity (% of total)
iSilo/iSilo 3	40%
Doc	18%
HanDBase	12%
Mobile DB	8%
Fire Viewer	
LIST	4%
Tome Raider	
BDCity	
LIT	
Teal Info	2%
Teal Paint	
Smart List	

[a]Note: Some documents are available in more than one format.

that differences between iSilo and iSilo3 are fully outlined at the end of this chapter.)

This breakdown shows that iSilo and Doc documents win the popularity contest. That's a good start but doesn't tell the whole story. The iSilo reader and Doc readers (including Aportis and Teal Doc) meet a broad general-purpose need with a broad range of applications. Other programs, such as BDCity and other database-like programs, excel at a narrower range of documents including medical dictionaries. Happily, all these programs offer some kind of trial period. You won't lose money if you don't like a program, just time and energy.

Graphics representation is a final document reader niche worthy of comment. As listed in Table 10.2, 2 of the top 50 medical documents (4%) found at www.memoware.com were in the Fire Viewer format. The actual titles were "Visible Human Cadaver Dissection Movie" and "Graphical Medical Formula Images." With handheld screen quality improving, chip speeds up, and memory size increasing (the cadaver dissection movie is a 1365-KB file!), the potential for useful graphical documents at the point of care grows brighter. Imagine showing patients pictures right on your handheld, instead of running to the office for a book.

Fire Viewer also includes a desktop program that converts most graphical formats for viewing on Palm OS handhelds (JPEGs, GIFs, TIFFs, BMPs, RLEs, PNGs, AVIs, MOVs, and HTML). You don't have to wait for more postings on the Internet—you can scan in your own photos and carry them in your handheld.

Check out Chapter 4 for more medical Internet sites where you can download documents.

Online Documents

The World Wide Web serves up an overwhelming number of documents via a surprisingly intuitive interface, the Internet browser. Search engines like Google make the over 3 billion available Web pages easily accessible. And, hyperlinks allow quick navigation between related items.

When it comes to medical information, the "more is better" rule usually holds true. With more resources available, the likelihood of finding an answer to your question goes up. Placing lots of medical documents on the Internet works great. There's room for volumes of literature, and online, the info seems more manageable. Publishers can update online media at lesser expense than printed media, so they tend to update more often.

Someday all the documents we access electronically will probably reside at central locations. These electronic libraries will be huge, we'll browse through them wirelessly, maybe with handhelds, and the world will be wonderful. We talk about current wireless capabilities later in Chapter 15. Suffice it to say that, for now, wireless technology has some way to go. Two significant limitations to widespread access remain. Cost is a big one. Compared to dial-up access, the cost of wireless service and equipment runs two to four times more expensive. At the same time, the bandwidth, or speed of data transfer, is almost always slower. The importance of bandwidth depends on what kind of data you're downloading. Text documents don't require too much bandwidth. However, even small black-and-white photos, like those you find in medical textbooks, demand much more.

Despite these limitations, lots of handheld users try wireless Internet browsers and like them. If you're a rabbit, then go for it! Buy the latest wireless-ready handheld, sign up for wireless service, and knock yourself out. If you're more of a turtle and like to take things at a slower pace, a very attractive option exists. In a word, it's caching.

Caching means temporarily copying Web pages into computer memory for access later (from memory and not from the Internet). Once cached, Web pages are no longer dynamic. They're like any other file on your computer and, sadly, are no longer updated. On the upside, you can still navigate between cached Web pages using hyperlinks.

If you pick the right software on your handheld, you can schedule caching at regular intervals. If a Web site of interest changes significantly every day, set your handheld to update the cache with every synchronization. If changes are rare, as for an online textbook, update only as needed.

In terms of both popularity and usefulness, the top two Web caching programs are AvantGo and iSilo, and fortunately both run on Palm OS and Pocket PC handhelds. We've already introduced iSilo as a popular document reader. Believe it or not, its usefulness for Web page caching is even more impressive. These programs are brilliantly conceived—you can't help but tip your hat to the developers—and work well on both platforms. They're powerful tools. We'll discuss both in detail and show you how to use them.

Medical Applications with AvantGo

AvantGo is easy to use. Just connect your desktop computer to the Internet, synchronize your handheld, and voila—it downloads small, pocket-sized versions of preselected Web sites right to your device. If you surf to www.avantgo.com and follow the online directions, you can probably subscribe (it's still free!), load it on your handheld, and browse a few "Auto Channels" without breaking a sweat. To make life really, really easy, we'll go through the steps here to get you started.

HANDS-ON EXERCISE 10.1. PUTTING CONTENT ON YOUR HANDHELD USING AVANTGO

First, go to www.avantgo.com and follow the links for "My AvantGo Consumer Service." AvantGo also offers "Enterprise Solutions" that companies

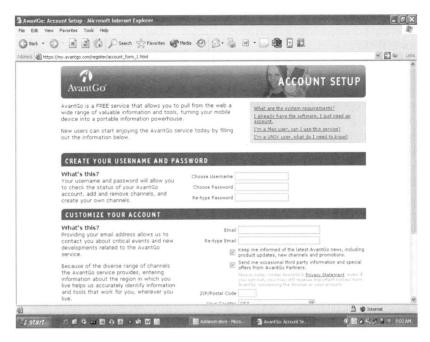

FIGURE 10.4. AvantGo Online Account Setup. (Reprinted with permission from AvantGo.)

can use to disseminate information to employees. If you've never been to AvantGo before, you should be prompted to create a new account. It's free. If you don't receive that prompt, try typing this link into your browser: "https://my.avantgo.com/register/." Figure 10.4 shows the account setup screen.

After completing a questionnaire about your interests and demographic information, you'll get to the good part—downloading and installing AvantGo on your handheld. You can't proceed without completing the questionnaire. If you love Internet spam, make sure you sign up to receive the "latest news and promotions" and the "occasional third-party information." Better yet, list your household income as "over $150,000." If you don't like spam (if you're sane), AvantGo does let you opt out.

Next, you pick your handheld device as in Figure 10.5 and download the software. You actually download a 3-MB installation file that runs on your desktop computer. As suggested by AvantGo, make sure you download the installer to an easy-to-find place like your Windows Desktop. Double-click the installer icon. The installer will run and then launch your browser back to the AvantGo Web site where you select the "channels" you'd like on your handheld. You'll have to synchronize your handheld several times before all is said and done, but overall the process works well.

In the AvantGo lingo, "channel" equates with "Web site." AvantGo offers a series of channels they term "AvantGo Auto Channels." These are prese-

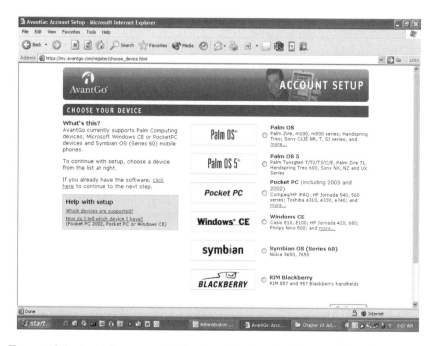

FIGURE 10.5. AvantGo supported devices. (Reprinted with permission from AvantGo.)

lected to look good on smaller handheld screens. AvantGo has become so popular that many Internet entities, such as Yahoo.com, and other media outlets, such as the New York Times and CNN, offer custom Web content just for AvantGo. My favorite nonmedical Auto Channels are Yahoo.com and the Wall Street Journal. If you have a "My Yahoo" account, this channel will show your local movie times complete with reviews, in addition to your stocks and other localized news and information. What a great service! AvantGo offers previews of most channels that show how they look on a handheld (as in Figures 10.6 and 10.7).

With AvantGo, as with iSilo, hyperlinks still work even without an active Internet connection. There's a practical limit to how far hyperlinks will go: this is called "depth." The higher you set the depth, the larger the number of Web pages included. And more Web pages translate into more memory on your handheld. Figure 10.8 summarizes how link depth corresponds to the architecture of a typical Web site.

You can sometimes control hyperlink depth as well as other attributes using the online Configure page as shown in Figure 10.9. In this case, the Link Depth is preset at 1 and cannot be changed. A 1 level deep Auto Channel makes for a more compact design. Other attributes include maximum channel size, whether or not to include images (which take up lots of memory), and whether or not to include offsite content. You also decide how often to refresh the Web content cached to your handheld. At

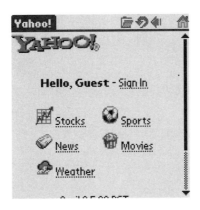

FIGURE 10.6. Yahoo on AvantGo. (Reprinted with permission of Yahoo! Inc. © 2004 by Yahoo! Inc. YAHOO! Inc. and the YAHOO! logo are trademarks of Yahoo! Inc. Reprinted with permission from AvantGo.)

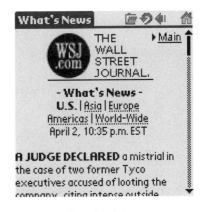

FIGURE 10.7. Joke-A-Day on AvantGo. (Reprinted with permission from AvantGo and The Wall Street Journal.)

first, "on every sync" is a good option. You'll find with time that certain channels take a particularly long time to download. Change these to intermittent channel refresh to save time when synchronizing.

When last checked, AvantGo offered 31 Auto Channels for health professionals, including several in Spanish and French (see Table 10.3 for a sample). Unfortunately, you'll still find more news content than peer-

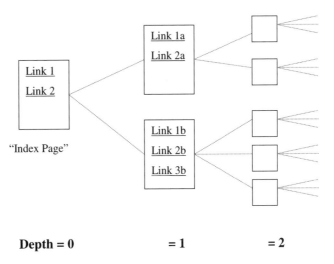

FIGURE 10.8. Hyperlink depth.

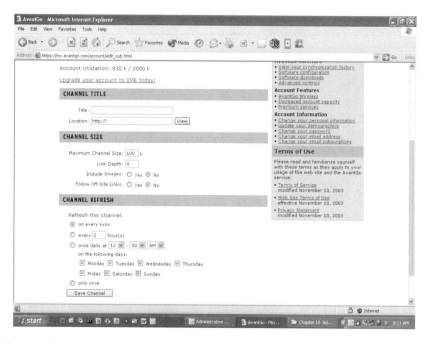

FIGURE 10.9. AvantGo Auto Channel configuration. (Reprinted with permission from AvantGo.)

TABLE 10.3. AvantGo auto channels for health professionals.		
Featured channel	Size (kilobytes)	Summary
A–Z of clinical medicine: Mobile GP Notebook (www.gpnotebook.co.uk)	100	"UK's leading clinical reference resource aimed at generalists"
Air Heart Professional	400	"Cardiology headlines, abstracts, and selected articles"
Clinical Evidence	850	"Best available evidence about common and important clinical questions"
CollectiveMed.com Mobile Medical Channel	30	"Helping physicians and healthcare professionals maximize their PDA hardware and software with tips, news, and reviews"
drcooper.palm	50	"A bilingual handheld-friendly Web site designed by a family physician"
Health News Digest	60	"Current and breaking news on the health industry"
Pocket Doctor	300	"Quality medical information and services wherever you are, including a full health encyclopedia"
pdaMD	40	"pdaMD.com is a lively community of healthcare professionals sharing information about how handheld and wireless technologies enhance their practices"

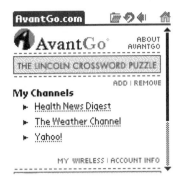

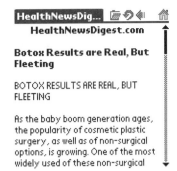

FIGURE 10.10. AvantGo with Palm OS. (Reprinted with permission from AvantGo.)

FIGURE 10.11. AvantGo Health Digest News. (Reprinted with permission from AvantGo and Health News Digest.)

reviewed journals. Also, available sites change often. Figure 10.10 shows what AvantGo looks like on an actual Palm OS handheld. Figure 10.11 shows how a news article appears in Health News Digest. They look exactly the same on a Pocket PC handheld.

Pocket PC users will notice that AvantGo doesn't have its own application icon. You launch AvantGo from within Internet Explorer.

Refreshing AvantGo channels can more than double the time it takes to synchronize. Limit the number of channels you add to your subscription at first. Then, pick and choose different channels until you find the right mix of usefulness and practicality. A free subscription limits you to 2000 KB, but that's more than enough, all things considered. You will find that AvantGo occasionally adds some advertising to the Web content on your handheld, which was not originally the case.... Although annoying, it's not a deal breaker for most users. It's just the price you pay for a "free subscription."

Great medical Internet content exists on sites without AvantGo Auto Channels. For some, you can create an AvantGo Custom Channel, as we discuss in Hands-On Exercise 10.2. Sites that change often, but aren't too big, work well with Custom Channels. A very big site will quickly overwhelm the 2000-KB limit. You're in luck, however, because that's where iSilo really shines. Keep reading and we'll get there shortly.

HANDS-ON EXERCISE 10.2. CREATING CUSTOM CHANNELS FOR AVANTGO

AvantGo Custom Channels are easy to set up but hard to master. You have to pick Web sites that adapt well to the small screen. Hyperlinks, usually depicted as underlined text, convert better than drop-down menus. Fancy Web pages with lots of animation may not work at all. In the end, you can't always predict which will work the best, and it comes down to trial and error.

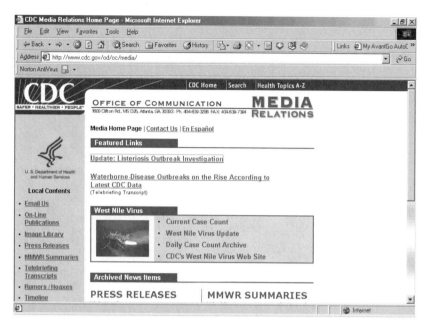

FIGURE 10.12. CDC News Update Web site.

As an example, let's look at the Center for Disease Control (CDC) news update page. You get there by going to www.cdc.gov on your Internet browser and clicking the hyperlink "In the News" at the left margin. The resulting Web page is shown in Figure 10.12.

So, what do you think? Would this make for a useful custom channel on AvantGo? The answer is yes and no, so we'll give it a try and learn as we go. A few links connect to pages with many, many more links, making for a bloated channel even with the depth set to 1. Clicking the link "MMWR SUMMARIES" opens the Web page shown in Figure 10.13. If the MMWR Summaries interest you, you'd be better off making a separate custom channel, starting on the page in Figure 10.13 and linking, with link depth set to 1, to the listed reports.

Once you pick a Web page to try, go to the AvantGo "Create Custom Channel" Web page shown in Figure 10.14. You get there by signing into your account at the AvantGo Web site, clicking the "My Account" tab, and clicking the "Create a custom channel" hyperlink. This page looks exactly like the Auto Channel attributes page already discussed.

As shown in Figure 10.14, copy the link for the desired Web page from your Internet browser (see Figure 10.12) to the Channel Title "Location," including "http://". Pick any title you want for the Channel Title "Title." Initially, a maximum channel size between 100 and 200 KB will suffice. You can fine-tune the size later. Unless images play a key role in the site content,

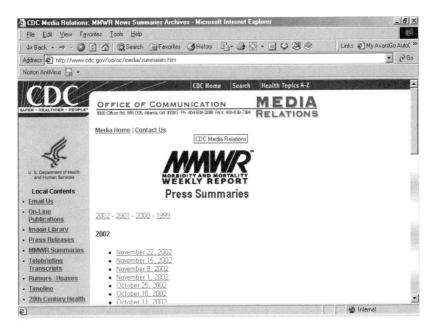

FIGURE 10.13. CDC *Morbidity and Mortality Weekly Report* Web site.

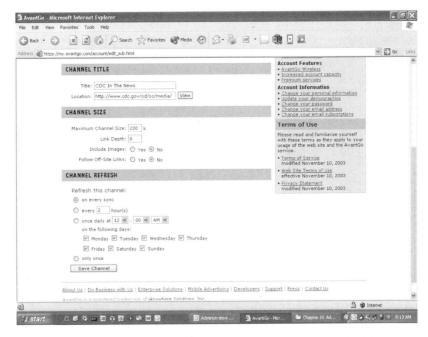

FIGURE 10.14. AvantGo Custom Channel configuration. (Reprinted with permission from AvantGo.)

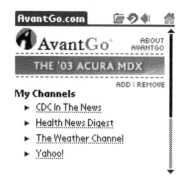

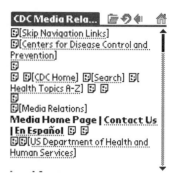

FIGURE 10.15. AvantGo Custom Channel on handheld. (Reprinted with permission from AvantGo.)

FIGURE 10.16. AvantGo Custom Channel: "CDC in the News." (Reprinted with permission from AvantGo.)

which they don't here, set "Include Images" to "No." Always set "Follow Off-Site Links" to "No": these mostly link to advertisements. You can always change this later if you find an offsite link useful.

Link depth is big issue. Set Link Depth to 1 initially in most cases, as increasing depth leads to exponentially increasing channel size. The truth is that properly selected sites work extremely well with a depth of 0.

Once you complete the Custom Channel form for your CDC In the News channel, click the "Save Channel" button at the bottom of the screen. If all goes well, the next page you see will declare, "Channel added successfully!" Next time you synchronize, the custom channel content will be added to AvantGo on your handheld. Figure 10.15 shows a Palm OS handheld screen with this custom channel added. The new channel is titled "CDC In The News." Tapping the link goes to Figure 10.16. Although we are using Palm OS screenshots in this example, the steps and resulting screens are virtually identical using a Pocket PC handheld computer.

Yikes! Lots of garbage and broken links . . . That's the downside of a custom channel over an Auto Channel—with Auto Channels, the formatting looks better. If you scroll down a bit, you'll reach the main page content as in Figure 10.17. Tapping on the link "West Nile Virus", "Current Case Count" connects nicely to the page shown in Figure 10.18. Remember, this all happens without an active Internet connection, wireless or otherwise, and the data are as up to date as your last synchronization! As it turns out, clicking on the link "Update: Update Outbreak of Gastrointestinal Illness" in this example (Figure 10.17) gives a "Size Limit Exceeded" error as shown in Figure 10.19.

It just so happens that this "Update" Web page contains a particularly long text article that AvantGo cannot handle. The next time you refreshed

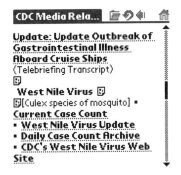

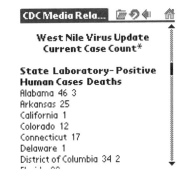

FIGURE 10.17. AvantGo
Custom Channel: "CDC in
the News" (continued).
(Reprinted with permission
from AvantGo.)

FIGURE 10.18. AvantGo
Custom Channel: "West Nile
Virus Update." (Reprinted
with permission from
AvantGo.)

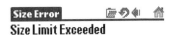

FIGURE 10.19. AvantGo Custom Channel: "Size   The requested file's size is too large
Limit Exceeded."   to be sent to this device.

the channel, by synchronizing, new content might appear and the error
resolve. So, expect to run into occasional bumps along the way while using
AvantGo. You'll probably find much more you like, though, than you
dislike. All in all, AvantGo Custom Channels offers a clever tool that greatly
expands the usefulness of AvantGo to health professionals.

Medical Applications with iSilo

Simply put, iSilo is the "big daddy" of Web page caching. iSilo works well
as a document reader but really shines when it comes to caching HTML
Web pages. The main reason is that iSilo doesn't limit the size of cached
sites the way AvantGo does but, using the free converter software, is just
as easy to use. With iSilo, you also avoid the advertisements encountered
with AvantGo. Finally, iSilo claims high text compression of up to 60% of
the original memory size.

The principal downsides of iSilo are two. First, you have to pay for the
software, and second, it's a bit more labor intensive. All iSilo downloads are,
in effect, custom channels. You can download prepackaged documents as
already discussed. For most Web content, though, you have to set up the

channel and manually refresh it when desired. By the way, don't even bother with "iSilo free." This version is in fact free, but the hyperlinks are nonfunctional. Hyperlinks make this program the star that it is, so don't waste your time.

An important twist to using iSilo has come up lately. The newest version, dubbed "iSilo3," is not completely compatible with older versions. Here's the difference. The old iSilo converter software turned all Web pages into one narrow but very long column. In other words, different columns, such as hyperlinks at either margin, were all lined up vertically. (You scrolled up and down through the page content, but never side to side.) iSilo3 more closely preserves the original HTML formatting. The handheld screen acts like a small window opening onto the Web page. (You scroll both up and down and side to side.) iSilo3 does read old iSilo documents in their original format, but the older version of iSilo can't read iSilo3 documents (created with iSiloX as in Hands-On Exercise 10.3).

Power User Tips: Old-Style Formatting with iSilo3

You might ask, which format is better, old iSilo or iSilo3? iSilo3 does offers pretty page layout and color. On the other hand, it necessitates both horizontal and vertical movement to fully view a page. This turns out to be a cumbersome process, because you can no longer get by with only the up–down mechanical buttons like you could with the old iSilo. You may, however, revert to the old-style layout if you prefer. Just open iSilo3, choose "Options" from the program menu, choose "Display" from the drop-down menu, and set the "Tables" property to "Single column." Consider Figures 10.20, 10.21, and 10.22 showing the same Web site, CDC "Health Topics A–Z," converted and viewed on a handheld screen. Figure 10.20 shows the

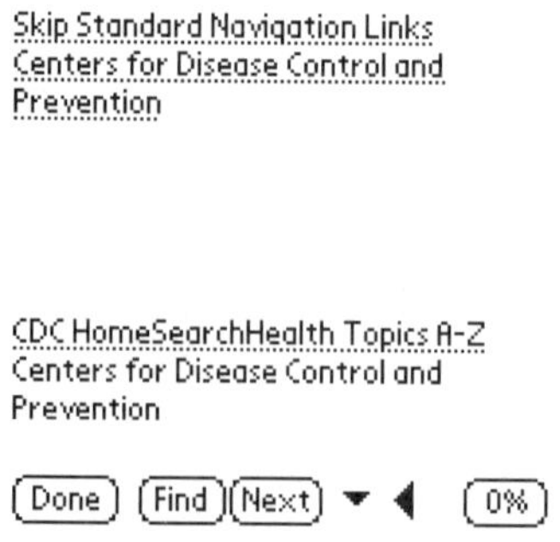

Skip Standard Navigation Links
Centers for Disease Control and Prevention

Health Topics A to Z

Health Topics A to Z provides a listing of disease and health topics found on the CDC Web site. It is not yet a complete index of the site. New topics are added on an ongoing basis.

CDC HomeSearchHealth Topics A-Z
Centers for Disease Control and Prevention

|A B C D E F G H I J K L M N O P Q R S T U V W X Y Z|

• Acanthamoeba Infection
• Acute Care

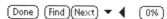

(Done) (Find)(Next) ▼ ◀ (0%)   (Done) (Find)(Next) ▼ ◀ (6%)

FIGURE 10.20. iSilo: "CDC Health Topics A–Z." (Reprinted with permission from iSilo.)

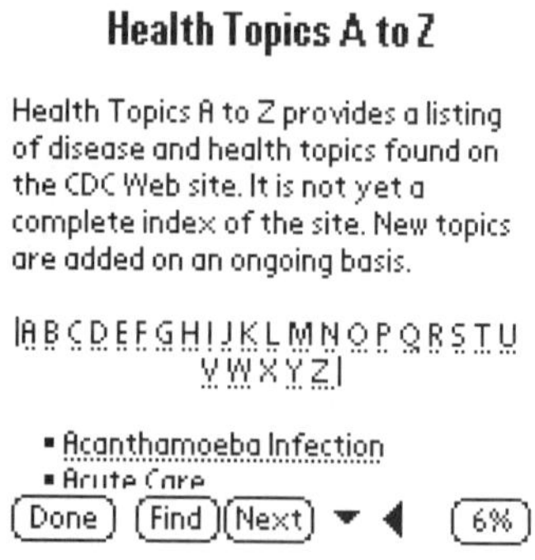

FIGURE 10.21. iSilo: "CDC Health Topics A–Z" (continued). (Reprinted with permission from iSilo.)

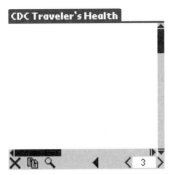

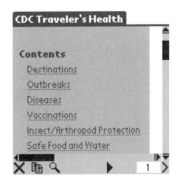

FIGURE 10.22. iSilo3: "CDC Health Topics A–Z." (Reprinted with permission from iSilo.)

FIGURE 10.23. iSilo3: CDC Home Page. (Reprinted with permission from iSilo.)

cached Web site as created using the old iSilo converter software. You intuitively scroll down until you find the information you want. Or, tap on the link "Skip Standard Navigation Links" to jump to the content shown in Figure 10.21. Figure 10.22 shows how the same Web site appears when cached and viewed using the new software. In this case, the information reads better setting the Tables property to single column. Other iSilo3 pages look great with multicolumn tables. Figure 10.23 shows another page from the CDC Web site as an example.

Caching and converting Web sites with iSilo, like most technical discussions, will make much more sense with a hands-on example. Let's dive into one right now.

HANDS-ON EXERCISE 10.3. CACHING A WEB SITE WITH ISILO

As with AvantGo, the first trick to using iSilo is picking the right Web site. We'll use the CDC Web site on Traveler's Medicine as our target. The content here represents the best information available in the United States on this topic. You'll love having this on your handheld! To get there, set your Internet browser to www.cdc.gov/travel/ (Figure 10.24).

You'll find travel destinations listed in a drop-down menu. Although this looks nice on your desktop, it flops with iSilo. Remember, iSilo needs hyperlinks to create links between pages. Similar problems crop up often, so you have to be creative. In this case, the solution comes easily. Just click the link "Destinations" to go to www.cdc.gov/travel/destinat.htm. You'll move to the Web page shown in Figure 10.25.

This page is perfect! Each hyperlink connects to a separate Web page covering that topic. With a depth of 1, you'll capture everything you need. Now it's time to download the iSilo converter software, iSiloX. If you haven't already done so, you'll also have to install iSilo on your handheld

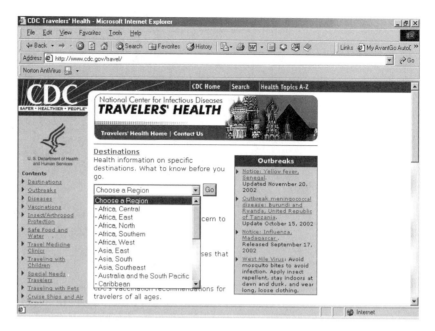

FIGURE 10.24. CDC Traveler's Health Web site with drop-down menu.

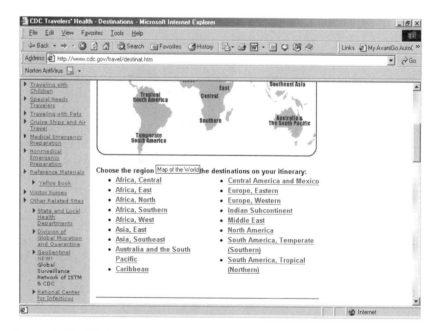

FIGURE 10.25. CDC Traveler's Health Web site with hyperlinks.

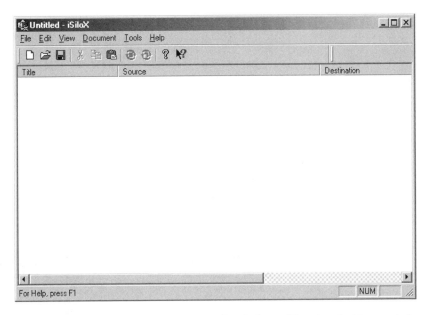

FIGURE 10.26. iSiloX Web page converter for desktop. (Reprinted with permission from iSilo.)

to complete the exercise. That's to say you use iSiloX, a program on your desktop computer, to cache a Web site and turn it into an iSilo document. Then you use the iSilo program for your handheld to actually view the document you've created.

The iSilo software is available at www.isilo.com. iSiloX is a 1.2-MB file. Installation is straightforward following the online instructions. The desktop program is shown in Figure 10.26.

To create an iSilo "document," click "Document" on the toolbar. Then, click "Add" on the drop-down menu. A dialog window will open (Figure 10.27). You supply the title as with AvantGo.

At this point, you have two options. You can click "Next" and follow the continuing instructions. Type in "http://www.cdc.gov/travel/destinat.htm" when prompted for a Web address. By using the wizard, you accept certain default values including link depth. A better option is to check "Go to document properties dialog next" before clicking "Next." Then you'll see the dialog window shown in Figure 10.28. The first step with this option is the same. Click the "Add URL/File . . ." button and type in your Web address.

Don't let the multiple tabs intimidate you. You can learn them as you go. We'll focus on three tab options. Click the "Links" tab as in Figure 10.29. Set "Maximum Link Depth" to 1 and deselect "Follow off-site links" and "Include unresolved link detail" as shown. We only want the CDC content. Off-site info would take up space without adding useful content. Also,

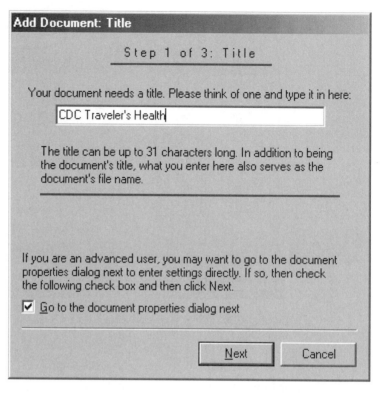

FIGURE 10.27. iSiloX conversion wizard step 1. (Reprinted with permission from iSilo.)

you can change this later if desired. Next, click the "Images" tab (Figure 10.30). Deselecting "Include images" will decrease the size of your final cached file.

Finally, the "Destination" tab (Figure 10.31) allows you to specify where the newly created document will go. You can specify multiple users and both Palm OS and Pocket PC devices. Also, you can choose to save a copy of the document to a file for backup purposes. When the document is created, iSiloX will place it in the installation folder of any intended users. The document will thus be installed at the next synchronization operation.

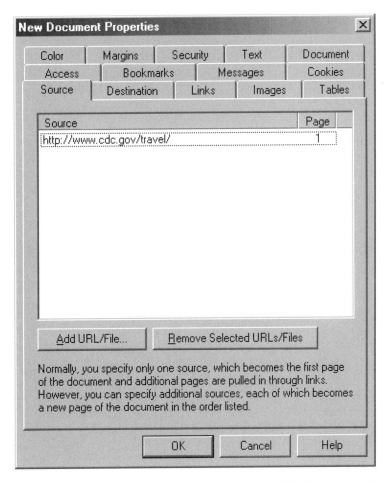

FIGURE 10.28. iSiloX Document Properties dialog: Add URL. (Reprinted with permission from iSilo.)

Power User Tips

An additional tab available is the "Security" tab. This option allows you specify a password needed to access certain web content. Although unnecessary in this example, it's sometimes required. For example, a physician with a Medscape account might want to cache Medscape content for personal use at the point of care. Without a password, iSiloX would be unable to retrieve any content. Entering the password here works like a peach.

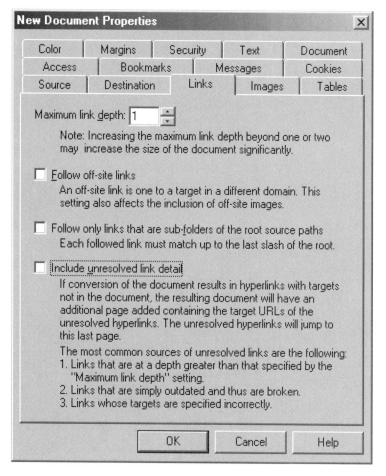

FIGURE 10.29. iSiloX Document Properties dialog: Setup links. (Reprinted with permission from iSilo.)

When you've finished with the above options, click "OK." You'll see the document information as shown in Figure 10.32. To convert the Web content to an iSilo document, make sure your desktop computer is connected to the Internet. Then, click "Document" on the toolbar and select the option "Convert" or "Convert All."

If all goes well, you'll see a dialog window that describes the steps taken as iSilo converts the Web content specified to a document for the handheld. iSilo literally parses through every link on the first Web page indicated by the supplied Web address shown in Figure 10.28. In turn, it goes to every

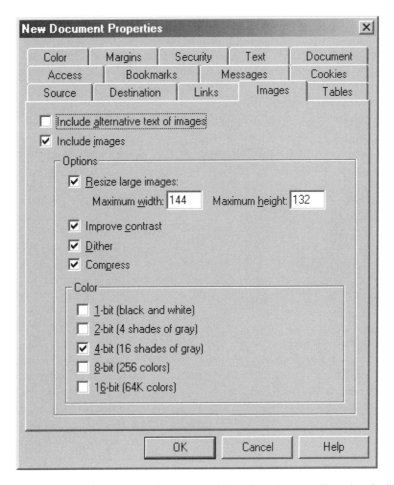

FIGURE 10.30. iSiloX Document Properties dialog: Setup images. (Reprinted with permission from iSilo.)

new Web page referenced by these links and adds that content to the document.

If you're not careful, this process can take a long time. Table 10.4 summarizes the relative conversion times and final document sizes using Link Depths of 0, 1, and 2. Going from a depth of 1 to a depth of 2 takes 15 times more memory and more than 20 times more time to complete! (Link Depth 3—forget about it!) These times were achieved using a single-channel, Integrated Services Digital Network (ISDN) connection. That's about twice as fast as a dial-up connection but much slower than a cable modem or DSL

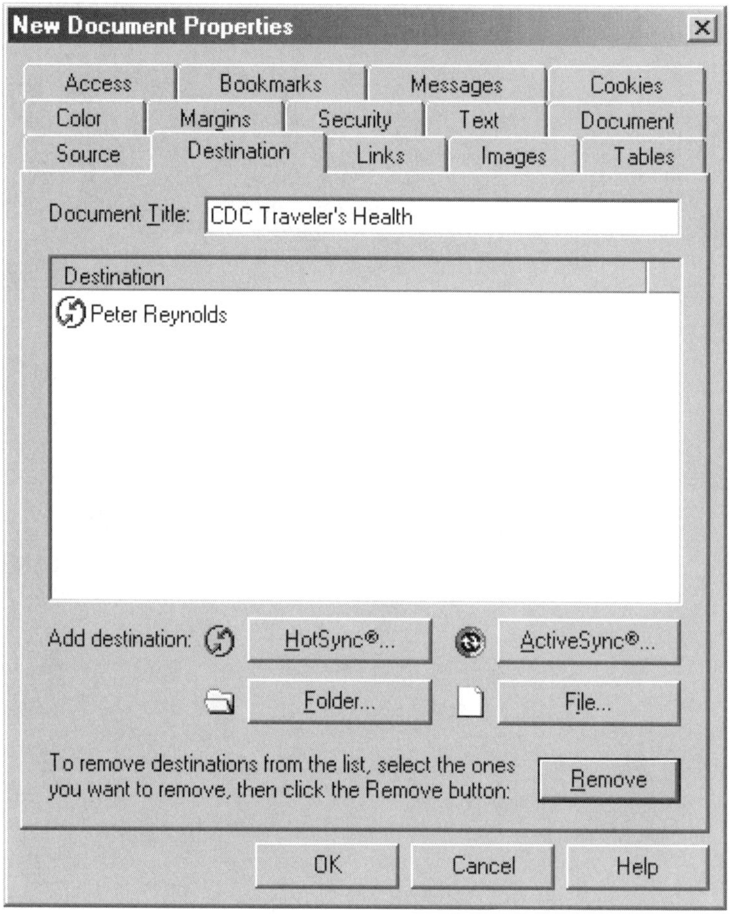

FIGURE 10.31. iSiloX Document Properties dialog: Choose Destination.
(Reprinted with permission from iSilo.)

TABLE 10.4. Comparison of iSilo conversion times and document size.

Depth 0	1	2
Total size, 5 KB	Total size, 125 KB	Total size, 1883 KB
Time, 30 sec	Time, 2 min 30 sec	Time, 60 min

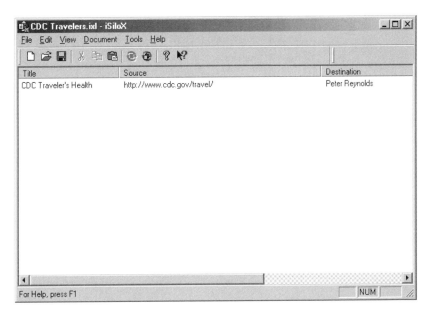

FIGURE 10.32. iSiloX conversion completed. (Reprinted with permission from iSilo.)

connection. If you ever run into a situation that calls for a Link Depth greater than 1, consider creating two documents with a depth of 1. You'll save lots of time and memory space.

When finished, synchronize your handheld and open iSilo from the Application Launcher. You should see the document title listed as in Figure 10.33. Tap on the title and follow destination links, as shown in Figures 10.34

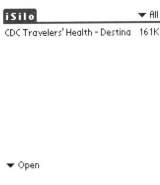

FIGURE 10.33. iSilo on handheld: Startup screen. (Reprinted with permission from iSilo.)

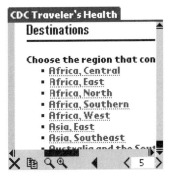

FIGURE 10.34. iSilo on handheld: "CDC Traveler's Health." (Reprinted with permission from iSilo.)

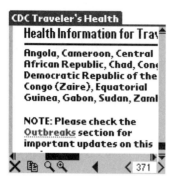

FIGURE 10.35. iSilo on handheld: "CDC Traveler's Health" (continued). (Reprinted with permission from iSilo.)

and 10.35. You did it! Now you can access information on vaccinations required and malaria prophylaxis for any destination in the world at your fingertips. Are you ready to open your own travel clinic?

Summary

In this chapter, we've discussed multiple ways to store and retrieve medical documents. From simple text memos to cached Internet content, handheld computers have opened a new frontier for portable medical documents. Using document reader software, you can bring vast stores of medical information to bear on point-of-care decision making as never before.

Reference

1. Slawson DC, Shaughnessy AF, Bennett JH. Becoming a medical information master: feeling good about not knowing everything. J Fam Pract 1994;38:505–513.

11

Capturing Life in the Palm of Your Hand: Getting Rid of the Yellow Stickies by Using a Handheld Database

JAMES M. THOMPSON, SCOTT M. STRAYER, AND MARK H. EBELL

Welcome to Handheld Computer Databases

How many times have you written down CME (continuing medical education) hours on a "yellow sticky" or put a patient label on an index card to track a procedure you just performed? Is this how you keep track of your billing? Now think a minute . . . just how many of these go through the laundry each week, or get lost in the trunk of your car? Be honest now! Imagine being able to track all these important daily activities on your handheld computer. Even better, you can beam the information to colleagues (such as a weekend coverage list), or have it synchronize with your desktop computer to use powerful database programs such as Excel and Access.

Handheld computers are ideal tools for maintaining and sharing electronic databases of information. It takes minutes for you to build and start using a personal database for tasks like logging personal medical education activities or tracking patients on rounds. At the high end, a hospital could build very complex handheld databases for collecting and deploying information among its staff.

In this chapter, we describe handheld database software products. We explain what databases are all about and guide you through the features you might want to consider if you decide to purchase a handheld database program.

In Chapter 17, we show you step by step how to build a database for logging clinical procedures performed by residents and staff physicians. We will refer to that example throughout this chapter too, because it seems to be a common use of handheld databases by physicians.

What Exactly Is a Database?

Databases Have Tables, Fields, Records, and Forms

A *database* is an organized collection of electronic data. The word "database" has several specialized meanings, which can be confusing.

This chapter refers to a special type of handheld computer database software in which the word "database" refers to a software family that displays information in *forms* showing *records* that contain data in *fields*. For example, a form might be used to gather information such as CME events you attended. Each record would correspond to a specific CME event, and the fields would have information such as the date, number of hours, and so on. In a database program, you could have one form for CME events and another for procedures you perform (and perhaps the all-important golf score form to document your progress or lack thereof).

A *table* is a collection of records in which each record has the same fields, but of course the data within each field might vary from record to record. Database software allows users to view, sort, edit, enter, share, and print data by manipulating the fields and records in a database.

People commonly call the various handheld software database products "databases" for short. HanDBase, MobileDB, Jfile, and Pendragon Forms are popular database products for Palm OS handhelds. In the Pocket PC world, similar software includes HanDBase, Visual CE, abcDB, db anywhere, Sprint DB, Pocket Database, Pocket DB, Wireless Database, db2Hand, Data Anywhere, and Data on the Run (Table 11.1).

Some people call each table a database. A software purist might call all the tables, forms, reports, queries, and other parts that are designed to work together for a specific data task a database, the way Microsoft Access does. It doesn't matter, so long as *you* understand what you mean for a specific project.

Key Points

1. Databases are *tables* containing *records* made up of common *fields*. A CME database might be a table where each record is one CME event, and the fields describe the date, number of credit hours, location of the event, and type of event.
2. A *form* is the software that displays the database data on the computer screen.
3. People also use the term database to refer to software products used to make databases. Illogical, but don't tell Spock that we all do it anyway.

TABLE 11.1. Handheld database products.

Palm OS

   List: http://www.magma.ca/~roo/list/list.html
   PDA Toolbox: http://www.pdatoolbox.com
   DbNow: http://www.pocketexpress.com
   JFile: http://www.land-j.com/jfile.html
   HanDBase: http://www.ddhsoftware.com/
   MobileDB: http://www.handmark.com/products/mobiledb/
   Pendragon Forms: http://www.pendragon-software.com/
   Satellite Forms: http://www.pumatech.com
   Marietta DB: http://www.mariettasystems.com
   FileMaker Mobile: http://www.filemaker.com
   IBM DB2 Everyplace: http://www.ibm.com
   Sybase UltraLite: http://www.sybase.com
   Oracle Lite: http://www.oracle.com

Pocket PC

   Data on the Run: http://www.biohazardsoftware.com/start.htm
   HanDBase: http://www.ddhsoftware.com/
   VisualCE: http://www.syware.com
   abcDB: http://www.pocketsoft.ca
   DB Anywhere: http://www.handango.com
   SprintDB Pro: http://www.kaione.com
   Pocket Database (by Surerange): http://www.surerange.com/database.html
   Pocket Database (by Pocket Innovations): http://www.pocket-innovations.com/Products
   Pocket DB: http://members.aol.com/doanc/dbce.html
   Satellite Forms: http://www.pumatech.com
   Wireless Database: www.kelbran.com
   db2Hand: http://www.smartidz.com
   Data Anywhere: http://www.smartidz.com
   Oracle Light: http://www.oracle.com

Flat File Versus Relational Databases

You cannot escape learning some new language when you start using databases. Two other very important terms are "flat file" and "relational." They refer to the way tables in a database do or do not relate to each other.

A *flat file* database consists of a single table of records, with data organized in records composed of fields common to all records in the table. Beginners usually start building single-table flat file databases. The table has no connection to any other table that might exist on your handheld.

As an example, you can create a simple HanDBase database (www.handbase.com) to log Continuing Medical Education hours on your handheld (see Chapter 17 for details on building your own custom-designed databases). The great thing about HanDBase is that it can be used on both Palm and Pocket PC handheld computers. You can view either a number of records in the table (Figures 11.1, 11.2; the "table view") or all the detail for one record (Figures 11.3, 11.4; the "record view"). Notice that in this

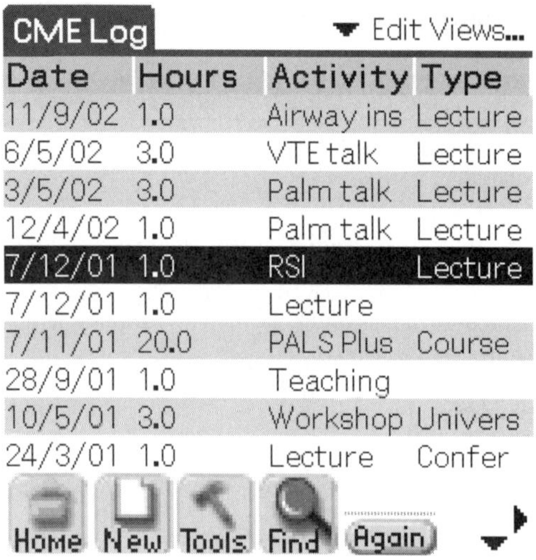

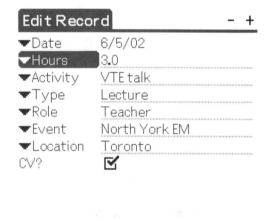

FIGURE 11.1. Logging CME hours: List of records (Palm OS).

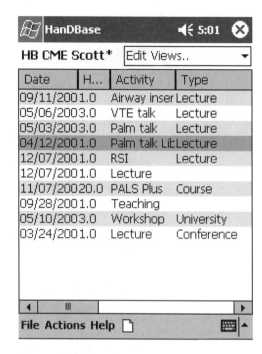

FIGURE 11.2. Logging CME hours: List of records (Pocket PC).

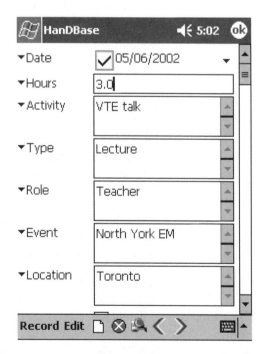

FIGURE 11.3. Logging CME hours: Detail for one record (Palm OS).

FIGURE 11.4. Logging CME hours: Detail for one record (Pocket PC).

particular example all the details for a single record happens to fit on one screen in the record view, but to see all the records in the database in the table view, you tap the navigation arrow to move the screen view to the right to see more of the data. Because screens for HanDBase are nearly identical on the Palm and Pocket PC models, the rest of this chapter uses Palm OS screenshots only to avoid duplication. There are a few different buttons and conventions (between the Palm and Pocket PC versions) that can be quickly learned and are very well documented in the HanDBase user manuals.

Relational databases consist of multiple tables linked to each other in structured relationships. Relational database design is very common because it creates powerful opportunities for automatically managing data. Relational designs save many screen taps and much Graffiti-writing. Most handheld database products contain features that allow varying degrees of relational database design. When you start using databases you might soon come to appreciate some simple relational features in your database software.

In Chapter 17 we show you how to build a simple flat file, single-table database for logging procedures. Later in that chapter we show you how to upgrade that flat file design to a relational design by creating a separate table for listing all the procedures and linking that table to the procedure log table. That way you can create links between the tables to look up all the information for a certain procedure, such as a billing code or dollar value, and return those bits of information accurately to your procedure log table. This is much better, because then you can maintain separate procedure tables for each specialty, or you can modify the dollar values for each procedure when you get a raise by simply editing the procedure list table.

Key Points

1. A flat file database is a single table, a useful design for simple tasks like logging CME hours.
2. Relational databases are two or more tables linked together for more efficient data management, such as maintaining subdatabases of procedure lists for each specialty.

"Hey, What About Me?" Spreadsheets Are Databases, Too

"Spreadsheet" software is a different family of software that displays data in rows and columns. Spreadsheets can also be called databases in one sense, but there are some key differences between spreadsheet programs and the kind of database programs we are talking about in this chapter.

In spreadsheets, the location of a piece of information in the database is defined by a unique row and column number combination, or "cell." This format differs from database programs such as HanDBase, where the location of a piece of data is not restricted to a certain location but is stored instead in a specific field in a specific record. In the kind of database products we are talking about in this chapter, fields can be placed anywhere on the screen, and data can be located in a more flexible way by the user. Records can be selected by searching for data in fields, for example. That's not so easy in spreadsheet products.

Spreadsheet software is less useful for viewing, entering, and editing most database data on handhelds. The small screen makes it difficult to view more than a few cells of the data. Spreadsheet software does not permit the user to design forms for displaying the data in a variety of ways. Spreadsheets have handier uses for manipulating smaller amounts of data, so this type of software might suit certain projects better than the kinds of database products we are talking about here.

Pocket PC users can easily put a Microsoft Excel spreadsheet on their handheld computers by simply transferring the file to the Pocket PC and using the already included software, Pocket Excel. To show you how Pocket Excel files look on the Pocket PC, we used the same CME log from our previous example, and created it in Excel and transferred it to the Pocket PC (Figure 11.5). Similar programs that allow reading Excel files on Palm handheld computers include Documents To Go ($69.95, www.dataviz.com); MobileDB ($29.95, www.handmark.com); and QuickOffice ($39.95, www.cesinc.com).

Key Point

1. Spreadsheet software displays data in rows and columns, so isn't nearly as flexible for many database projects as proper database software.

Convince Me: Why Would I Want to Spend Time and Money on a Database Program for My Handheld?

Database software allows you to organize, access, and manipulate data easily. Here are some healthcare provider uses for this kind of software:

• Creating references, such as lists of billing or diagnostic codes, oncology drugs or antibiotics, or immunization indications.
• Recording patient billings, such as house calls or operating room procedures.

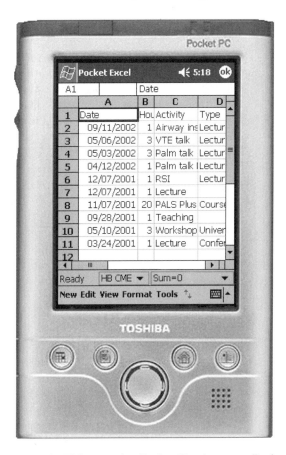

FIGURE 11.5. Logging CME hours using Pocket Excel on your Pocket PC.

- Collecting data from your physician or nursing group for a research project.
- Tracking clinical procedures that residents perform during their rotations.
- Tracking hospital inpatients during rounds.
- Maintaining inventory on nursing wards or in medication carts.
- Deploying patient records and daily visit schedules to home care nurses, and then collecting the results of home visits.
- Tracking your personal collection of music compact disks, logging your vehicle maintenance events, or keeping an inventory of your boat's hardware. We all have private lives that need attention.

How to Log Your CME Credits Without All Those Loose Scraps of Paper

I use a simple database to log my CME credits. I made it one day during a coffee break. First, I built a simple database with a few fields to capture the essential information (see Figures 11.1–11.4). Then I collect information about my CME events on my handheld wherever I am. Back at the office I let the synchronization software automatically back up the database to my desktop computer for security. I also have a little utility on my handheld that automatically backs up the database to an expansion memory card in the handheld every morning. Another utility could allow you to print basic reports from the handheld to a printer, but I open the database on my desktop with other software to print reports from there instead.

As we already mentioned, in Chapter 17 we explain step by step how to build a database to log clinical procedures, and you can apply that knowledge to build the CME database we just showed you as well. Those are probably two of the most common uses of handheld database software among physicians.

Most database applications come with a bundled or optional desktop companion program. The companion program allows the user to open databases on his or her desktop computer to view, edit, and print data on the larger screen. I use HanDBase's Windows companion program to maintain my CME log sometimes. The larger screen is easier to work on than the handheld's small screen, but the handheld is handier (no pun intended) when I am on the move away from my desk.

These desktop companion programs allow the user to share data manually with other desktop software by importing and exporting a common file type, typically the "comma separated values" file format ("csv" extension). I use the desktop companion to export my CME data to an Access database, where I can print fancier reports. It doesn't take long to learn how. We also explain in Chapter 17 how to use the HanDBase desktop to do this for the procedure log database.

Key Points

1. It only takes a few minutes to build a simple database on your handheld for logging your CME hours.
2. Desktop computer programs that come with handheld database products make it easy to maintain the database on either platform.
3. You can use the companion desktop program to export the data on your desktop computer to a format that can be used by other software for analyzing or reporting your data.

I Log My CME Credits with Access and Excel Already: What Have You Got to Say About That?

Many database products come with utilities that allow users to synchronize databases automatically between their handheld and an entirely separate program on their desktop computer, such as Microsoft Access or Excel. These utilities are *conduits* that connect the databases through software code with the HotSync process. When the user synchronizes their handheld with the desktop, the conduit uses HotSync to update the database on both devices automatically. This allows you to take advantage of much more powerful features for manipulating and reporting the data using desktop database programs like Access, Excel, FoxPro, and many others.

Pendragon Forms is a specialized Microsoft Access database designed to support handheld databases. Macros behind the scenes help you to design tables and forms without requiring you to know computer programming. The forms automatically load onto your handheld, where you enter and edit data. The tables stay on the desktop computer in Access. At each HotSync the data flow into the tables in the Access version of the database on your desktop computer. A similar program for the Pocket PC platform is Visual CE by Syware ($129, www.syware.com). Also, HanDBase can synchronize with Access databases, which are available for Pocket PC and Palm handheld computers as previously mentioned.

Key Points

1. Handheld databases can easily be linked to software on your desktop computer.
2. You can make changes to the data on either computer, and then synchronize it to the other machine. So take your CME log with you everywhere, and then cut and paste the data into your curriculum vitae or your expense refund claim when you return to the office.

Linking the Whole Practice into One Big Happy Electronic Family: Multiple Users and Networking

Databases can be made to synchronize over networks with multiple users throughout an organization. Each user's handheld can share tailored parts of the database with the rest of the organization, and vice versa. Solutions for this kind of databasing range from reasonably simple to very complex. Even though inexpensive handheld database products provide tools to enable this kind of networking, you should consider hiring a software engineer if you need this kind of networking capability for your database project.

The Mount Sinai Department of Surgery in Toronto, Canada, used JFile to develop a procedure log for tracking their residents' operating room experiences. Their paper describing this early experiment is worth reading if you want to get a feel for the issues involved in a project like that.[1]

Key Point

1. Consult a software engineer who is familiar with your institution's network before trying to deploy a handheld database over the network to multiple users.

Where Do I Get a Database for My Handheld?

You have several options if you want a database for handhelds, such as making a procedure log for the residents and physicians in your clinical group:

1. Write the program in a low-level computer language like C++ and then compile it for the Palm operating system. Programs written this way certainly are fast, efficient, and completely customizable to your needs, but they are very expensive to build in dollars and time, and require highly skilled programmers. Most users prefer a cheaper compromise solution.
2. Purchase a custom-built database from a software engineer who uses high-end database design software. Sometimes this is an appropriate option, especially for fitting the database into existing software infrastructure, but it is still expensive and you would still have to hire a consultant software engineer.
3. Buy a ready-made database that someone else developed for his or her own use; this can be a little expensive, and almost always you will want to tailor the program for the way your staff works anyway.
4. Buy a database software product (see Table 11.1) to make your own database. That's what this chapter is all about. This option makes most sense for the majority of users. All these products require compromises compared to building a completely customized program with high-end tools, but they work fine for most projects.

Key Point

1. Handheld database software is so simple to use that usually it is easiest to build and customize your own database.

I Downloaded a Database, But Where Did It Go?

Beginners commonly make a simple mistake. They download an interesting database from the Internet, install it to their handheld, and then cannot find it on the handheld. The reason is simple: databases can only be opened by their parent application. A database written for HanDBase can only be used with HanDBase, for example, not with other database software products.

Similarly, desktop companion programs written for a given product will only open databases made by the related Palm program. All of them can import or export data to and from other applications to varying degrees, however, so there are ways to share data between database products. We'll explain that later.

Key Point

1. You can only open a handheld database with the software product it was written for. Open HanDBase databases with HanDBase, and JFile databases with JFile, for example.

I'm All Confused About the Variety of Handheld Database Software Products on the Market

Database applications were among the first third-party software products written for both Palm and Pocket PC operating systems when they came out in the mid-1990s, so there are a variety of products from which to choose. Also, they are continually evolving, which makes it kind of hard for the beginner consumer. Search the Google Web site at http://www.google.com to find more than a couple of dozen Palm OS and Pocket PC database applications (see Table 11.1), ranging from very simple and free to very complex and expensive. In this chapter, we explain the feature sets typical of handheld database software, and show how they vary from product to product.

More Complex Databases Cost More and Take More Time to Learn, But They Allow You to Do More

Database software functionality ranges from simple to complex. You pay more for more functions. But do you need a more complex database program? To simplify this a bit, we classified available database software into light-, middle-, and heavyweight categories, like boxers. This makes it easier for me to make sense of the bewildering differences between products, so maybe it will help you, too.

Lightweights

The simplest database is a single table, and these handheld database programs allow users to do little more than enter or edit one or two data types in a flat file table. The lightweight products have few features and tend to be quite limited, but even these products can be very useful. Palm OS examples include List (www.magma.ca/~roo/list/list.html), dbNow, and Trans/Form, although the latter products have a few added features. An example of a simple list manager for the Pocket PC and Palm platforms is ListPro ($19.95, www.iliumsoft.com).

As simple as it is, List is a basic prototype for handheld database products. List allows only two 120-character-label fields and one 4-KB note field (Figure 11.6). Physicians in Ontario, Canada, share List databases of fee codes and diagnostic codes for looking up information while recording billings (Figures 11.7–11.9).[2]

List is about as basic as a database product can be. It is free, so if you have never used handheld database software, then I recommend that you download it from the Internet (see Table 11.1) and give it a try.

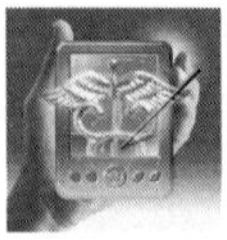

HANDS-ON EXERCISE 11.1. TRY CREATING A FEE REMINDER DATABASE WITH LIST

First, you give the database (table) a name, and then name the fields (Figure 11.6). Then, you open a new record form and enter data (Figure 11.7).

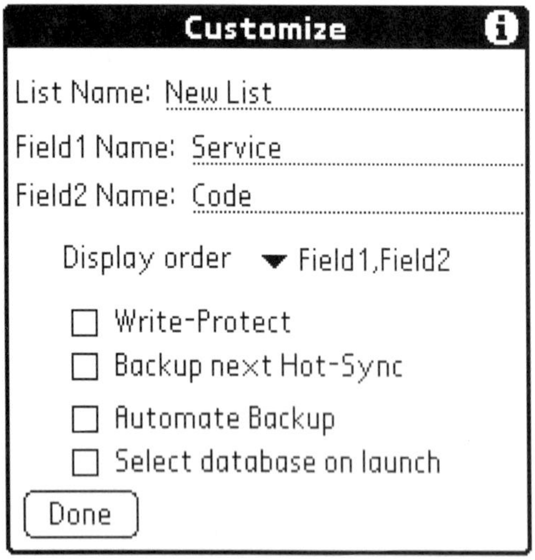

FIGURE 11.6. Design screen in the database program called "List."

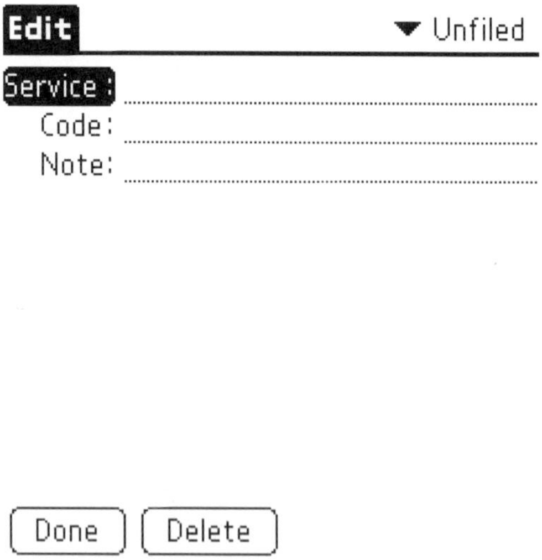

FIGURE 11.7. New record form in a fee reminder List database.

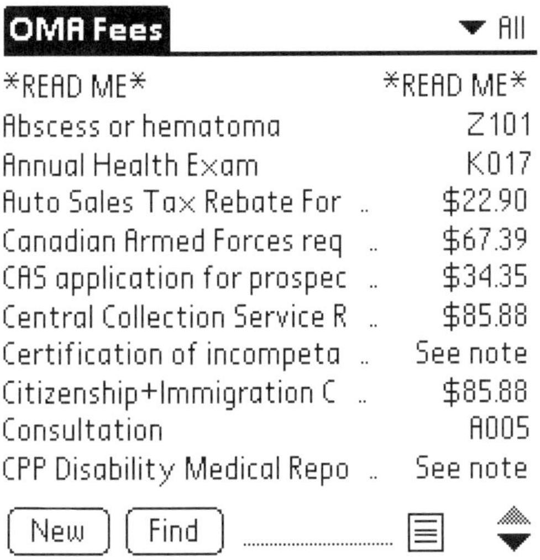

OMA Fees	▼ All
READ ME	*READ ME*
Abscess or hematoma	Z101
Annual Health Exam	K017
Auto Sales Tax Rebate For ..	$22.90
Canadian Armed Forces req ..	$67.39
CAS application for prospec ..	$34.35
Central Collection Service R ..	$85.88
Certification of incompeta ..	See note
Citizenship+Immigration C ..	$85.88
Consultation	A005
CPP Disability Medical Repo ..	See note

(New) (Find) .... ☰ ♦

FIGURE 11.8. List database of fee reminders.

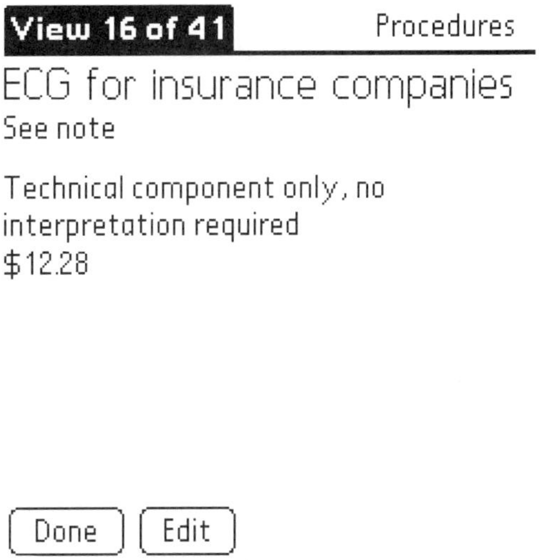

View 16 of 41	Procedures

ECG for insurance companies
See note

Technical component only, no
interpretation required
$12.28

(Done) (Edit)

FIGURE 11.9. Record detail in the List fee
reminder database.

TABLE 11.2. Middleweight databases for Palm OS.			
Database	HanDBase	JFile	MobileDB
Version reviewed	3.0	5.04	3.01
Footprint	464 KB	201 KB	36 KB
Base price (U.S. $)	$29.99	$24.95	$19.99
Desktop companion	Yes	No	Yes
Limits	200 databases; 65,000 records per database; 100 fields per database	120 databases; 16,000 records per database; 50 fields per database	No limit to number of databases or records per database; 20 fields per database
Field types	Text, Note, Date, Time, Integer, Float, Popup, Check Box, Unique, Image, Link, Linked, Heading, DB Popup, Calculated, Relationship, Conditional, External	String, Date, Time, Integer, Floating Point, Checkbox, Popup, Calculated Field	Text, Date, Time, Number, Checkbox, List, Sequence

After entering some records, you can open a screen that lets you view two of the three fields for as many records as will display on one screen, often called the "list view" (Figure 11.8). Or, you can open a form to view all the data for a specific record, often called the "record view" (Figure 11.9).

Chances are you will soon want more functionality than List provides. For example, you couldn't create a very useful procedure log with List, because it only allows you to have two fields for each record. What would be the point of just recording patient name and procedure, without the date too? Your handheld is a powerful computer for automating tasks, so why not put that horsepower to work?

Middleweights

Popular mainstream database applications like HanDBase, ThinkDB, Jfile, and MobileDB (see Table 11.1) have been around for years and are becoming increasingly sophisticated. They are inexpensive (about US $20–40), very easy to use, reasonably powerful, and well supported by their developers. These products have larger feature sets than the lightweights (Table 11.2), but not as much programming power as the heavyweights. The middleweights have rudimentary form design, simple relational features, and basic desktop companion programs. They can handle enterprise projects that require two-way synchronization with a network of users. Of note, HanDBase is one of the few programs that runs on both Palm and Pocket PC handhelds. It even allows beaming between the two platforms without any third-party software! Other middleweights for the Pocket PC include Visual CE lite and Sprint DB (Table 11.3).

Most of the middleweight database programs allow you to design a database right on your handheld. They are flexible enough to allow you to build almost as much complexity into your database as most users are likely to want, including links to a variety of desktop database software, and even networking your database with groups of people.

All these middleweight products require you to make compromises. You can have complete control over a database project if you program it from the ground up with a basic computer language like C++, but most of us cannot afford the time or money to hire someone to do that kind of software construction. The middleweights are evolving steadily, however. For example, HanDBase and ThinkDB offer "plug-in" technology, where you can connect your middleweight database to software utilities that can do fancier things with the data, if you really need that capability. All the middleweights can be made to synchronize with desktop database programs to varying degrees, using optional third-party utilities.

Most healthcare providers will be satisfied with one of the middleweight products, and might only need to consult a software engineer when they start networking, or if they want to link to external desktop databases in more than basic ways. But even then the middleweights can be useful.

TABLE 11.3 Middleweight databases for Pocket PC.				
Database	HanDBase Plus	HanDBase Pro	Visual CE Lite	Sprint DB Pro
Version reviewed	3.0	3.0	7	1.7a
Footprint	700–750 KB	700–750 KB		850–900 KB
Base price (U.S. $)	$29.99	$39.99	$19.99	$19.89
Desktop companion	Yes	Yes	No, but can synchronize to ODBC databases (i.e., Access, Lotus Approach, Sybase, Oracle, Visual Basic)	No
Limits	200 databases; 65,000 records per database; 100 fields per database	200 databases; 65,000 records per database; 100 fields per database		65365 records per per database; 256 fields per table
Field types	Text, Note, Date, Time, Integer, Float, Popup, Check Box, Unique, Image, Link, Linked, Heading, DB Popup, Calculated, Relationship, Conditional, External	Text, Note, Date, Time, Integer, Float, Popup, Check Box, Unique, Image, Link, Linked, Heading, DB Popup, Calculated, Relationship, Conditional, External	Text, Note, Date, Time, Dropdown lists, Popup, Check Box, Integer (with number pad), Images, Digital Ink, Time (stopwatch) capture, Tabs, Calculated, Relational, Calculated	Text, Integer, Double, Memo, DateTime, Yes/No, Small Integer, OLE Object
Comment		Adds Sync exchange with Access, desktop Forms designer, multiuser synchronization	Capable of real-time wireless access to server data with mEnable product	Support Forms/SubForms, macro script engine, and database functions

Heavyweights

The middleweight products are quite powerful, but still cannot match the complexity of desktop programs like Microsoft Access, FileMaker, or Oracle. Examples of heavyweight tools for creating high-end handheld databases for the Palm OS include Pendragon Forms, Satellite Forms,

FileMaker Mobile, Marietta PDE, IBM DB2 Everyplace, Sybase UltraLite, and Oracle Lite (see Table 11.1). On the Pocket PC, examples include the professional or enterprise versions of Visual CE, Satellite Forms, and Oracle Lite. Some of these products are designed to work only with a single parent product, such as Oracle Lite and Oracle. These tools are for professionals, not beginners. Keen amateurs can make them work too.

For sophisticated databasing projects, you might have to turn to one of these tools. If you do, then you might need to hire a software engineer. In fact the process might be reversed; you might decide to start by finding a database programmer, who in turn will have their own favorite program for developing handheld databases.

You cannot design a heavyweight database on a handheld computer. Instead, the programmer uses the heavyweight desktop computer programs to build a database on the desktop, freezes the design, and deploys the design to a handheld computer along with a small "run-time" engine that enables the extra functionality to work when the handheld's user uses the database. The handheld version of the desktop database is much "lighter" than the desktop version, but still has more functionality than is possible with the middleweights.

Pendragon Forms is an example of this group. You work within a specialized Microsoft Access database to design Access forms that are converted to a Palm file for use on a Palm handheld.[3] Satellite Forms is a similar heavyweight database program that uses a special designing application on the desktop, and then files are converted for use on either Palm or Pocket PC handhelds. Unlike the middleweights, which allow the user to build databases on the handheld, Pendragon Forms and Satellite Forms databases have to be built on the desktop. You cannot modify the database design on the handheld, however.

These sophisticated database systems utilize programming languages like SQL (structured query language) to build queries to manipulate data. There are no software products that allow users to build and redesign this kind of database on a handheld. However, it is possible for programmers to use desktop software like Pendragon Forms, Satellite Forms, Marietta DB, IBM DB2 Everywhere, Sybase UltraLite, and Oracle Lite Consolidator to build databases that have complex query functionality built in. The database design has to be "frozen" and converted to a programming language that the handheld can run.

Over time, distinctions between the middle- and heavyweight database products are narrowing. Third-party utilities increasingly supplement the middleweights to offer some of the functionality previously provided only by the heavyweights. However, the heavyweights remain the best choice for very complex database projects.

Key Points

1. Lightweight database software products let you build very simple databases, but they soon become too limited for most users.
2. Middleweight products satisfy most beginner and intermediate users, and can be made to handle quite complex tasks if you wish.
3. Middleweight products are so cheap, at less than $50, that the biggest problem is deciding which of them to buy.
4. Heavyweight database products tend to be reserved for specialized or high-end databasing projects.

I'm Less Confused, But What Exactly Do I Look for When I'm Deciding on a Database Product for My Handheld?

Distinctions between handheld database software products have blurred considerably since the first products appeared in the mid-1990s. Developers continually add new features to their products to upstage competitors, and third-party developers continue to write utilities that enhance the basic product. All this constant evolution and marketplace variety can be bewildering when you go shopping for a database program.

- Consider the type of project you want to build. If you simply need a single-table, flat file database to store some reference data, use one of the light- or middleweights. If you plan to print regular reports or enter new data regularly, use a middleweight. Consider the heavyweights if you want to deploy databases to multiple users across networks, although the middleweights can handle some of those tasks too.
- Anticipate features you will need. The feature set you need depends on how you will use the product. If you want only two fields for simple databases and intend to use the database only on your own handheld, then a lightweight such as List probably will do. But if you want to build databases with more fields, and want to be able to open, view, and edit your databases on your desktop, then consider the middleweights. If your project demands very precise and complex data management, consider a heavyweight solution.

Key Point

1. Use a middleweight database product if you think you will also use the database on your desktop computer.

Use the Web, Read the Directions, and Try a "Demo" Version: They're Free!

Carefully evaluate the latest version of these products to see if one of them will provide the features that you want for your database project. Most users will be quite content with simple flat file designs, or the basic kind of relational features offered by the middleweights. All the light- and middleweight products come with free demonstration versions. The "demo" software is usually limited, but gives you a good feel for the product.

We recommend that you try the latest product versions posted on the developers' websites before buying one. Most vendors publish their product's manuals online too, which is another good way to compare products.

Key Point

1. Evaluate a database software product by trying the free demo version and reading the product's user manual.

Start by Thinking About the Type of Projects You Will Be Working On

Simple Flat File Databases for Just Yourself

If you will be the only user of your databases, and all you want to do is make simple flat file databases to track simple sets of information, then start with any of the light- or middleweight products, like List (see Figure 11.6) or HanDBase (see Figure 11.1).

If you like to use a desktop program like Access, Excel, or a similar program to print out reports, then pick a middleweight product that comes with a desktop companion program. Then you can export or import data to and from the handheld and desktop database versions. Or, purchase a utility that allows you to set up a conduit that automatically synchronizes your handheld and desktop databases.

For example, say you want to audit your interpretation of head CT scans that you interpret during shifts in the Emergency Department. You need to convince the Department Chief to let you do preliminary CT interpretations at night without waking the radiologist. If this works out, all your colleagues might want to join in by using the database on their handhelds too. Figure 11.10 shows what a HanDBase data collection screen would look like on your handheld for this project (these are illustrated with Palm screenshots, but Pocket PC screenshots are virtually identical, just like the previous CME log example). You don't have a lot of time for entering data on the handheld during shifts, so the idea is collect just enough data to make it easy for your secretary to pull charts and fill in the rest of the data on a desktop computer. Figure 11.11 shows how to speed up data entry by providing a pop-up list of possible diagnoses.

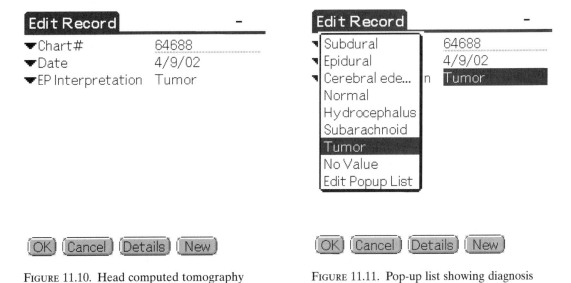

FIGURE 11.10. Head computed tomography (CT) audit data collection screen.

FIGURE 11.11. Pop-up list showing diagnosis choices.

Each time one of you synchronizes your handheld to your computer, the data flow from the HanDBase database on the handheld over your office's Local Area Network to a corresponding Access database on your secretary's desktop. Then, your secretary can open the database in Access to generate an electronic report to e-mail to Medical Records for the charts. When the charts arrive, they can open a Microsoft Access form on the desktop computer to enter the missing data. Figure 11.12 shows what the form looks

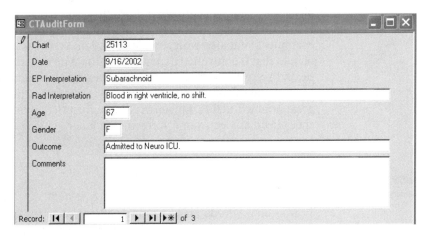

FIGURE 11.12. Head CT audit data modification screen on the desktop (Microsoft Access).

like on the desktop. When your staff finishes entering the data you need, you can use either Access or Excel to analyze the data and complete the audit, mightily impressing the Chief with your ability to interpret head CT's safely in the middle of the night—and your ability to use handheld computers.

Key Point

1. Handheld database software features like pop-up lists make it easy to collect data when you're in a hurry.

Sprucing Up Your Database with a Few Simple Relationships

As you become more familiar with databasing, you might want to design some simple databases that allow you to retrieve information from fields in linked tables—a basic relational database design. Most of the middleweight products have limited relational features that should be adequate for most projects. The CT audit database could be made much more useful by linking the data collection screen to a subdatabase listing standard ICD diagnostic codes, for example.

Relational Databases for Multiple Users

The real power of handheld databasing becomes obvious when you think about collecting data from whole groups of people. The middleweights can be made to work within groups such as a residency program or a group of physicians in practice together. It is fairly easy to share the HanDBase head CT audit among all the physicians in an Emergency Department, for example. Databases with complex relational designs and bidirectional flow of data that is controlled depending on the type of user require more sophisticated software. Group databasing over a network is challenging and can require expert software engineering. The heavyweight products offer much greater functionality for networking enterprises, but they usually require specialized advice from a software engineer.

Key Points

1. Middleweight database products allow you to build simple databases for just yourself to use, or you can share them within a whole group too.
2. Handhelds can be used for a wide range of database projects, from just yourself to sharing data over a network with a whole group.

3. Hire a software engineer for heavyweight database products and more complex projects that involve networking; otherwise, you might founder on unseen rocks.

Make Your Choice Based on the Database Features You Want to Use

The following topics give you a rundown of the specific features you might want to have in a database software product. The computing software term is "feature set." (Kind of like "horsey set," or "tennis set," but less glitzy.) You might not be able to impress anyone at the polo match or "the club" with your knowledge of handheld database feature sets, but this should make it easier for you to decide on a specific product.

Key Point

1. Draw up a list of possible features that you think you will want to have in your database software from the following pages and pick a product that will work for you.

What Types of Fields Can I Have?

All mainstream products support a basic set of field types such as *text* (shorter string of words), *memo* or *note* (longer blocks of words), *number* (integer or floating), *date*, and *time*. Products vary in the number of more specialized field types that they contain, but developers continue to add to their field types over time. The problem for the developers is trying to keep the software compact and simple enough, so they have to trade away some features contained in really powerful, complex desktop computer database software. Most middleweight products seem to be converging on sets of field types with similar capabilities (see Tables 11.2, 11.3). The heavyweight products are capable of quite complex programming and have few limitations such as field types.

The following specialized field types are available in most of the middleweight databases:

- Calculated fields: fields that show the result of a calculation based on previously entered data or data already collected in the database.
- Check boxes: fields that allow the user to enter "yes/no" or "on/off" type of data with the tap of the stylus.
- Relational fields: fields that allow users to link databases and tables.

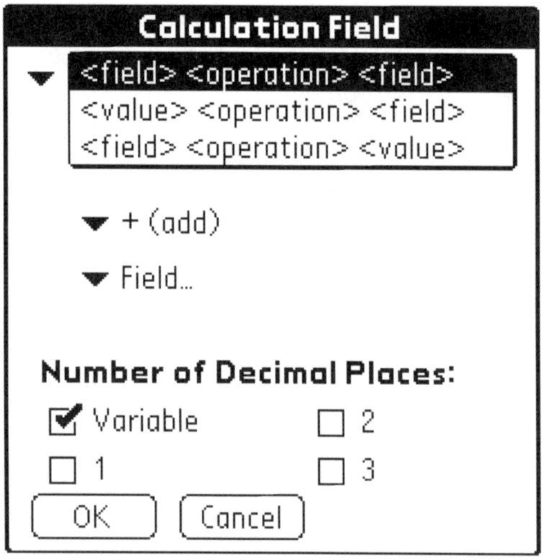

FIGURE 11.13. Creating a calculated field in JFile.

Tell Me More About Calculated Fields: How About Adding Up My Billings?

The middleweight products offer limited calculation capability in the database on the handheld. You can multiply the billing for a procedure by the duration to get a total billing for the session, or you can add up the number of patients you've seen on hospital rounds in a week.

Their simplest implementation works like JFile's calculated field (HanD-Base has very similar functionality for the Pocket PC and Palm platforms; see following). Here are three ways you can combine data to generate a single number with JFile:

⟨field⟩ ⟨operation⟩ ⟨field⟩: example: field 1 + field 3
⟨field⟩ ⟨operation⟩ ⟨value⟩: example: field 1 + 5
⟨value⟩ ⟨operation⟩ ⟨field⟩: example: 8.2 − field 4

Figure 11.13 shows the screen for creating a calculated field in JFile. It's really quite easy to tap on the various down arrows and then select the options you want. Other middleweight programs have slightly different screens for the same task.

HanDBase allows you to build calculated field expressions using up to five different fields or number values, not just two; this gives you a lot of flexibility. Pendragon Forms allows you to build more sophisticated calculated fields using scripts that you write in the advanced properties button of the Forms Designer, using the desktop computer.

The heavyweight products provide the greatest flexibility for programming calculations into databases. Chances are, however, that the middleweight's compromises won't hold you back significantly. Handheld databases do not often require the user to look up calculated results that require complex programming.

Key Points

1. Different products let you create different types of fields.
2. All the middleweight products offer similar basic sets of field types.
3. Some specialized field types available in desktop database software are not available in handheld software.

Designing Pretty Screens: Using Forms

Forms are software layouts that define how the data look on your handheld's screen. Basic default forms in all the products display either several records on the screen in rows with fields in columns (list view), or a single record with field labels in the first column and field contents in the second column (record view). The light- and middleweight products currently do not give users options for changing much more than field order and column width on these default forms.

Here are two examples of record views for the Procedure Log database: one for HanDBase, and the other for ThinkDB. In the standard HanDBase record view (Figure 11.14), note how the fields simply line up in two columns: a label on the right, and the data on the left. All you can do is change the order of the fields, and widen or narrow the data column. The user has to page down to see all the fields in the record. This two-column look is a pretty standard for the industry at present, but there are other options.

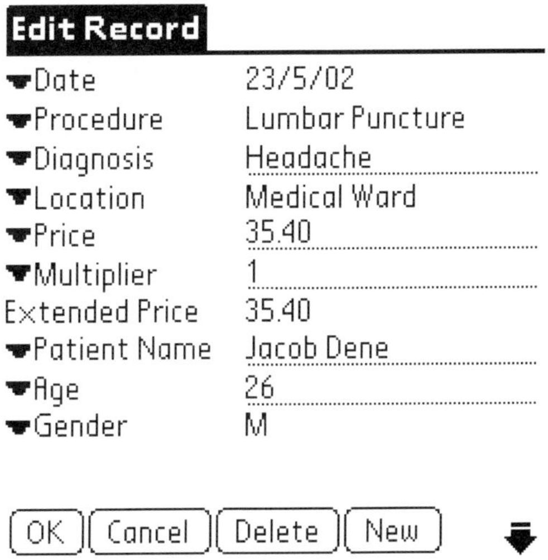

Edit Record

▼Date	23/5/02
▼Procedure	Lumbar Puncture
▼Diagnosis	Headache
▼Location	Medical Ward
▼Price	35.40
▼Multiplier	1
Extended Price	35.40
▼Patient Name	Jacob Dene
▼Age	26
▼Gender	M

(OK)(Cancel)(Delete)(New)   ⬇

FIGURE 11.14. Basic HanDBase two-column record view.

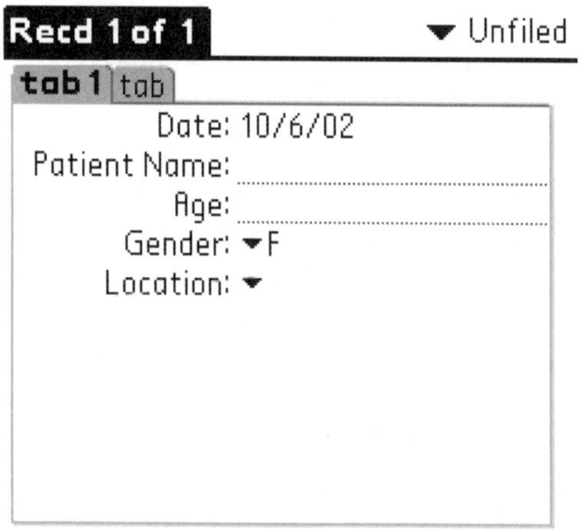

Recd 1 of 1   ▼ Unfiled

tab 1 tab

```
            Date: 10/6/02
Patient Name: ............................
         Age: ............................
      Gender: ▼F
    Location: ▼
```

FIGURE 11.15. Tabbed record view in ThinkDB.

Record views in ThinkDB are only two columns, but notice in Figure 11.15 how I was able to group fields using *tabs*. I put all the patient-related information on Tab 1 and all the procedure-related information on Tab 2. Some users might like this slightly higher level of organization better than paging up and down in other products.

Users get used to a particular form layout once they start using a database. Users who plan to deploy their databases to other people might want more control over form and record view designs, however, because some users might need more "intuitive" screen layouts than the more limited standard two-column record views that these products have provided in recent years.

In 2002 HanDBase version 3.0 introduced much more flexibility over form design. An extra 70-KB utility called "Forms" (what else?) allows you to make customized forms on your handheld. It includes tab capability too. You can also make the forms on your desktop computer using a desktop version of the utility, and then upload the forms to your handheld. On either the handheld or the desktop you can drag and drop fields around the screen, and then let them go where they look best. And you can customize the field labels too. If you have a color handheld then you can choose different colors. Anybody who has version 3 of HanDBase can view the data using your custom forms.

Key Points

1. The basic two-column record view forms in most handheld products work well for most people.
2. Until recently customizing screen forms has required highly specialized programming, but now products like HanDBase make custom form design possible for the masses too.

Can I Enter and Edit Data in Views Other Than Individual Records?

Most light- and middleweight products only allow users to enter and edit data at the individual record level on the handheld. The user taps a virtual button on the screen to open the record, and then enters data in the fields. Some products allow users to enter and edit at least some data types in a list view that shows several records at once. HanDBase, for example, allows users to check or uncheck checkbox fields in list view showing multiple records.

You can use desktop computer programs to set up more flexible data entry and edit mechanisms, if you need that kind of computing power or convenience.

Finding the Edge of the Envelope: What Are the Product's Limits?

Handheld databases can only be so big. In the early days of handheld software, databases were very limited in the number and size of records they could support. Today, however, even middleweight programs can support larger databases than most users will ever need, typically up to 65,000 records.

Handheld memory and processing limitations will constrain some database projects. Users will get frustrated if they have to wait long seconds or minutes for the device to search through a long lookup list. For example, rather than building a lookup table containing the thousands of diagnostic codes, a group should select out the diagnostic codes most relevant to their practice.

All database software restricts the sizes of various elements. For practical purposes most users will never bump into the limits of the middleweight products, although it is wise to check ahead if your project looks big. At the time we wrote this, HanDBase allowed 200 tables (the vendors often call them "databases"), ThinkDB allowed 200, and JFile, 120. Similarly, the number of fields per table is limited: HanDBase 100, ThinkDB 80, JFile 50, and MobileDB 20. However, even the lower limits imposed by these programs will be more than ample for most users. See Table 11.3 for similar technical specifications on the Pocket PC middleweights.

Users are more likely to encounter limits in the number of characters allowed for various field types. Database names in HanDBase can only be up to 19 characters long, for example. Text fields in some product are limited to 254 characters, so use a note or memo field if you anticipate longer text.

Key Point

1. All database software has limitations for all features. Be certain that the product can handle your database design, although the limits in this day and age are so large that most users won't bump into them.

Can I Share My Databases? "Beam Me Up, Colleague!"

Imagine being able to beam your list of patients to your colleague who's stuck covering the weekend! Forget about tediously writing out the list, let alone the chance (slim to none) that he or she will be able to read your writing. Handhelds are a healthcare provider's dream in this scenario, because you can simply beam the database invisibly to your colleague's handheld, eliminating the need for a scrap of paper containing all those valuable data.

Most of the middleweight products contain a Beam function so that you can select a database and beam it through the infrared ports to someone else's handheld. HanDBase even lets you share databases this way between Palm OS and Pocket PC handhelds, if both users already have HanDBase on their handhelds. Or, you can simply e-mail your database to someone else's desktop computer from yours.

Although some products allow you to share your databases, others don't. Some products might require you to purchase special run-time licenses to distribute your databases to other handhelds.

Key Point

1. There are many easy ways to share electronic databases with colleagues, from beaming to e-mailing.

Can I Sort Data on My Handheld to View It Differently?

All the middleweights allow users to sort records, typically using up to three to five fields in a hierarchical order; this usually is more than ample. Figure 11.16 shows how I sorted a HanDBase procedure log on the Procedure field, for example, so that all like procedures are grouped together in the resulting list view (Figure 11.17). With a sort like that you can simply count up the number of times you did a lumbar puncture in the past year. During daily rounds you are more likely to sort the records by fields such as date or patient name.

Can I Filter Data on the Handheld to Show Certain Records and Hide the Rest?

All the middleweights allow users to view selected records, typically with up to five levels of logic. Most products call this "filtering." All you do is tap on the "Filter" button, then select a field from a drop-down list, enter a search string of text or numbers, then tap "Done." The resulting view is a list of all the records containing the search string you entered for the field you selected. You might filter records for a specific date or a patient's name.

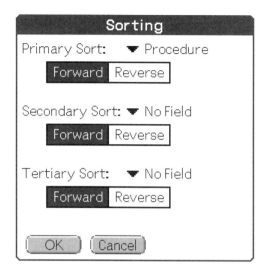

FIGURE 11.16. Sorting records in HanDBase.

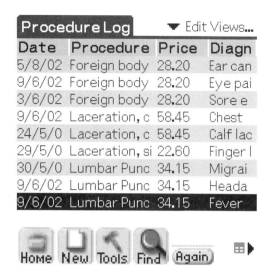

FIGURE 11.17. Records sorted on the procedure field.

In Figures 11.18 and 11.19, we filtered the HanDBase procedure log database to show only "lumbar puncture" in the procedure field. Other products work in a similar way, although their exact procedures and screens are slightly different.

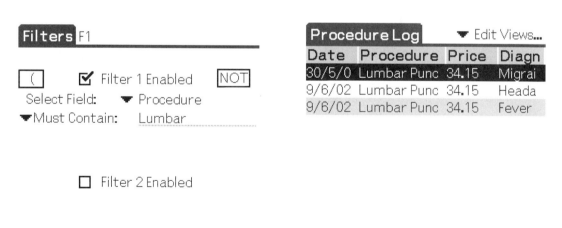

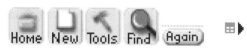

FIGURE 11.18. Filtering for "Lumbar" on the procedure field.

FIGURE 11.19. Records filtered on the procedure field.

Can I Use SQL Language to Automate My Databases?

This is going to be one of those "Do I really need to know this?" sections for a lot of readers, but eventually most people who play with handheld databases need to know what "SQL" means. SQL (structured query language) is a standard language that programmers use to talk to databases. If you want to automate some custom database tasks, or create queries to view your data in more complex ways than the simple (but powerful) default filters provided in simple database software, then SQL is a common way to go.

None of the Palm OS middleweight database products yet allow you to build SQL queries and scripts, but similarly priced Pocket PC products do allow this. Some of the heavyweight Palm OS products allow programmers to build SQL scripts into the database on the computer, and then they freeze the design before uploading it to Palm OS handhelds. Once again, this is an area where paying a programmer, or at least an IT professional, a few bucks to help you out may enhance your project.

Can I Build Relational Features into My Database to Link Tables Together?

This section might be another "Do I really need to know this?" for most of you. Many users will be satisfied with simple, single-table flat file databases. With experience, you might want to exploit some basic relational database capabilities. For some projects, you will have no choice.

For example, you might want to maintain a second table of information, go out from the first table to look up data from the second table, and then return data from selected fields to specified fields in the first table. You can use pop-up lists for short lists of one-column information, but often it is more convenient to maintain the options for a field in a different table entirely. Also, pop-up lists are quite limited in most products, often allowing you to enter only a few dozen items (only 60 pop-up items are allowed in HanDBase, for example). This is a common reason why people start learning how to build relational databases.

In Chapter 17 we show how to build this basic type of relationship into a HanDBase procedure log. First, we build a table to log the patient encounters where we did a procedure. Then, we build a second table containing all the procedures, along with their billing and coding data. Finally, we link the first table to the second, so all you have to do is tap on the procedure's name in the second table to bring all the related data into your log, without laboriously entering it all by hand every time. Except for JFile and MobileDB, the middleweight Palm OS products allow for that simple type of relational lookup capability.

Because of software, operating system, and hardware constraints, relational features on handhelds tend to be more limited than the more powerful kinds of relational functions possible on desktop computers. A handheld computer typically is used to collect or view a subset of the data in a more restricted way than is possible on the desktop, perhaps using some simple relational features such as looking up information for one table from another table on the handheld. Then, after the handheld's data are synchronized to the desktop computer, a database management system can be used on the desktop to set up more complex relationships among the data elements. Thus, although some simple relational features are possible on the handheld, it is best to think of the handheld database as a simpler version of an associated desktop database when planning and using complex relational databases.

The relationships between database components can be much more complex than simply looking up data in another table. Eric Giguère's book describes relational database issues in more detail.[4] He describes how to use a Sybase product called UltraLite to build sophisticated relational database designs that can be used on a Palm or Pocket PC handheld. Database products of this type are beyond the scope of our book, however, and require knowledge of programming tools like SQL (structured query language).

Relational features that work on the handheld might not necessarily be maintained on the desktop after synchronizing. If you need that kind of functionality, then check the product carefully.

Key Points

1. The middleweight database products have limited features for supporting relational database designs.
2. Although some simple relational features are possible on the handheld, it is best to think of the handheld database as a simpler version of an associated desktop database if you intend to use complex relational databases.

Can I Print a List of Patients from My Handheld?

Say you want to print out a paper list of all your inpatients for the coming weekend. You already have a database on your handheld where you record your patients every morning during rounds. What now?

All the Palm middleweight products support printing from handhelds using third-party utilities like PrintBoy; several Pocket PC products like SprintDB Pro and abcDB offer printing-enabled versions that cost $10 more than the standard version. Visual CE requires the purchase of Report CE for an additional cost of $49 for the personal edition. HanDBase supports printing from Palm and Pocket PC handhelds via either infrared, network, or bluetooth using add-on software such as PrintBoy. They work by sending the report through an infrared port to an infrared port on a printer, or through a wire attached to the handheld's serial port connection. So all you have to do is point your handheld at a printer's infrared sensor and tap "Print"!

Reports made directly from the handheld tend to have limited formatting, but they are adequate for simple jobs, such as printing the essentials of a patient's encounter or printing your billings for a session in the operating room.

My Handheld Is Stuffed with Software, So Can I Use the Database on an Expansion Card?

This is a tricky question. RAM (random access memory) capacity is limited in handheld computers. Long before handheld models started coming out with lots of memory, the software that healthcare providers were interested in using soon exceeded the storage memory that was available on existing models.

Expansion memory cards like Secure Digital, Compact Flash, and Sony's Memory Stick are popular with physicians for storing large electronic references (see Chapter 1 for descriptions of the various types of memory cards). But, they are not perfect memory extenders. The memory on these devices does not work the same way that RAM memory does, which means that developers have to program work-around solutions.

All the mainstream handheld database products are evolving to take advantage of handheld expansion memory. They have succeeded to varying degrees. JFile, for example, is VFS compliant (Virtual File System). The main JFile .PRC file and JFile databases can be kept in expansion card memory. JFile shows a "chip" icon beside each database name. Tapping on this icon drops down a list of available cards, allowing you to move the database to one of them. Figure 11.20 lists two cards because my HandEra device has both compact flash and secure digital card slots.

JFile invisibly moves the database from the card's memory to RAM memory for editing and viewing, and then stores them back on the expansion card when finished. This means that there must be enough free RAM memory on the handheld to permit these operations. At the time of this writing, JFile's developers were researching a way to get around having to

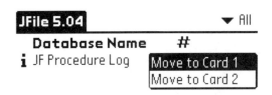

FIGURE 11.20. JFile detected that my HandEra 330 had two cards inserted.

move the database to and from RAM, which will speed operations and free up RAM.

Pendragon Forms uses VFS to allow users to secure databases by backing up individual records to expansion memory cards. HanDBase allows you to both move the main program and databases to an expansion card. But if you do, then the HotSync conduit will not synchronize the databases to the desktop computer automatically. And, like JFile, you must have enough free RAM memory so that HanDBase can silently copy the stored database into RAM when you use it. You should check each product's documentation carefully before using it on the expansion card, whether you have a Palm or Pocket PC handheld computer. This area is also evolving rapidly.

Key Points

1. Database software works on handheld expansion cards, but there are important limitations that you must understand.
2. Expansion card memory does not work like the memory on your computer's hard drive or floppy disks. Not yet, anyway.

Can I Share My Handheld Databases with Others?

Most databases that people write are useful only for themselves or the group they designed them for. But, users often like to share their database designs or content with others. You can modify someone else's database design for your own purposes, for example.

The middleweights allow users to share their databases for free, including both content and design, but typically each user must own their own copy of the parent program. For the Palm OS, each database (table) is stored as a separate PDB file on the handheld and can be backed up as a separate PDB file to the desktop during a HotSync operation. Then you can either beam the PDB file to someone else's handheld, or e-mail the PDB from your desktop computer through the Internet. HanDBase also works this way for Pocket PC handhelds. Visual CE requires purchase of the Enterprise or Professional editions if you want to distribute databases that you create in the program, and SprintDB Pro databases can be distributed using the form file (.raf) and Pocket Access file (.cdb).

The heavyweights vary on this point. Some of these products produce stand-alone software applications that require a run-time version to work on other handhelds, and you might have to pay a royalty to the company when you distribute copies. Or, you might have to license the software for a certain number of users. There are a variety of multiuser solutions. Be sure to check into this before buying if you intend to share your databases with other users.

Can I Run My Databases on Both Palm OS and Pocket PC Handhelds?

Healthcare providers are a mixed group: some use Palm OS handhelds and some use Pocket PC handhelds. So if you do a lot of work to develop a nice database that your group might find useful, will it work on either platform?

Not all handheld database products are cross-platform capable. HanDBase is a market leader in this area. You can beam a HanDBase database from a Palm OS handheld to a Pocket PC through their infrared ports, and the database will open on platforms. And the HanDBase desktop companion program can open either type of database too. Satellite forms is a heavyweight database solution that is available for both Palm and Pocket PC handhelds as is Oracle Lite. Other products might have cross-platform solutions, so if this is an important feature then check out the various products carefully.

That Little Screen Is Pretty Small: Can I Open My Databases on My Desktop Computer?

All but the simplest handheld database apps typically come with companion Windows programs for viewing, editing, printing, and importing or exporting the handheld's databases after they are synchronized to the desktop computer during the HotSync process. Figure 11.21 shows a procedure log database opened in HanDBase's desktop program on my office computer.

Depending on features programmed by the developer, companion programs generally allow the user to do all these tasks:

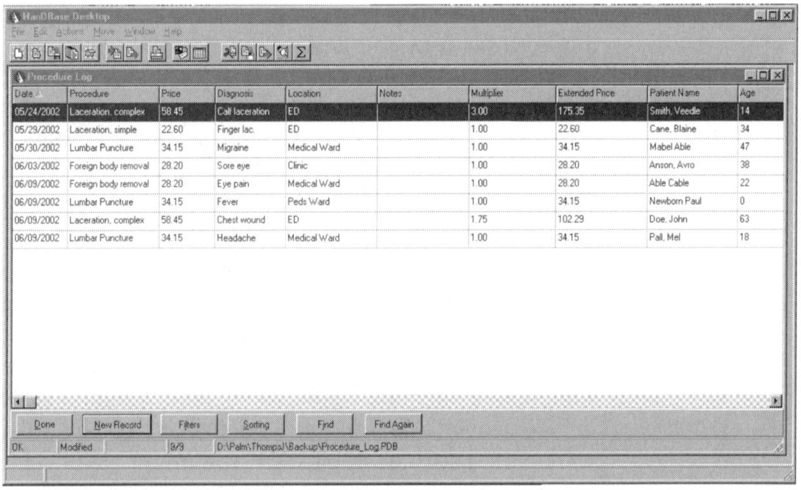

FIGURE 11.21. Procedure log database opened in the HanDBase desktop computer companion program.

- Edit and create database designs, then upload them to the handheld.
- Edit and create database content, then synchronize the changes with the handheld.
- Print reports. Note that reports from these companion programs tend to be very basic, and the user usually has limited or no control over the look of the reports.
- Import and export data to generic formats, typically the CSV (comma separated variable) and TXT (tab separated) file types. Some products can convert to proprietary formats required by popular external desktop programs.
- Export directly into a Microsoft Access database. (HanDBase can do that with a mouse click, for example.)

Although both the database's data and structure can be changed on the desktop, it is not always possible for you to make simultaneous changes on platforms at once. Ensure that the product you use allows for simultaneous bidirectional synchronization, if it is required for your projects.

Not all desktop companion programs preserve relational features on the desktop that work on the handheld. If you need that capability, then check out the products carefully. HanDBase preserves the relational features. Pendragon Forms is a special case. Pendragon's desktop product is a specialized Microsoft Access database that you use to create and modify databases for the handheld. Changes to the database structure (forms) can be made only on the desktop, not on the handheld.

Can I Synchronize My Data on Both My Handheld and My Desktop?

All handheld database programs usually update a copy of their handheld databases on the desktop computer each time you synchronize. Do not assume this most basic synchronization process is happening automatically, however. Always check.

Databases are much more useful if you can make changes to a database on both the handheld and the desktop computer. There are two types of synchronization: one-way and two-way (bidirectional). As an example, let's imagine you create a charge capture database that has a desktop and handheld database (there are several versions already made; these are described earlier in Chapter 8). If your office staff is entering all the office visits on the desktop, and you are out rounding in the hospital and entering your hospital visits . . . what happens when you synchronize? If it is one-way, you will lose data entered on one of the databases (depending on the synchronization rules of the product). But, if the database product has two-way synchronization, the charges entered by the office staff and those entered on your handheld will all synchronize and appear in both databases.

One-way synchronization means that one copy, usually the handheld's, overwrites the other, usually the desktop. When you synchronize your handheld, the software copies the database from your handheld to your desktop computer, or vice versa. Changes to the database on the second device are not uploaded to the first. Usually you can control the way the software works by changing settings in a synchronization control window. This limited type of synchronization might be useful in specialized circumstances.

Bidirectional synchronization means that changes on either the handheld or the desktop are copied to the other device during the synchronization process. There are two forms of bidirectional synchronization.

1. In partial bidirectional synchronization, you can make changes on either the handheld or the desktop copy, and then at synchronization one copy overwrites the other. If a product only supports this level of synchronization, then you have to be careful to make changes in only one version at a time.
2. In complete bidirectional synchronization, you can make changes to the database on either device, and then during synchronization the changes are reflected in both copies at once. When changes have been made to a single record on both devices, you will be given an opportunity to integrate the records manually. HanDBase offers complete bidirectional synchronization, but this feature increasingly is available in other middleweight database products.

As with all the other features that you might wish to have for your database, some projects could require bidirectional functions that can only be achieved by doing specialized programming using one of the heavyweights.

Can I Link My Handheld Database to Access, FileMaker, and Other Desktop Software?

Companion desktop programs that come with handheld database products are useful, but they are not as flexible or sophisticated as full-featured desktop database software like Microsoft Access, Excel, DBase, or File-Maker. But, oh joy!—the handheld version of a database can be linked to one of these external programs, and then you can manipulate or report the data from it. Different products achieve linkages to external database products in different ways.

All the middleweight databases can be linked to external desktop database programs at least semiautomatically by using optional software utilities. Some of these linking utilities are produced by the parent company, others by third parties. Usually the linking process requires a degree of manual intervention by the user each time a connection is made, but automatic linkages are available for some products.

HanDBase's desktop computer program allows you to export your data to and from Microsoft Access by clicking on a menu item, but you only get this capability if you purchase the slightly more expensive package that contains that add-in utility.

MobileDB's Access link is a desktop computer program called MobileDB-Access. The user selects a handheld version of the database, and then presses a button to create an Access version. Their utility works the other way too, to convert from Access to handheld. HanDBase works in a similar manner.

Pendragon Forms databases are directly integrated with Microsoft Access. In fact, the user designs a Pendragon database directly within a special Access database on the desktop. Once the user finalizes his or her design, Pendragon's software automatically creates appropriate forms for uploading to the handheld. Data then flow automatically between the handheld and desktop databases at each HotSync.

Even more flexible and sophisticated connections between database programs are possible. These solutions typically require the services of a consultant software engineer. For example, Sybase' UltraLite synchronizes to an external database on the desktop computer using a specialized Sybase conduit that streams the data to and from a server program (MobiLink) on the desktop.[4] The MobiLink server then synchronizes data to and from any ODBC (open database connectivity)-compliant relational database.

The other Pocket PC middleweight database programs, Visual CE and SprintDB Pro offer connectivity to desktop databases like Microsoft's Access. See their product literature or try out the demo for full details.

Can I Link My Handheld Database with ODBC? (What the Heck Is That, Anyway?)

"ODBC" stands for "open database connectivity." ODBC is a software standard for sharing data between programs. A dynamic link library (DLL) file enables the software to gain access to a data source. Each database program (such as Microsoft Access or dBase) or database management system (such as SQL Server) requires a different driver.

Most handheld database developers are working on or already offer ODBC utilities to connect their programs with external desktop programs. ODBC links, once they are configured and running, allow automated updating between the two software systems. A user enters new data on a handheld and synchronizes. The synchronizing software copies the database from the handheld to the desktop computer in the usual fashion. Then, ODBC software streams the data to and from the other program automatically.

Here's how this can work for you. You might want to use an ODBC link when you routinely prepare reports from your handheld database. Say your scheduling clerk at the clinic wants a nicely formatted Microsoft Word report of the inpatients you have in hospital. Then, he or she can compare that list with your bookings for the day to see if any of the inpatients might be taking up an appointment slot that can be freed for someone else that day. Word is ODBC compliant, so you can build an automated link to Word from your handheld database. When you synchronize your handheld after you get back to the clinic from morning rounds at the hospital, the ODBC link peels off the relevant data and plunks them into the corresponding Word file. Your scheduling clerk opens the file by clicking on its icon on the desktop, and presto! there is a current list of inpatients. Assuming, of course, that you updated the database during rounds. (You did do that, didn't you?)

ODBC software can invisibly automate both data and database structure tasks, offering programmers very powerful options for integrating handheld databases. A handheld database can be integrated with an ODBC-compliant word processing or spreadsheet program, automatically updating a document with the new data, or vice versa.

Can I Secure My Database from Prying Eyes and Fiddling Fingers?

Security means controlling the level of access that users have either to data (viewing, entering, and editing) or to database structure on the handheld. When databases contain sensitive patient data, security is a prime concern.

The middleweights offer varying levels of security. The simplest forms of security are choosing whether the database can be viewed or whether it can be edited (enter or change data). Higher levels of security include features such as preventing some users from viewing or changing data in certain fields, or from changing the underlying database structure, and from printing, beaming, or copying data from the handheld. Some products, such as JFile and HanDBase, allow you to encrypt databases.

Heavyweight products provide the greatest flexibility for security features, because a programmer can build databases nearly from the ground up.

Choose a product that will provide enough control over security for your project. Most individual users probably will not need complex security settings for their own use, but when a group shares a database then the risk of accidental damage to data or the database structure increases. Security problems increase considerably when databases are shared over a computer network. It would be wise to consult a software engineer for larger network projects.

How Do I Network My Database over Multiple Computers in Multiple Offices?

A group of obstetricians might want to share a database containing all the patients with pending deliveries, together with a brief clinical summary on each patient. That way the obstetrician on call can look up a patient's essentials during the night when they are covering for the others. Or, a group of family physicians might want to share similar information about nursing home patients (or their own OB patients) when going on call for the group. Or, a clinic group might want to transmit their billing data for hospital rounds to the billing clerk in their office.

You Can E-Mail Databases over the Internet or Copy Databases over a Network

The simplest way for a group to share databases (but not necessarily the most elegant method) is to e-mail them to the head office where someone manually uploads them to a computer, merges the records with a central repository, and then redistributes the revised database to the group. Or, you can copy them from one computer workstation to another over a network connection. This isn't the kind of automated networking we usually think of with computers, because it requires a lot of manual work at both ends, but it does work.

Obviously there are problems with this simplistic method. Changes would have to be in one direction at a time, unless the merging software could handle synchronization in a more sophisticated way. Users couldn't make changes to their databases in the field while waiting for the group's revised database to be sent out from the head office, for example. And users would have to do the manual labor of copying their databases on a regular basis. Human interaction like that runs the risk of introducing errors.

You Can Synchronize Databases over a Network

Small local area networks (LANs) are common now, so users might want to run their handheld database automatically over a network (see Chapter 15 for more on LANs). An individual user might want to be able to synchronize the database to his or her own workstation by physically synchronizing their handheld at different workstations around the workplace, or even from home. Or a small group of physicians might want to share a central database by synchronizing from several workstations throughout the workplace.

Networking a database is feasible for amateurs, but can be challenging. This is a very attractive market for software designers, so options are rapidly increasing, and even the middleweights offer at least some network capability. In most cases, however, it is wise to employ a software engineer when setting up a handheld network database.

Most middle- and heavyweight products offer solutions for automatically synchronizing databases over a network. HanDBase, for example offers an Enterprise version for both Palm and Pocket PC operating systems that can synchronize multiple users to an ODBC-compliant database such as Microsoft Access.

Summary

So now that we've told you how to create and use databases on your hand-held computer . . . watch out! It's addictive. You will find yourself making databases for everything from your car's last oil change to your relatives' birthdays. The many medical uses will make your professional life simpler, and maybe give you more time to enjoy it.

We have categorized available software products into light-, middle- and heavyweight categories based on their feature sets to help sort out all the issues of picking a product. We provided guidelines to help you choose an appropriate product based on the type of project you might be contemplating, or on the feature set that you think you might need. We did not attempt to review all the database products that are on the market. We gave you a way to make your own choice. We described examples from the more popular middleweight database products to explain how this type of software works. We explained that you could share databases by beaming, e-mail, or networking. Finally, we explained that you could link handheld databases to more powerful desktop computer database software for more extensive data management than is possible on a handheld.

References

1. Fischer S, Lapinsky S, Weshler J, Howard F, Rotstein LE, Cohen Z, Stewart TE. Computerized procedure logging using handheld devices. Mount Sinai Hospital, Toronto, Ontario, Canada. http://www.infiniq.com/products/industry/surgery%20Review%20Final.pdf. Retrieved from the World Wide Web on July 26, 2003.
2. Higgins G. List database of physician fees. http://palmdatabases.tripod.com. Personal communication, used with permission.
3. Sancho D, Phillips I. The Official Pendragon Forms for PalmOS Starter Kit. New York: M & T Books, IDG Books Worldwide, 2000.
4. Giguère E. Palm Database Programming: The Complete Developer's Guide. New York: Wiley, 1999.

12

Software for Nursing: RNs Are Mobilizing

JENEANE A. BRIAN, DANIEL S. BRIAN,
SYLVIA SUSZKA HILDEBRANDT, AND YVONNE STOLWORTHY

It's "nurse Newbie's" first day on the job and Doctor-I-have-the-worst-handwriting-in-the-world leaves an order to administer Z*&^^#(* every day for patient Hackie's I'm-going-to-hack-out-a-lung-with-a-fever disease (yes, you guessed it, she's related to Hattie and Hallie in Chapter 9). The writing is undecipherable except for the Z. Is it Zaditor, Zagam, Zantac, Zebeta, Zerit, Zestril, Zemplar, Zarontin, Zaroxolyn, Zemuron, Zenapax, zanamivir, zafirlukast, Ziagen, zaleplon, Zinacef, Zinecard, Z-max (who's got time to write it out?), Ziac, Zocor, Zofran, Z-pak, Zonegran, Zonalon, Zostrix, Zosyn, Zovia, or Zovirax?

Well, if you guessed Zithromax, you're probably right, but wouldn't it be nice to look it up quickly and effortlessly on a handheld computer, to quickly confirm this with Doctor-I-have-the-worst-handwriting-in-the-world who is also known as Doctor-I-have-bad-phone-manners when called by the nursing staff? And even better would be having Doctor-I have-the-worst-handwriting utilizing a handheld to beam his order regarding patient Hackie directly to nurse Newbie's handheld during patient rounds. This solution would certainly eliminate those daily eyestrain headaches along with those testy calls to the provider for clarification.

Gone are the days when newly graduated nurses were armed with the information they would need for a lifetime of practice. Good nursing practice requires tools to extend the human mind's limited capacity to recall and process large amounts of relevant variables. Handheld computers provide the solution to data access needs and help support the nurse's clinical practice at the point of care.

An even more compelling reason is the opportunity presented by handheld computing to enhance patient safety and care. When the entire healthcare team adopts handheld technology, the elusive improved efficiencies and patient record keeping promised by a standardized knowledge management system might be realized. After all, even Florence Nightingale was known as a "systems person," compiling and analyzing statistics about patient care so effectively that she helped to reduce the mortality rate for hospitalized soldiers from 38% to 2% during the Crimean War. Just imagine how much easier her job would have been if she had a handheld computer!

Clinicians have taken it upon themselves to adopt mobile computing. It is a grassroots movement initiated by physicians when they realized that handheld computers are particularly well suited for data collection, drug reference access, and various medical calculations at the point of care. Handhelds are currently experiencing significant growth in health care. These tiny, powerful computers are being used to support information management, general administration, and clinical practice.

Nurses began to notice the ubiquitous use of handhelds at the bedside by physicians and especially medical students. Their curiosity was piqued. Nurses wanted to know just what was on that electronic organizer that was so clinically useful at the bedside.

The adoption of handhelds for clinical practice by nurses lagged behind physicians by approximately 2 years. As recently as March 2000, conducting an Internet search with the search criteria: "Nurse + Palm", would yield: nurse Jane Doe who lives in Palm Springs. Modifying the search to: "Nurse + Handheld + Computer" returned equally useless results. Why would a nurse want to hold the hand of her computer?

The movement to adopt Personal Digital Assistants (PDAs) in nursing practice closely parallels the adoption of PDAs by physicians insofar as it is a grassroots movement. Web site articles on handheld computers in nursing are starting to appear online, and research on the use of mobile computing in nursing is beginning to be published. Mobile Nursing Informatics will be at the core of nursing in the twenty-first century. Ready access to data and analytical tools will fundamentally change the way practitioners of the health sciences practice, take care of patients, conduct research, and approach and solve problems. Integrating mobile information systems into the practice of health care will add value by helping to decrease costs, increase efficiency, and enhance patient and clinician satisfaction. These mobile computing devices will transform data into valuable information at the point of care. Handheld applications are recognized as significant tools to assist the clinician at the point of care. They support clinicians as does a colleague or a textbook, enhancing their training, experience, and common sense.

Currently, handheld computers are experiencing rapid adoption by nurses. Many of the handheld applications that were developed or adopted by physicians are also useful to nurses. The majority of data collection applications meet the needs of both physicians and nurses. These applications are probably adaptable to other healthcare professionals as well. The same can be said for many of the reference and drug database applications. Yet, nursing is different from medicine, and nurses have different software needs than physicians. As a result, responsive vendors are making nursing references available in handheld format.

Health care is renowned for collecting lots and lots of information. Nursing has its own data collection forms. After collecting this information nurses then need to decide, within their scope of practice, what is wrong with their patients and what they can do to help them. This brings us to nursing diagnoses with specific nursing interventions. In addition to nursing interventions there are medical interventions, physical therapy interventions, dietary interventions, respiratory interventions, and so on. Social work and clergy may also be involved in the care of the patient. Did any of these interventions do anything for the patient or not? Was the intervention a good thing?

To enhance our constant striving for improvement of quality care while participating actively to impact issues related to medication errors, documentation redundancy, and the current nursing shortage, we need to utilize the technologic advances that are at our disposal and those to be developed in the coming years. Nursing-specific handheld applications are needed to augment the care and assessment provided in a wide variety of settings.

Nurses have truly become the "corridor cruisers" of the twenty-first century. Broadly defined, this means any setting where care is provided away from the home base of operation. The common denominator for nursing is documenting patient assessments, interventions, and out-comes. Health care is, and will remain, the most information intensive of all industries.

Lighten Your Load: Use Your Money for Technology, Not Sticky Notes

Imagine all the paper that could be saved if hospitals and healthcare professionals didn't need to buy sticky notes anymore (Figure 12.1). Nurses need one-time data entry that produces usable information and provides legal documentation. A searchable format that allows faster responses

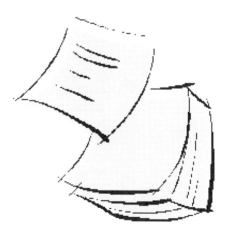

FIGURE 12.1. The ubiquitous sticky notes.

to client needs while providing timely availability of critical information to perform necessary nursing care in any setting is of great value. We need to manage data and information that supports our clinical practice, education, and administration—the value being to support clinical practice management, increase our efficiencies, and decrease costs associated with patient care while providing and improving quality. The data can be transformed at the point of care into valuable information and knowledge along with research through the electronic data collection methods afforded by the use of handhelds.

And what about the student nurses? A student nurse in the 1980s carried around a drug book that easily fit into a uniform pocket and had less than a quarter of the pages contained in today's nursing drug guides. Also in the student nurse's pockets were several file cards that contained information related to each patient assignment. Today student nurses arrive in the clinical area with their arms full of books and calculators! They have nursing drug guides, diagnostic test texts, and enormous medical-surgical textbooks. Do you have any idea just how much those med-surg books weigh?

As the number of drugs and diagnostic tests continues to grow, students cannot possibly be expected to remember the salient features of each. This is most challenging when new orders are written and students need to quickly prepare to continue to provide safe patient care in an ever-changing environment. Even experienced nurses find themselves frequently consulting the pharmacy department, texts, handbooks, and the Internet for information as a result of the rate at which new drugs are being introduced.

Novice nurses will need to carry an armload of resources similar to that of students to accomplish safe and efficient patient care while trying to remain sane. At this time of nursing shortages and shortened orientation programs for new nurses, newly hired nurses need to be extremely self-directed and resourceful. In addition to general resources, they may need several resources that provide information related to the specialty area they may be working in.

Handheld computers shine as a tool for student, novice, and seasoned nurse. In addition to phone numbers and shift schedules, a wide variety of relevant clinical resources can be stored on handheld computers.

Nursing uses for handhelds include but are not limited to recording patient data; drug references and medication dosage calculation; time management; calculation of body surface areas; creatinine clearance rates; chemotherapy regimens; patient satisfaction data collection; evidence-based pathway documentation for diagnosis; risk factor calculators specific to patient assessment and interventions; pain assessment and tracking; and research data collection. The use of handhelds for monitoring individual patients with chronic diseases like asthma and diabetes ultimately could enhance care management and patient teaching and also assist in tracking patient progress, all integral factors in providing quality patient care.

Data Collection Software: How to Get Rid of Your Index Cards and Scraps of Paper

We have all used those sticky notes, index cards, file cards, or organization-made paper scraps (usually recycled forms no longer in use that are cut, stapled, or glued) to record those valuable notes specific to our patients. Now you can keep those same notes, shift change reports, to do items, or what-have-you by using the memo and to do functions built into the handhelds (see Chapter 2: Getting to Know Your Handheld). You may not want to "beam Scottie up," but beaming those notes, addresses, or tasks to the next shift, on-call partner, or peer to share information is a real time-saver.

Documentation software needs to match information in your employer's paper documents, and any efforts to replicate standard institutional paper records usually requires a great deal of time and effort to get official approval. However, there are several software applications that enable nurses to collect information and then transcribe it into the paper documents which make up the health record. These programs allow nurses to enter patient identifiers plus the location of the patient. The program can then be set up so that vital signs and other physical assessment data can be recorded.

Reference Software: Avoiding Shoulder and Back Trauma by Carrying the Dreaded "Med-Surg" Textbook Electronically

More and more references are available in handheld computer format. There are references for medical-surgical information, nursing diagnoses and interventions, and laboratory results and interpretation. Some of the most frequently used references include drug references and medical calculators. Handheld versions of drug references for nurses include the essential elements found in paper versions (Figure 12.2), such as assessment, administration, monitoring guidelines, and patient education. In today's fast-paced world, there is little time at the point of care to make rapid decisions when the reference book tucked into your pocket is outdated or is at the main nursing station. The handheld has become the "cool tool" of choice for rapid deployment of current references on medication administration and monitoring.

Are you feeling like a cat drowning after its first bath (Figure 12.3) from information and work overload, tired of hunting for those outdated referencing texts that disappear when you need them most or all the PC's are in use? Then help is just a pocket away with the handheld and a few clicks of your stylus!

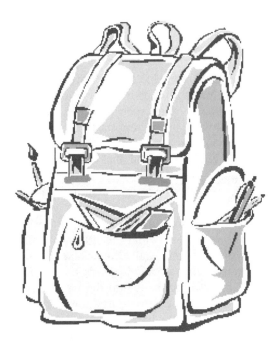

FIGURE 12.2. The heavy way to carry needed references.

Help in the Palm of Your Hand

The following applications represent some of the best available for nursing today. Help is available. With a few clicks and taps on your computer to download (see Chapter 3 for downloading and installing software), you will have the power of information in your hand.

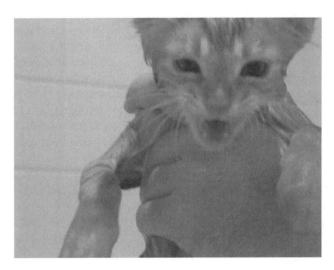

FIGURE 12.3. Bezoar after a bath.

Beginning the Odyssey into Nursing Handheld Computer Informatics

After purchasing and becoming familiar with your dream handheld, begin by downloading some of the free applications that abound on many Web sites. Practice accessing the wealth of information. When you have become familiar with this, and this will not take a great deal of time, think about your needs in relation to your employment setting.

Medication references are a great starting point. Many have 30-day free trial downloads that allow you to "try before you buy." Some of the drug references provide regular updates to help you keep up to date with new drugs and new information about currently used drugs. This is an enhancement over the paper version; purchase of the updated book on an annual basis is required. With the handheld version you get the update as soon as it is available—no waiting. Also, cost should decrease over time because electronic copies are less expensive to produce compared to firing up the old printing press for traditional references.

Many current applications require a minimum of 2 to 5 MB of memory (especially drug references and text books). It will not take long to use the 8 MB that come with the least expensive handheld models. Preplanning can and will save your funds in the future, by purchasing a model with expansion capability (see Chapter 1 for a full discussion on selecting a handheld computer).

Programs You Can Use in Practice (Florence Nightingale Would Have Been Envious)

Nursing Lexi-Drugs (http://store.lexi.com/, $50, or Lexi-Complete for $225) (Palm OS, Pocket PC)

Note: Lexi-Complete includes Lexi-Drugs Platinum, Lexi-Drugs for Pediatrics, Griffith's 5-Minute Clinical Consult, Lexi-Natural Products, Lexi-Poisoning &Toxicology, Lexi-Infectious Diseases, Lexi-Diagnotic Medicine, Lexi-Interact, and Lexi-Drugs for Nursing.

Many nurses have carried and accessed Lexi-Comp's Drug Information Handbook for Nursing. The company astutely provided the identical information for handhelds that is available for both the Palm OS and Pocket PC. Purchase of the product allows the complete application and updates for 1 year from the date of purchase, and 4780 medications are available, with information on administration (oral, I.M., I.V., etc.). Patient Education, Assessment, Pregnancy Issues, Lactation, and Geriatric Considerations are included (with up to 34 data fields depending on which version is purchased). Lexi-Comp (http://www.lexi.com) is the first to offer IR (infrared) printing capability for their product through the use of a patient advisory leaflet, in addition to offering translation into alternative languages.

After opening the application (which will occupy a spot on your hand-held's list of applications), the usual choices are an alphabetical listing, or categorical or therapeutic classification. If you are uncertain, always choose the alphabetical listing. Once the medication is chosen, the data fields, such as generic name, dosage parameters, mode of administration, and contraindications, are accessible via a drop-down list on the left-upper screen. Simply choose what you want to review. A screen tap anywhere will take you back to the beginning of that drug description.

After opening the application screen, choose the alphabetical listing and enter the drug name. Tap the stylus on your drug choice where you will see the information available for further investigation. Nurses will be particularly interested in the administration, warnings, precautions, pregnancy implications, contraindications, and ethanol/nutrition/herb interactions as well as the patient teaching information (Figure 12.4).

For example, consider the medication amphotericin B (Figure 12.5). Now just what did Dr.-I-have-the-worst-handwriting want? the conventional or amphotericin B Cholesteryl, Deosycholate, or the lipid based? For simplicity's sake, let's look at amphotericin B because the patient is being treated for the antiinfective/fungal effect. Besides the usual information you want to review, administration types are important.

Knowledge of special warnings and precautions is an integral function of nursing. These are noted under the fields by tapping the down arrow next to General. Your "choose list" includes these subfunctions (Figure 12.6).

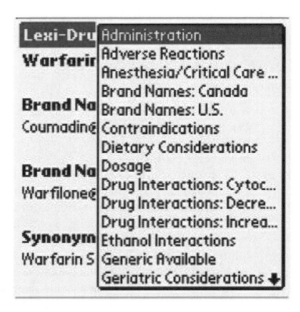

FIGURE 12.4. Lexi-Drugs: category selector (Palm). (Reprinted with permission from Lexi-Drugs.)

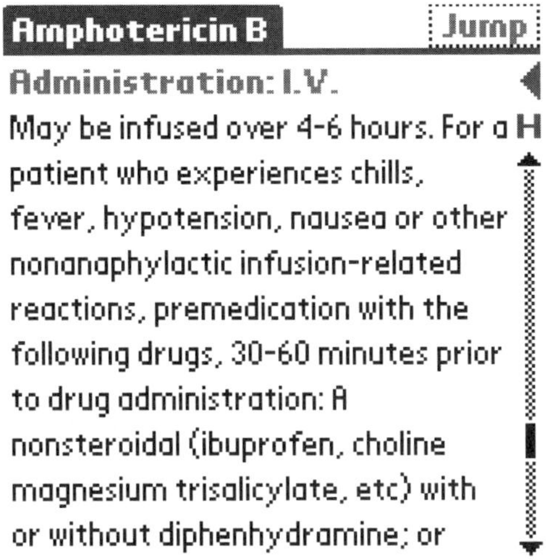

Amphotericin B   Jump

Administration: I.V.   ◀

May be infused over 4-6 hours. For a H
patient who experiences chills,
fever, hypotension, nausea or other
nonanaphylactic infusion-related
reactions, premedication with the
following drugs, 30-60 minutes prior
to drug administration: A
nonsteroidal (ibuprofen, choline
magnesium trisalicylate, etc) with
or without diphenhydramine; or

FIGURE 12.5. Lexi-Drugs:
Amphotericin B—
Administration. (Reprinted
with permission from Lexi-
Drugs.)

Amphotericin B   Jump

Warnings/Precautions   ◀

Avoid additive toxicity with other H
nephrotoxic drugs. Monitor BUN and
serum creatinine, potassium, and
magnesium levels every 2-4 days,
and daily in patients at risk for
acute renal dysfunction. I.V.
amphotericin is used primarily for
the treatment of patients with
progressive and potentially fatal
fungal infections. Topical

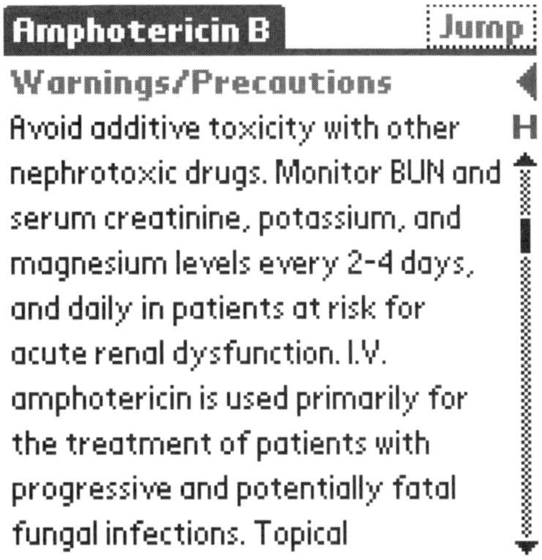

FIGURE 12.6. Lexi-Drugs: Amphotericin B—
Warnings/Precautions. (Reprinted with
permission from Lexi-Drugs.)

Another closely related task is physical monitoring and assessment of the patient (Figure 12.7). Patient education is as critical as assessment. Nurses need this information to be available on the spur of the moment, relevant, and current with the approved FDA recommendations (Figure 12.8).

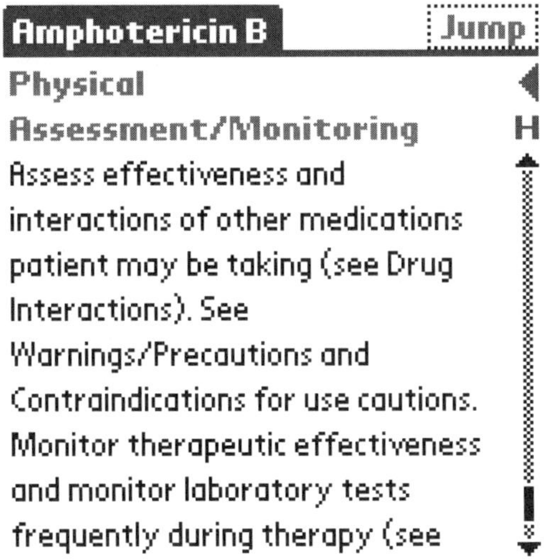

Amphotericin B   Jump

Physical   ◀
Assessment/Monitoring   H

Assess effectiveness and
interactions of other medications
patient may be taking (see Drug
Interactions). See
Warnings/Precautions and
Contraindications for use cautions.
Monitor therapeutic effectiveness
and monitor laboratory tests
frequently during therapy (see

FIGURE 12.7. Lexi-Drugs: Amphotericin B—
Physical Assessment/Monitoring. (Reprinted
with permission from Lexi-Drugs.)

Amphotericin B   Jump

Patient Education   ◀

Take/use as directed; complete full H
regimen of treatment (most skin
lesions may take 1-3 weeks of
therapy). Maintain adequate
hydration (2-3 L/day of fluids
unless instructed to restrict fluid
intake). You may experience
nausea, vomiting, or anorexia
(small frequent meals, frequent
mouth care, sucking lozenges, or

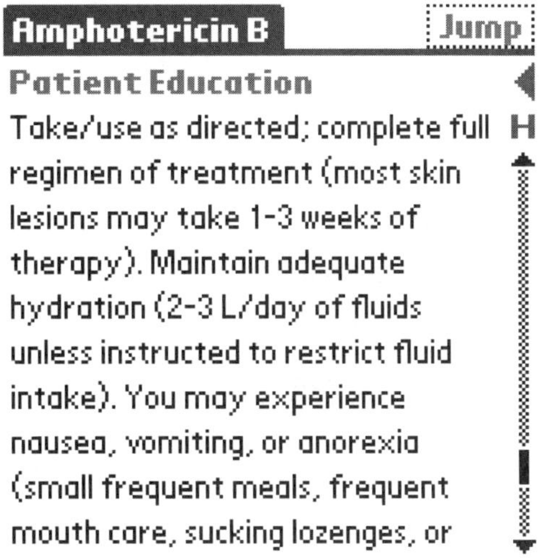

FIGURE 12.8. Lexi-Drugs: Amphotericin B—
Patient Education. (Reprinted with permission
from Lexi-Drugs.)

Davis Drug Guide for Nurses (http://www.skyscape.com/, $49.95) (Palm OS, Pocket PC)

This handheld reference provides a detailed, up-to-date, and practical resource for Palm OS, and Pocket PC handheld devices. It has more than 1000 drug monographs covering more than 5000 trade and generic drugs as well as herbal products. There are more than 150 drug classifications covering both therapeutic and pharmacologic. In addition, there are more than 500 commonly used combination drugs, including the dosage amount of the active generic ingredient.

Also available from F.A. Davis Company (http://www.fadavis.com) for Palm OS, and Pocket PC handhelds is the oft-used Tabers Cyclopedic Medical Dictionary. Figure 12.9 provides a sneak peek of the available options after opening the application.

The Table of Contents screen contains specific choices from drug monographs, combination drugs, and naturopathic, pharmacologic, and therapeutic classifications (Figure 12.10). Each medication has numerous field searches, as indicated by the drop-down list shown in Figure 12.11.

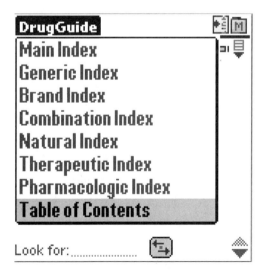

FIGURE 12.9. Davis Drug Guide: Available options after opening the application. (Reprinted with permission from F.A. Davis Company.)

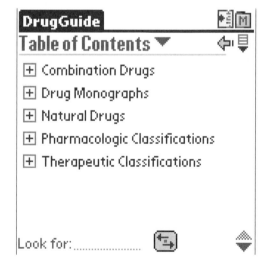

FIGURE 12.10. Davis Drug Guide: Table of Contents. (Reprinted with permission from F.A. Davis Company.)

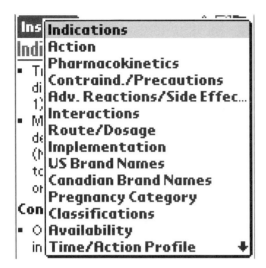

FIGURE 12.11. Davis Drug Guide: Field drop-down list. (Reprinted with permission from F.A. Davis Company.)

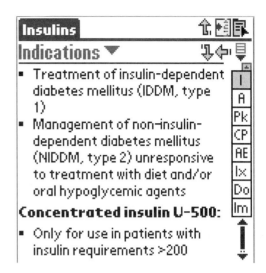

FIGURE 12.12. Davis Drug Guide: Insulins. (Reprinted with permission from F.A. Davis Company.)

If you choose to preview the indications for a specific drug such as insulin, the following information will be shown on the handheld screen (Figure 12.12).

General Reference Applications

PEPID RN (http://www.pepid.com, $59.95–$139.95, subscription 6–24 months) (Palm OS, Pocket PC)

For the price of a daily latte, you too can have a first-class point-of-care reference tool nicknamed the 5-minute clinical consult for nursing.

This database contains 1500 nursing presentations combining clinical content (complete with Nursing Considerations) on diseases and conditions, with weight-based dosing and body surface area calculators, health and wellness teaching guides, and a complete drug database to assist clinical nurses with the problems and decisions encountered in the normal course of treating and planning care for their patients. Labeled the Clinical Nurse Companion, its strengths include applicability to daily practice and the convenience of having a comprehensive, portable database available wherever and whenever additional information or decision support is needed. Also included are the nuclear, biological, and chemical weapons information along with an integrated dosing calculator for weight-based and body surface area-based dosing. Access is at http://www.pepid.com.

On opening the application, the Table of Contents will be visible (Figure 12.13). Choosing General Nursing from this list allows further separation of search functions (Figure 12.14). Choosing Pain Management provides separate fields to allow specific subsets to be reviewed and utilized with patient care and teaching (Figure 12.15).

In addition to the aforementioned functions, nurses can alphabetically search individual diagnoses (Figure 12.16). There are certainly numerous

PEPID RN
Table of Contents

Index
General Nursing
System And Specialty Nursing
Health & Wellness
Drug Reference
Toxicology
About PEPID

GENERAL NURSING

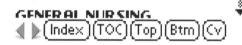

FIGURE 12.13. PEPID RN: Table of Contents. (Reprinted with permission from PEPID RN.)

GENERAL NURSING

Procedures
Pain Mgmt
Electrolyte Imbalances/ABG's
Drug Interactions
Vascular Access Devices
Equations, Formula, Normals
Medicolegal

SYSTEM AND SPECIALTY NURSING

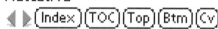

FIGURE 12.14. PEPID RN: General Nursing selected from Table of Contents. (Reprinted with permission from PEPID RN.)

PAIN MANAGEMENT

General Principles and Definitions
Pain Assessment
Pain Interventions
High Risk Patients
Special Circumstances
Patient Teaching/Discharge Instructions
Legal and Regulatory Considerations

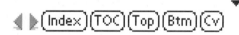

FIGURE 12.15. PEPID RN: Pain Management selected from General Nursing. (Reprinted with permission from PEPID RN.)

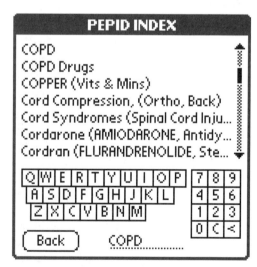

FIGURE 12.16. PEPID RN: Alphabetical Diagnosis search function. (Reprinted with permission from PEPID RN.)

[REL. TOPICS]

Crohn's vs. Ulcerative Colitis (Differentiation)

95% of Crohn's can be distinguished from UC by following factors (i.e., Crohn's has following and UC does not):
1) Small bowel involvement
2) Rectal sparing
3) Absence of rectal bleeding
4) Segmental or symmetrical

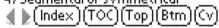

FIGURE 12.17. PEPID RN: Related topics for the chosen set of field entries. (Reprinted with permission from PEPID RN.)

[REL. TOPICS] [INRX]

Dopamine (Intropin)

Dosing
- Adult:
  - Low dose: 0.002-0.005mg/kg/min IV 🔲
  - Medium dose: 0.005-0.015mg/min IV 🔲
  - High dose: 0.02-0.05mg/kg/min IV 🔲
  - Titrate to response

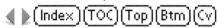

FIGURE 12.18. PEPID RN: Find quick information on treatments and medications. (Reprinted with permission from PEPID RN.)

medical diagnoses with similar symptoms where some comparison would be beneficial. The top-right corner always affords the opportunity to view related topics for the chosen set of field entries (Figure 12.17).

There is also the ability to find quick information on treatments and medications (Figure 12.18). The screen shown in Figure 12.19 illustrates options for treatment of infections.

Besides offering a special section on biological warfare symptoms and treatments, PEPID has made special calculators available in the application. Begin with the conversion for weight (Figure 12.20). Enter the appropriate number (Figure 12.21). Click "Calculate," and a wealth of options is displayed, such as the example of Dopamine IV with the appropriate amounts by weight in solution (Figure 12.22).

Nursing Care Plans (http://www.handheldmed.com, $45) (Palm OS, Pocket PC)

Comprehensive guidelines for nursing care plans encompass total patient needs, including the physical aspect as well as cultural, sexual, nutritional, and psychosocial needs. Available for Palm OS or Pocket PC handhelds.

Nursing Diagnosis (http://www.pdacortex.com/) (Palm OS)

Nursing Diagnosis is a quick reference guide to search the nursing diagnosis; it is compiled according to the North American Nursing

Treatment/Disposition

1) Bedrest

2) IV antibiotics x 2wks, then PO x 4wks (choice of Abx depends on suspected route of infection & similar to those for Osteomyelitis, Acute)

3) Broad spectrum coverage first then narrow as culture & sensitivity available (Vancomycin plus Cipro OR Nafcillin or Oxacillin PLUS Cipro)

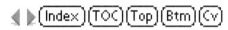

FIGURE 12.19. PEPID RN: Options for treatment of infections. (Reprinted with permission from PEPID RN.)

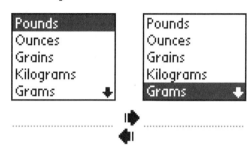

PEPID Conversion Calculator

▼ Weight

Pounds		Pounds
Ounces		Ounces
Grains		Grains
Kilograms		Kilograms
Grams		Grams

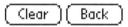

Tap on arrow to convert value.

(Clear) (Back)

FIGURE 12.20. PEPID RN: Conversion Calculator. (Reprinted with permission from PEPID RN.)

Drug Calculation

Dopamine

To obtain proper dose will require:

weight

If you don't know weight, (Calculate it)

▼ Weight   80|

☐ kg   ☑ lbs

(<- Back) (Calculate)

FIGURE 12.21. PEPID RN: Drug Calculation. (Reprinted with permission from PEPID RN.)

Drug Results   Back

Dopamine

0.005 - 0.15 mg/min/kg; incr. heart

Patient wt: **36.28 kg**   (Recalc)

0.181–5.44 mg/min

IV

2.3-70 mL of 40 mg/500mL

1.1-35 mL of 80 mg/500mL

0.55-17 mL of 160 mg/500mL

FIGURE 12.22. PEPID RN: Drug Calculation Results. (Reprinted with permission from PEPID RN.)

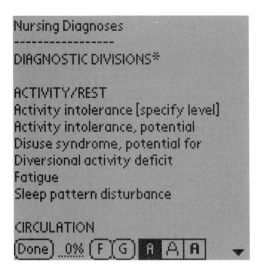

FIGURE 12.23. Nursing Diagnosis: Diagnostic Divisions.

Diagnosis Association (NANDA) list. This is a freeware program by Man King Kwong and requires the iSilo reader that is available from http://www.isilo.com (Figure 12.23).

Red Book 2003 (http://aapredbook.aappublications.org, $149.95) (Palm OS, Pocket PC)

Nurse change-a-job works for Dr.-I-always-forget-the-recommendations-for-the-catch-up-schedule-for-DTaP. Patient Sally has a parent who has moved frequently during her young lifetime; she is now entering kindergarten next week and there are only two listed immunizations, at ages 2 and 18 months. Doctor forgetful passes you her chart saying "Give her what she needs to begin school next week." Luckily you are a technology-savvy nurse and can pull out your handheld to check the current recommendations for catch-up immunizations for this age group.

Red Book 2003 is the American Academy of Pediatrics' guideline for control of infectious diseases in children. This book contains a composite summary of current AAP recommendations concerning infectious diseases in and immunizations for infants, children, and adolescents. This application is fully indexed for rapid retrieval of data and features a Summary of Major Changes to assist clinicians in assimilating those changes from previous recommendations. The subscription price also includes on-line access to the text.

The following applications (also see Chapter 7 for download locations.) contain useful information for nursing-specific references. The Merck

Manual contains references for vitamin and mineral deficiencies plus toxicity along with specific information on diets.

Merck Manual

The Merck Manual covers all subjects expected from a leading internal medicine textbook and provides detailed information on a multitude of topics, including pediatrics, gynecology, psychiatry, ophthalmology, otolaryngology, and dental disorders.

HarrietLane

Any nurse practitioner will delight in having this reference available for the quick-and-easy format to search current diagnostic guidelines. This application holds all the practical information you need from The Harriet Lane Handbook in the handheld format. Use this best-selling medical reference at bedside for easy access to diagnostic guidelines, recommended tests, therapeutics, and dosage schedules. Skyscape (http://www.skyscape.com) creates innovative ways of navigating through this information so that you can access solutions to the treatment of children in seconds.

Continuing Education Tracking (http://www.pdasoftnet.com/mce)

For any certification maintenance in nursing, tracking classes and credits are no longer a nightmare of certificates and papers that are easily lost. Included functions are the ability to filter the record by date range, sort by course title/date, and display a running total for all your credits earned. There is also an extra notes field for entering additional info.

RNLabs (http://www.skyscape.com, $43.95) (Palm OS and Pocket PC)

RNlabs is an application based on the Nurse's Manual of Laboratory and Diagnostic Test by FA Davis and Skyscape. This handheld gem for nursing combines the background information and clinical applications data for hundreds of laboratory and diagnostic tests. Focus is geared toward care before, during, and after the performance of the tests.

Each test is covered in a single, integrated monograph with a description of the procedure, with reference values (adults, children, infants) in conventional and SI units. Indications, contraindications, and step-by-step procedure are included. Special "nursing alerts" call attention to clinical implications of tests.

Options from the initial screen on opening the application are as shown in Figure 12.24. Simply tap which section you want to open. Let's say you choose section 1. An alphabetical list appears. You would like more information regarding triglycerides. After choosing that option, the real fun

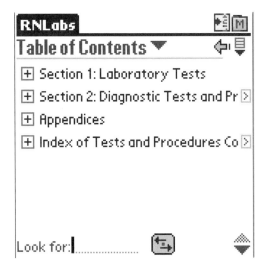

FIGURE 12.24. RNLabs: Table of Contents.
(Reprinted with permission from Skyscape.)

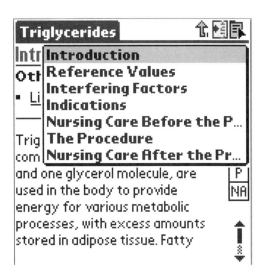

FIGURE 12.25. RNLabs: Test-related drop-down
list. (Reprinted with permission from Skyscape.)

begins with the ability to view individual sections of interest. Or, you can
scroll through the whole listing.

The field drop-down list contains the parameters for subsets that address
the nursing process and quality nursing care issues (Figure 12.25). Tapping
another choice would bring up the procedures information, where again
you can choose a single procedure for more in-depth information (Figure
12.26).

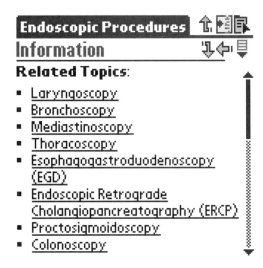

FIGURE 12.26. RNLabs: Procedures List. (Reprinted with permission from
Skyscape.)

RNDiseases (http://www.skyscape.com, $45.95) (Palm OS, Pocket PC)

This application, based on *Diseases and Disorders: A Nursing Therapeutics Manual*, contains complete information on 241 disorders providing a quick search to understand the disorder and effectively plan nursing care. This is an ideal reference for community health and clinical settings. Each entry begins with the Diagnosis Related Groups (DRG) covering causes, pertinent physical and psychosocial findings, lifespan considerations, and primary nursing diagnosis along with collaborative and independent nursing interventions. Special emphasis is on patient teaching and home care essentials, including documentation and discharge planning and teaching.

Unique to nursing is our diagnosis paradigm, along with how we get where we are going and why. This is your first day doing home visits, and your first patient has a multitude of diagnoses. Where do you begin your assessment? Pulling out your trusty handheld provided by the agency, you begin the process by looking at the Table of Contents (Figure 12.27), where you find the subcategories of the Nursing Process and Nursing Diagnosis. A sigh of relief. You are not alone: Skyscape's Nursing Diagnosis to the rescue!

Enter your choice from the table of contents for a specific DRG, and off you go again with the tap and choose functions (Figure 12.28). Individual nursing diagnoses can be searched for additional information for interventions within the subcategory. This function provides specific actions com-

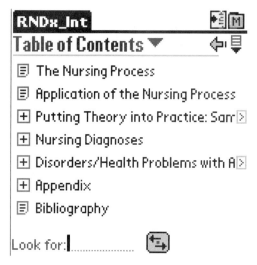

FIGURE 12.27. RNDx_Int: Table of Contents. (Powered by Skyscape. Reprinted with permission.)

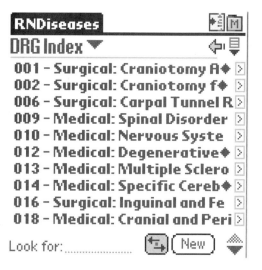

FIGURE 12.28. RNDiseases: DRG Index. (Powered by Skyscape. Reprinted with permission.)

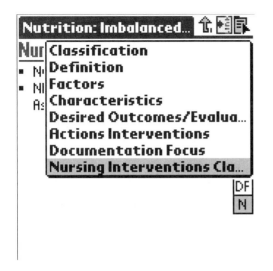

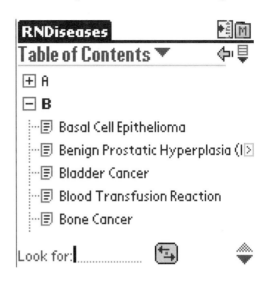

FIGURE 12.29. RNDiseases: Nursing Diagnosis-Related drop-down list. (Powered by Skyscape. Reprinted with permission.)

FIGURE 12.30. RNDiseases: Alphabetical listing of nursing-specific information. (Powered by Skyscape. Reprinted with permission.)

plete with the documentation necessary. Nutrition imbalance is a prime example of the needed nursing interventions you can provide to the patient and family (Figure 12.29).

Do you need additional nursing-specific information on a particular disease? The beloved alphabetical listing makes this an easy process. Scroll and tap your choice (Figure 12.30).

This application needs little practice to quickly extract and review the variety of fields for a complete picture of the process for evaluation and documentation of the nursing process complete with interventions that have been proven.

Calculators and Conversion Applications (Where Were These Gems in Nursing School?)

Individual practice areas need to be considered with regard to what is needed. The following are a few examples of tried-and-true applications. It is no longer prudent waiting for Dr. I-don't-have-time-to-answer-your-questions, when nursing decisions are needed immediately. This is an essential nursing function, especially in the ICU arena, whether you are the staff nurse, nurse practitioner, or head nurse for that service. These programs have been covered in the previous chapter on calculators and are mentioned here specifically for nursing's need to know. These applications are also reviewed by the docs in Chapter 6.

MedMath (http://smi-web.stanford.edu/people/pcheng/medmath/index.html, freeware, Palm OS)

MedMath is a medical calculator for the Palm Computing Platform. It is designed for rapid calculation of common equations used in adult internal medicine.

Most calculators and conversion applications are simply a matter of entering data, generally with a handy visible keyboard. Once the data are entered, tap the calculate button and the solution is processed with lightning speed (Figure 12.31).

MedCalc (http://www.palmgear.com, freeware, Palm OS)

This medical calculator runs on Palm OS handheld devices. The design is a rapid calculation of common equations used in internal medicine. Approximately 73 formulas are available. Specific to the variety of measurements used, generally one can enter either pounds or kilograms. Variety is the spice of life, and having at your fingertips the formulas needed for any practice arena is essential. Some of the choices available follow in Figure 12.32.

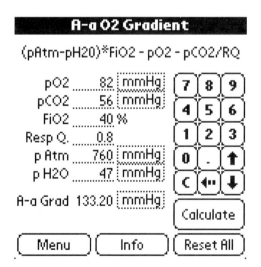

FIGURE 12.31. MedMath: Calculating A-a Gradient. (Reprinted with permission from MedMath.)

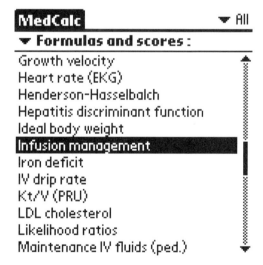

FIGURE 12.32. MedCalc: 73 formulas listed alphabetically. (Reprinted with permission from Mathias Tschopp, MD)

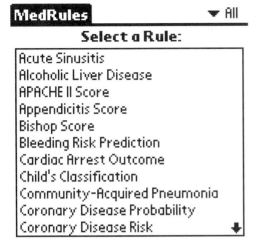

FIGURE 12.33. MedRules: Clinical prediction rules (educational tool). (Reprinted with permission from Kent E. Wilyard, MD.)

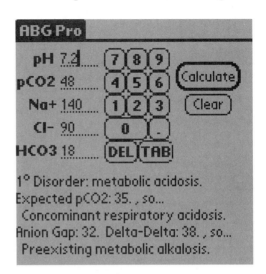

FIGURE 12.34. ABG Pro: Arterial blood gas analysis. (Reprinted with permission from StacWorks.)

MedRules (pbrain.hypermart.net, freeware, Palm OS)

This application features useful clinical prediction rules taken from the medical literature. Complete references for each rule may be found by clicking the question mark icon in the upper-right corner of the screen. *Note: This application is for educational use only. It should not be used to make decisions affecting patient care.*

Selecting rules for specific scores can save time and the eternal brain searches for the correct computational formulas (Figure 12.33).

ABG Pro 2.2 (http://www.pdacortex.com, freeware, Palm OS)

A program that will completely analyze arterial blood gases for you! No longer will you be confused by ABGs. Not only will the program tell you whether or not you have a metabolic or respiratory acidosis or alkalosis, but it will also calculate expected PCO_2 and expected HCO_3 when needed, and will then tell you if there is a concomitant acid–base disorder (Figure 12.34).

Doser 4.2 (http://www.pdacortex.com, freeware, Palm OS)

This is a program that calculates mcg/kg/min, mg/kg/hr, mcg/kg/hr, mg/kg/min. It is useful for calculating various drug infusions (Figure 12.35).

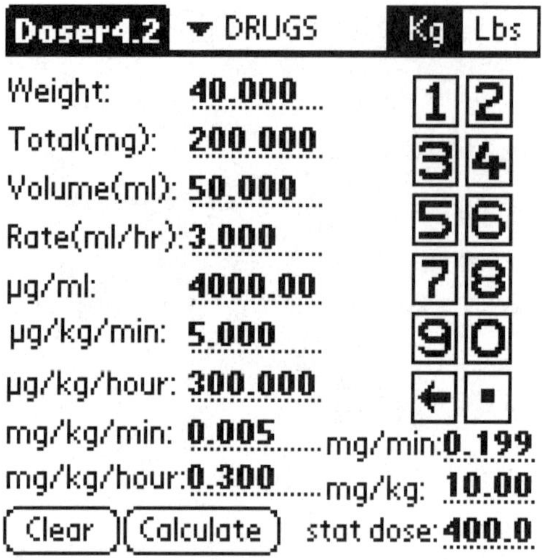

FIGURE 12.35. Doser: Calculate drug infusions.

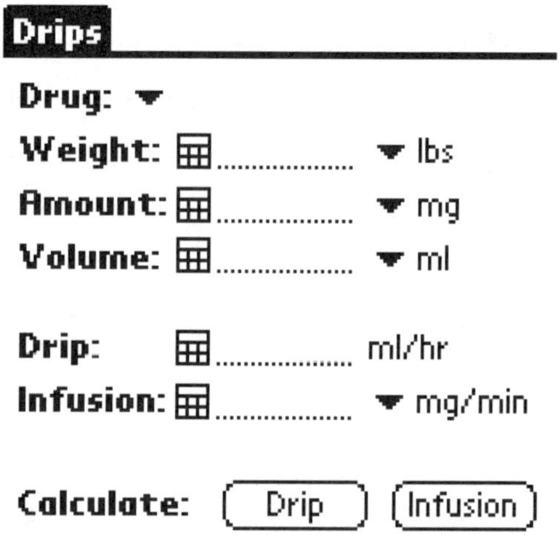

FIGURE 12.36. Drips: Calculate IV doses; save and beam frequently used calculations.

Drips (www.pdacortex.com, freeware, Palm OS)

An application that calculates I.V. doses for drugs, this allows use of multiple units, for example, lbs versus kg or mcg/kg/min versus mg/min. You can save frequently used patterns/drug mixes, and also beam them (Figure 12.36).

Numerous applications also have those highlighted down arrows, which when tapped give you additional choices for entering data.

RSI (http://www.pdacortex.com, freeware, Palm OS)

RSI (Rapid Sequence Intubations) is a program that Spiros Kontas, RN, developed for Medflight of Ohio. RSI is invaluable for any nursing professional working in a setting that would require intubations and quick access to the necessary information on medications for adults and children. RSI calculates drugs used in their rapid sequence intubation protocol (adult and pediatric), just by entering the weight (Figure 12.37).

PICU 3.0 (www.pdacortex.com, freeware, Palm OS)

You are working evenings, having been assigned to the Pediatric Intensive Care Unit, and a code is called for bed 2. As you are the designated recorder this evening, this application proves to be a lifesaver not only for the patient but also for your documentation of events.

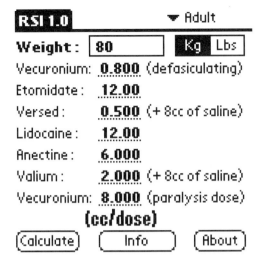

<table>
<tbody>
<tr><td>

RSI 1.0   ▼ Adult

Weight : [80]   Kg Lbs

Vecuronium: **0.800** (defasiculating)

Etomidate : **12.00**

Versed : **0.500** (+ 8cc of saline)

Lidocaine : **12.00**

Anectine : **6.000**

Valium : **2.000** (+ 8cc of saline)

Vecuronium: **8.000** (paralysis dose)

(cc/dose)

(Calculate)   (Info)   (About)

</td><td>

P.I.C.U. 3.0   ▼ Reanimation

Weight : [25]   Kg Lbs

Defibrilation : **50.000**

Adrenalin : **2.500**

Atropine : **1.250**

NaHCO3 : ....**25.000** **ML/DOSE**

Bretylium : **2.500**

Lidocaine : **1.250**

CaCl2 : **5.000**

D50% : **50.000**

(Calculate)   (Info)   (About)

</td></tr>
</tbody>
</table>

FIGURE 12.37. RSI: Rapid Sequence Intubation protocols.

FIGURE 12.38. PICU: Pediatric ICU calculator.

A rapid input of the patient's weight is all that is needed for this calculation to occur. The display is in ml/dose. In the Vasoactive section, the medications are calculated by mg/50 ml of solution. The concentrations were based on the Cardiac surgery protocol at Sainte Justine's Pediatric Hospital in Montreal, Canada. There are three main categories: reanimation, intubations, and vasoactive for calculation. Each category contains the needed drugs and solutions necessary for the category. This screen could also serve as a record for documentation and disposition of the patient. This is a well-thought-out application that responds to the situation at hand (Figure 12.38).

Patient Tracking

RN Floor (www.pdacortex.com, $14.99, Palm OS)

This is a comprehensive nursing application for tracking and planning patient care and recording information. It tracks patient demographics, diagnosis, previous history, MD info, medication schedule, tests, procedures, vitals, IVs, activity, nutrition, respiratory, fluid balance, dressings/drains, discharge planning and code status and last dose of meds. Set reminders for next dose of meds, vitals, blood glucose test, turns, dressings, procedures, and tests. Also includes GCS (Glasgow Coma Score), Apgar, and calculators for drip rate, drug dose, pediatric weight/vital signs, and pregnancy wheel. Areas to record continuing education, shifts, OT (overtime), expenses, passwords, and work-specific phone numbers are also included. Beam your info to coworkers at shift change. Other titles applicable to nursing are RN Obstetrics, RN ER, OB tracker, and PediTracker, available at http://www.palmgear.com.

Multipurpose Applications

CogniQ by Unbound Medicine (http://www.unboundmedicine.com/cogni.htm) is an enterprise subscription service for the mobile professional (this is also reviewed in Chapter 7 by the docs). Search journals, drug information through A–Z Drug Facts, Clinical Evidence, MedWeaver Diseases, Drug Interaction facts, and Medline through this service. This knowledge base will revolutionize the way you utilize and share content. Subscription information and changes are Web controlled on your PC. Each HotSynch will update current channels and conduct new searches for Medline journals.

The initial screen shows your current subscriptions (Figure 12.39). After selecting A–Z Drug Facts, the option is available for an alphabetical or therapeutic search (Figure 12.40). Entering to search the alphabetical subset brings up the list with additional methods to select your choice (Figure 12.41). Scrolling or simply using the "jump to" function allows quick search functions within the drug monographs. An extensive list is available for subsets within the drug monograph, as indicated next (Figure 12.42).

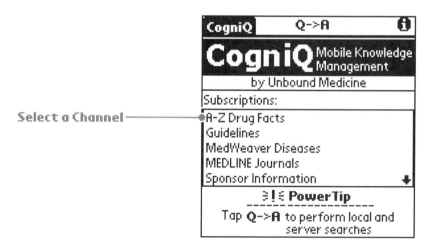

FIGURE 12.39. CogniQ: Main page. (Reprinted with permission from Unbound Medicine.)

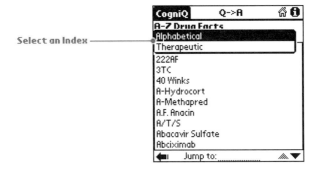

FIGURE 12.40. CogniQ: A–Z Drug Facts. (Reprinted with permission from Unbound Medicine.)

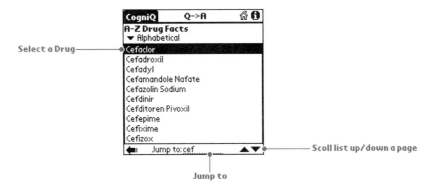

FIGURE 12.41. CogniQ: A–Z Drug Facts, alphabetical search function. (Reprinted with permission from Unbound Medicine.)

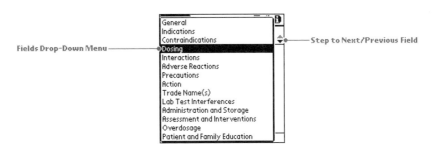

FIGURE 12.42. CogniQ: A–Z Drug Facts, extensive drug subset list. (Reprinted with permission from Unbound Medicine.)

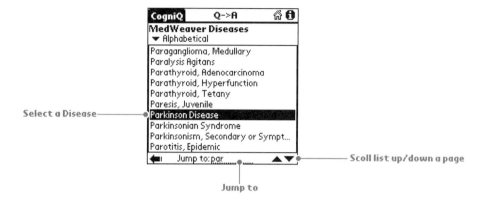

Select a Disease

Scoll list up/down a page

Jump to

FIGURE 12.43. CogniQ: MedWeaver Diseases. (Reprinted with permission from Unbound Medicine.)

MedWeaver Disease searches follow the pattern with the alphabetical listing (Figure 12.43). This includes a subset viewing choice for the example of Parkinsonian syndrome (Figure 12.44). An additional drop-down list provides further search categories (Figure 12.45).

For the nursing professional on the go, having the ability to perform Medline Journal searches is invaluable. One does not need to wait until back at the desktop to place a query. The journals are managed by your subscription home Web page at your desktop, which is then synchronized

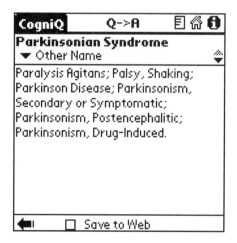

FIGURE 12.44. CogniQ: MedWeaver Diseases, Parkinsonian syndrome. (Reprinted with permission from Unbound Medicine.)

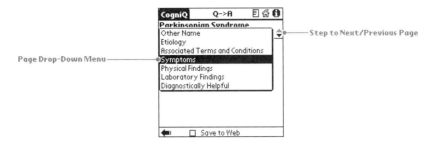

FIGURE 12.45. CogniQ: MedWeaver—Parkinsonian syndrome symptoms. (Reprinted with permission from Unbound Medicine.)

to your handheld (Figure 12.46). The handheld screen shows the journals you have chosen (Figure 12.47).

Queries are entered anywhere, anytime. Simply enter the keyword and any additional information you have, using either Graffiti or the keyboard function (Figure 12.48). After performing the synchronization, each query is downloaded with ability to "Find" or scroll through the added entries on

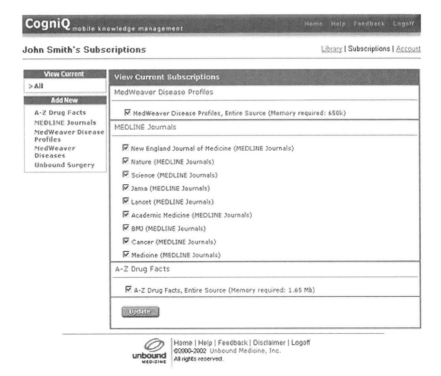

FIGURE 12.46. CogniQ journal subscriptions. (Reprinted with permission from Unbound Medicine.)

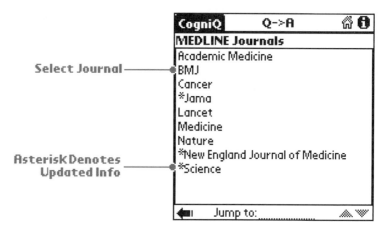

FIGURE 12.47. CogniQ list of Medline journals. (Reprinted with permission from Unbound Medicine.)

your handheld (Figure 12.49). The open screen for your query also contains those with abstracts available (Figure 12.50).

Each subscription also contains the ability to save the searches to your desktop, providing your own personal folders that are managed with your desktop. The popular operating systems (Palm OS and Pocket PC) are available.

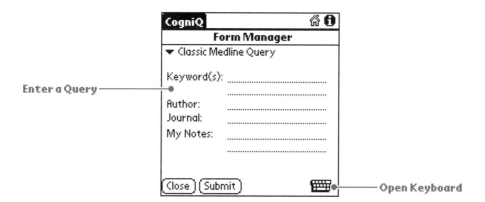

FIGURE 12.48. CogniQ query form. (Reprinted with permission from Unbound Medicine.)

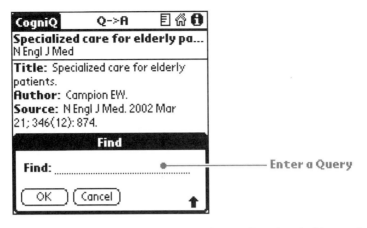

FIGURE 12.49. CogniQ query result: find added entry. (Reprinted with permission from Unbound Medicine.)

Summary

One reason handhelds are so appealing to nurses is that they can be tailored to meet each nurse's specific needs. As is probably evident from the small sample of software that is available and useful for nursing featured in this chapter, there is something for everyone! Nurses can have in their pockets the resources they need to provide efficient, effective, and safe patients care. The handheld can be tailored so that it will contain drug references, med-surg references, data collection forms, and calculators that are selected and modified according to personal and professional preferences.

A beginning nurse's handheld device will most likely look quite different from the more experienced nurse's handheld even when both nurses work on the same unit. The nurse with only 1 year's experience in the Inten-

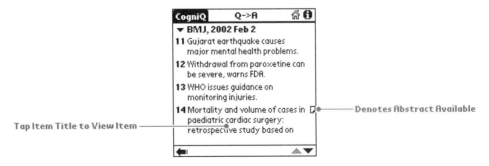

FIGURE 12.50. CogniQ list of journal articles: abstracts indicated. (Reprinted with permission from Unbound Medicine.)

sive Care Unit (ICU) will most likely have more handheld references than the nurse with 5 years experience in that same ICU.

There are strong indicators that nursing is moving quickly to adopt this new technology and utilize it to its full potential at the point of care. We anticipate the rate of adoption for mobile information systems within nursing to be rapid, and it will ultimately equal and perhaps exceed that of physicians.

The fact that nurses are picking up handheld devices and using them to solve clinical problems bodes well for the future of handhelds in health care. The grassroots origin of the movement toward handheld computing in health care holds great promise for the future of mobile computing at the point of care.[1,2]

References

1. http://www.PDAcortex.com
2. http://www.VNAHHS.com

13

Software for Other Healthcare Professionals: Hey, What About Me?

LAURA KOSTEVA, GREG SCHALLER, JENEANE A. BRIAN,
AND SCOTT M. STRAYER

If you're not a physician or nurse in the healthcare field, you might be asking at this point... "Hey, what about me?" Although many of the programs we have described so far can be used by different healthcare professionals, it certainly has been written from our doctor-centric perspective—we just don't know anything else! So we asked a speech pathologist, a physician assistant, and the CEO of a home health nursing agency to write about other uses of handheld computers in the healthcare industry.

Just as there are a plethora of different types of handheld computers in every shape, size, and color, there are an infinite number of uses for them in health care, and that's what this chapter is all about. We were pleasantly surprised by the creative uses that different healthcare professionals find for their trusty handheld companions.

Public Displays of Affection (My PDA): By Laura Kosteva, MS, CCC

I am a speech-language pathologist, and work in acute care at the University of Michigan Hospital in Ann Arbor, Michigan. My day is probably not at all what you might think. I rarely address "speech" disorders anymore because my focus is so predominantly on swallowing. Yes, that's right, swallowing. Eighty percent to 90% of my caseload involves swallowing disorders, otherwise known as dysphagia. It's not particularly engaging during dinner party conversation beyond the "What do you do for a living?" opener. Once the topic is out and on the table, people politely reply, "Oh, that's nice" and continue 'swallowing' their chicken wing-dings. The role of the hospital-based speech-language pathologist has changed significantly over the past 10 to 15 years. We now are required to have a thorough understanding of how cranial nerve and cortical dysfunction impacts the muscles involved in swallowing. The specialty of dysphagia also commands expertise in oral and tracheal suctioning and related tracheostomy and ventilator issues, as well as videofluoroscopic and fiberoptic-endoscopic examinations of the swallow. These valuable skills add to our traditional knowledge base of head and neck cancer, stroke, and head injury, while adapting to an ever-changing insurance industry.

In response to these many challenges, the acute care speech-language pathologist, not unlike most healthcare professionals, must be well equipped to offer comprehensive diagnostics and functional treatment in the least amount of time. Arriving on the scene in a timely manner is the array of electronic and computerized devices that serve to streamline paperwork, supplement treatment, and facilitate patient and family education. These devices store resources and references, enable slide show presentations, and, yes, even display instrumental evaluations of swallowing. As a result, my iPAQ 3850 has become one of the most efficient additions to my diagnostic and therapeutic repertoire. I have gone from a meek, mild-mannered professional to one who shamelessly flaunts and thoroughly enjoys PDA-related 'public displays of affection.'

Documents

Pocket Controller from Soft Objects Technologies, Inc. (www.soti.net) offers the ability to modify the iPAQ screen from my desktop keyboard. This "screenshot program" can, in turn, display an enlarged, desktop view of my iPAQ screen for those blurry-eyed, late-night hours. My iPAQ contains Pocket Excel and Pocket Word, in addition to Compaq's Foldable Keyboard, which allows on-the-road input. To be fair, my job involves more than dysphagia intervention. Throughout the course of an average day, I also see patients who have survived stroke (CVA) and traumatic brain injury (TBI) as well as patients with pulmonary, cardiac, and degenerative neurologic diseases. Rehabilitation of many of these patients takes place on the University of Michigan's Inpatient Rehabilitation Unit and, as expected in healthcare delivery today, documentation is a never-ending avalanche of reports, dictations, letters, and referencing.

My handheld provides me with report templates stored in Pocket Word for cognitive and language evaluations (Figure 13.1) and fiberoptic-endoscopic and videofluoroscopic swallow studies (Figure 13.2). With keyboard in tow, I can often get the first chunk of a report written upstairs, on the floors. This method becomes extremely efficient when I find myself waiting for my next patient to become available, a physician to complete rounds, nursing to pass meds, etc. It's not always practical to return to my office between patients, therefore writing reports on the fly has become an enormous time-saver. The next time I resync, my documents are ready for final editing, printing, or sending! I've compiled quick-lists of dysarthria differentials, aphasia types, their cortical and subcortical correlates, and cranial

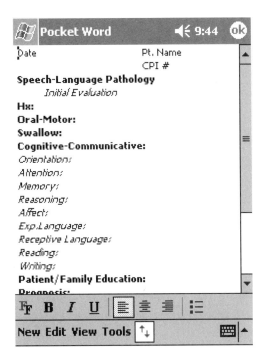

FIGURE 13.1. Speech-language pathology evaluation report template. (Reprinted with permission from Microsoft Corporation.)

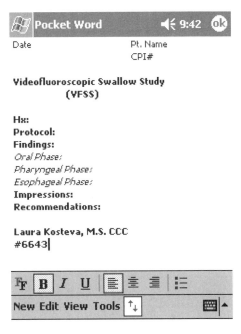

FIGURE 13.2. Video fluooscopic swallow study (VFSS) report template. (Reprinted with permission from Microsoft Corporation.)

nerve descriptions as well as an inventory of swallow-specific muscles should an unsuspected "senior moment" surface. I've also amassed a collection of frequently administered articulation, language, and cognitive age-equivalencies and norms for immediate referencing. The iPAQ's recording mode allows an audio attachment to Pocket Word documents and comes in handy for those reports that are left midstream. Audio recording can also be accomplished in Notes and, although not yet attempted, has the potential to link into Central Dictation for transcription.

References

Many professional journals (Figure 13.3) are now providing automatic e-mail delivery of their tables of contents. Through the University's Taubman Medical Library, full-text links are often available; this offers the convenience of reviewing titles (Figure 13.4) and reading journal articles on my own time (such as while waiting for my daughter's soccer practice to end). If I've downloaded an article for future reading, it's merely a matter of reaching in my pocket. Tabers 19th edition of the *Cyclopedic Medical Dic-*

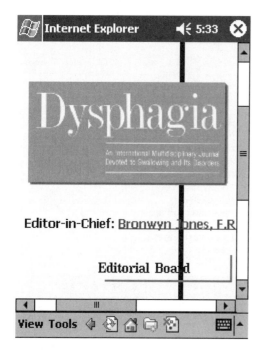

FIGURE 13.3. Downloaded *Dysphagia* journal. (Reprinted with permission from Springer-Verlag.)

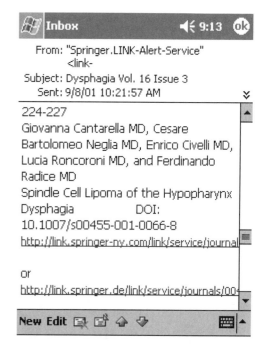

FIGURE 13.4. Automatically e-mailed *Dysphagia* journal table of contents with links to full text articles. (Reprinted with permission from Springer-Verlag.)

tionary (Figure 13.5) has also been a quick reference that has proven to be worth more than its weight in pixels.

Staff and Patient Education

It's surprising to me just how much of my job involves educating. An artist I am not. However, if I am up on the floors and a concerned family member asks questions necessitating impromptu, graphic illustration, I rise to the challenge. The tongue? The epiglottis? No problem. Now, I know the iPAQ is richly equipped, but it cannot put lipstick on a pig or make a ballerina of a linebacker, and it certainly can't make me an artist. The proof is obvious: yes, my drawing (Figure 13.6), which was proudly completed in the drawing mode of Pocket Word, falls painfully short of the illustrations found on GastroAtlas.com (Figure 13.7). However, although MDs, RNs, and PAs often relate better to the standard anatomic representation, somehow families and patients seem to enjoy and understand my version better. I do what I can for my patients, their families, and anyone else bold enough to ask.

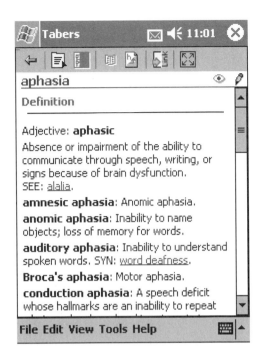

FIGURE 13.5. Taber's Cyclopedic Medical Dictionary, 19th edition (Tabers™). (Reprinted with permission from F.A. Davis Company.)

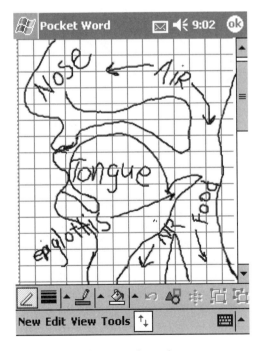

FIGURE 13.6. The normal oropharynx. (Courtesy of Laura Kosteva, unpublished drawing.)

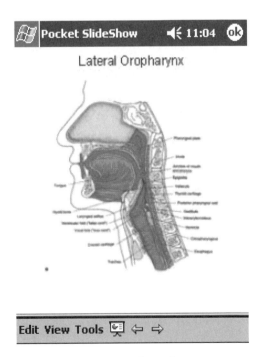

FIGURE 13.7. The normal oropharynx. (Reprinted with permission from Springer-Verlag.)

Movable Feast

Pocket SlideShow from CNetX (www.cnetx.com), a modified PowerPoint program designed for the handheld, has been invaluable to the patient, family, and staff education that I provide. I can illustrate normal and abnormal function and structure at the bedside, in rounds as well as in clinic. This program includes transitions, animations, and text formatting that can be added using a desktop version of PowerPoint. Currently, I have a few slides downloaded from GastroAtlas.com that detail lateral and anteroposterior (AP) views of the normal oropharynx, the cricopharyngeus, and esophagus. As illustrated in Figures 13.8 and 13.9, I also have slides of videofluoroscopic swallow studies (which boast laryngeal penetration, aspiration, unilateral pharyngeal paresis, cricopharyngeal prominence, and esophageal strictures) in addition to fiberoptic endoscopic evaluation slides. The benefit of walking around the hospital with my pocket-accessible slide shows not only addresses patient and family education, but also provides informal staff and faculty in-services. This has been a bona fide traffic stopper! Imagine, a walking slide show of swallowing! It doesn't get better than this!

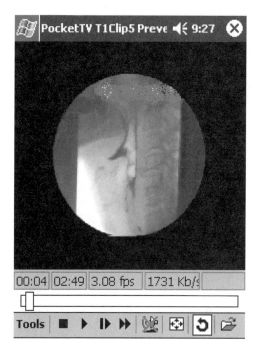

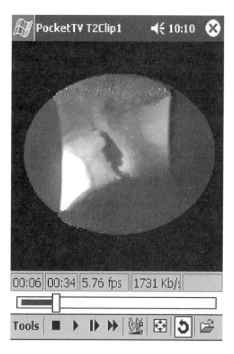

FIGURE 13.8. Videofluoroscopic image of laryngeal aspiration. (Courtesy of Laura Kosteva)

FIGURE 13.9. Videofluoroscopic image of cricopharyngeal prominence. (Courtesy of Laura Kosteva)

Presentations/Video

Radiologic, videofluoroscopic contrast studies, archived on analog video-tapes, are integral components of my work. I complete these studies in GI Radiology, whose technical ability to 'burn' these studies directly onto CD ROM is on the not-too-distant horizon. In the interim, our University's Media Center converts them to digital, video format (MPEG or Moving Picture Experts Group). Once this conversion is completed, viewing these studies on my iPAQ is pretty straightforward utilizing a program such as PocketTV from *MpegTV* LLC (www.mpegtv.com). Software choices capable of projecting these MPEG video clips or a Pocket SlideShow presentation include, among others, Presenter-to-Go from MARGI Systems, Inc. (www.margi.com) and Voyager VGA CF from Colorgraphic Communications, Inc. (www.colorgraphic.com). Although I have not yet made the purchase, these programs enable SlideShow displays to a monitor or directly from the handheld through a projector. The benefits and convenience of this feature during large-audience presentations will be immeasurable.

Calendar/Appointments

The most "no-brainer", yet critical feature of my iPAQ's cerebral cortex is the calendar. While my daily schedule, appointments, and agenda items are updated regularly via e-mail from our Administrative Assistant, I generally schedule my own GI swallow studies (Figures 13.10, 13.11) while away from my desk. With calendar in hand, I can easily avoid the inherent conflicts of coordinating these videofluoroscopic swallow studies around multiple appointments. With my next synchronization, the appointment is sent off to our department's Administrative Assistant for formal scheduling and notification.

Just Desserts

Clearly, my PDA is the object of my professional affection. It has been an exciting addition to my clinical practice, not to mention my busy life! By offering portable referencing, slide show presentations, short dictating capabilities, and the capacity to store novels or downloaded journal articles, my iPAQ has proven to be more useful than a Sherpa guide. Coupled with the obvious advantage of having a pocket calendar and daily schedule within arm's reach, I now enjoy the advantages and conveniences of a compact workplace that is always in my pocket. 'Waiting' is a thing of the past for me (soccer practice can now drag on as long as it needs to). As for those dinner parties: illustrating exactly how those wing-dings slide down can kick off quite the dialogue!

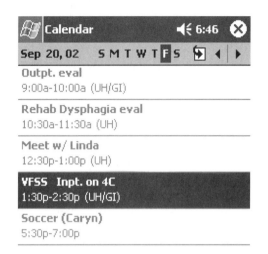

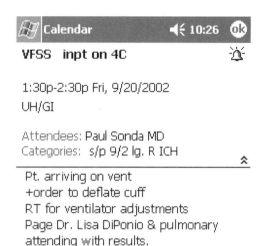

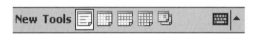

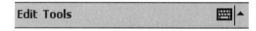

FIGURE 13.10. e-Mailed appointment, automatically entered into Calendar upon synchronization. (Reprinted with permission from Microsoft Corporation.)

FIGURE 13.11. The "Notes" details of the iPAQ's Calendar. (Reprinted with permission from Microsoft Corporation.)

From PDA Naïve to PDA Savvy: A Physician Assistant's Story: By Greg Schaller, MPA, PA-C

Learning Curve

Several years ago, in 1997, I purchased my first computer. I was one of those people who said: "I'm never going to get a computer." It wasn't long after hooking up to the Internet that I saw the computer light. All of a sudden, my access to information took a quantum leap. I distinctly remember coming across the term "Palm Pilot," when I was Web searching for some information about my computer modem, but I had no idea what a Palm Pilot was.

Flash forward to the year 2000, when I entered the PA (Physician Assistant) program at Eastern Virginia Medical School in Norfolk, Virginia. It was about that time that PDAs really started infiltrating American culture. Initially, there were only a few PDA-owning students. Within a semester, like popcorn popping, one student after another became a PDA owner. Watching my fellow students look up medications with ease in pharmacology class pushed me over the edge. During the winter of 2001, I became a PDA owner.

My first PDA was a Handspring Visor Platinum. I got a Handspring because that's what "everyone" was getting. Then the "form factor" (desirable physical characteristics) intervened, and I upgraded to a Palm m505 and then to a Palm m515. The m515 is my current PDA. It works very well for me, and it is a vital part of my personal organization system.

Initially it was hard to let go of my "old" paper and pen organizer. As I became trustful of the dependability of my Palm, and as I used more and more of its features, however, the Palm gradually took over all of the "old" organizer's functions. I found that the more I used my Palm, the more I used my Palm.

Acceleration

Before we get to the medical applications, let me tell you about some of the general Palm applications that I have found particularly helpful, including AvantGo (see Chapter 10), Address Plus (http://www.addressplus.net/, cost $8), DateBk5 (see Chapter 1), City Time (http://www.codecity.net, cost $14.95), SplashID (http://www.splashdata.com/splashid/index.htm, cost $19.95), Jot (http://www.cic.com/home.asp, cost $39), PalmReader (http://www.palmdigitalmedia.com/home.cgi, cost $14.95), and PhotoSuite (http://www.roxio.com, free with most newer Palm models).

AvantGo enables me to download a variety of websites onto my Palm. It's like working with Internet Explorer "offline." Address Plus (Figure 13.12) and DateBk5 (see Chapter 1) are highly tweaked-up, multifeatured upgrades to the standard built-in Palm address and date books. City Time is a world map/clock. With City Time, I can touch a location on the map, and it tells me the time there, very helpful because I often communicate across time zones (Figure 13.13). SplashID is a secured list of all the pass codes and numbers that are required for (my) life in the twenty-first century (Figure 13.14). Jot is a substitute for the Palm's Graffiti input system. With

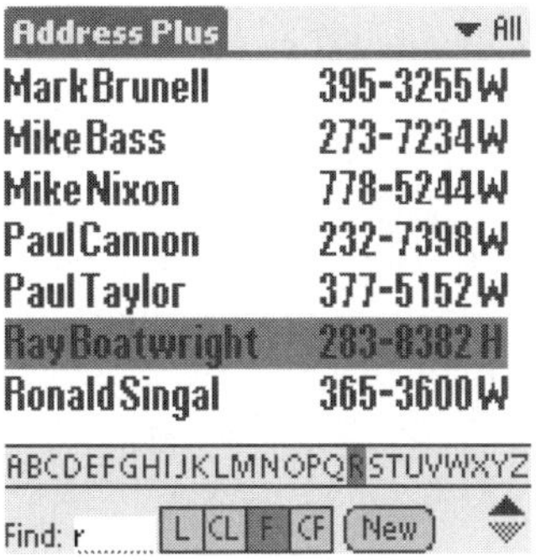

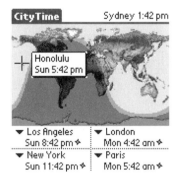

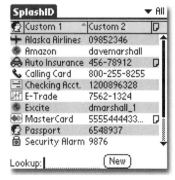

FIGURE 13.12. Address Plus for Palm handheld computers. (Reprinted with permission from PST Consulting.)

FIGURE 13.13. Touching the map displays the local time in that location in City Time. (Reprinted with permission from palmOne, Inc.)

FIGURE 13.14. SplashID for securing your pass codes and numbers. (Reprinted with permission from SplashData.)

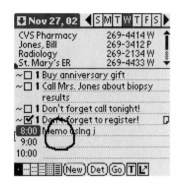

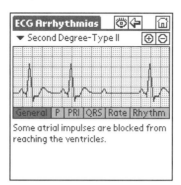

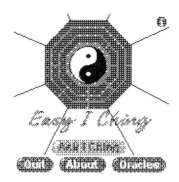

FIGURE 13.15. Write in your own handwriting using Jot. (Reprinted with permission from palmOne, Inc.)

FIGURE 13.16. Reading EKG's using PalmEKG. (Reprinted with permission from palmOne, Inc.)

FIGURE 13.17. Ancient Chinese advice using EasyIChing. (Reprinted with permission from palmOne, Inc.)

Jot, I can write in my own handwriting; I could never master or remember the strokes of Graffiti (Figure 13.15). PalmReader is Palm's book reader, allowing me to keep several books on my Palm, for reading during those in-between times. PhotoSuite is a Palm-based personal photo album.

There are a huge variety of medical applications available for the Palm. The ones I use the most include Griffith's 5 Minute Clinical Consult (5MCC) (see Chapter 7), ePocrates qRx and qID (see Chapter 7), MedCalc (see Chapter 6), and PalmEKG. 5MCC is an amazing A-to-Z list of diseases and how to diagnose and treat them. The ePocrates applications are constantly updated drug reference guides, which update through the Internet every time you synchronize your handheld computer. ePocrates has a notes section that enables addition of personal medication comments. MedCalc is a veritable gold mine of medical calculations: everything from body mass index to transtubular K gradient. PalmEKG is an excellent EKG trainer (Figure 13.16). Not a day goes by that I don't medically reference my Palm.

My Palm also has Quickword, enabling me to write a Word document on my Palm, with my Palm Portable Keyboard, BigClock (a timer/alarm clock), and Easy I Ching (ancient Chinese divinatory system) (Figure 13.17). As one can see, PDAs are inherently customizable: there is truly software for every need. For example, as my life is now requiring increasing project management, I soon will download Shadow Plan, a premier project/task management application. I'm not big into games, but there's no lack of PDA games!

Research

Being a Masters' program, my Physician Assistant program requires a research project. After several false starts, I developed a survey to evaluate PDA use among PAs in the Commonwealth of Virginia. My survey population consisted of all the members of the Virginia Academy of Physician

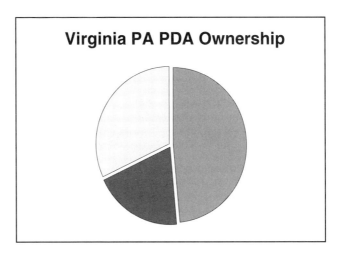

FIGURE 13.18. Virginia Physician Assistants' PDA ownership.

Assistants, about 43% of all Virginia PAs. The survey was completed in November 2001, with a 57.3% response rate.

There were two particularly notable research findings. One was that 48.5% of Virginia PAs were current PDA owners, with another 19.6% intending to purchase in the next 12 months (Figure 13.18). The second finding was that 76.8% of surveyed PA students owned PDAs, compared to 38.8% of working PAs. These findings predict two noteworthy events. One event is there are now a significant number of PDAs owning PDAs, while the second is a further doubling of use by working PAs, when the current "crop" of students graduate.

What about the nonowners? Reasons for nonpurchase were primarily "cost" (22%) and "lack of familiarity" (17%); 8.5% of respondents thought that they were "not helpful," and 8% were "waiting for new technology." Three percent of respondents stated that they were "intimidated" by the technology. As device costs go down, and as cultural knowledge increases, it can be predicted that PDA use will further increase.

What type of PDAs did Virginia PAs have? Survey results indicated that 96% of owners have Palm OS devices, with most being Palm or Handspring brand. Survey results further showed that although there were more owners younger than age 37 (59%) than over 37 years old, there were minimal differences in ownership by gender, with an almost 50–50 split.

Although 43.4% of respondents considered themselves to be "early adopters" of technology in general, early adopter status doesn't seem particularly important with regards to PDA ownership. Almost as many non-adopters (42.3%) as adopters own PDAs. Mean self-declared "computer literacy" of survey respondents was 6.5 on a 10 scale, with only 39.8% of those with below mean computer literacy owning PDAs compared to 56.4% of those of above mean computer literacy. Over half (53.5%) of surveyed

PAs had taken computer classes/workshops, but interestingly enough, 33.6% of those above mean computer literacy were self-taught. A majority (77.4%) of surveyed PAs expressed an interest in taking a class or workshop on PDA use in medicine.

What types of handheld applications were Virginia PAs using? Three top-ranked applications were listed by survey respondents. Ranking number one were drug information applications, such as ePocrates. Ranking number two were medical textbooks, such as 5MCC/2002. Ranking number three were personal information management applications such as date books, address books, and to do lists.

There seem to be differences among states. Two national surveys[1,2] of PAs done around the same timeframe as my survey showed a much higher rate of PDA usage by PAs nationally (68.29% and 64%, respectively) than the 48.5% use rate noted by this study. One can speculate that these state versus national differences indicate technology diffusion patterns across the United States.

Prognosis

Given these research results, it is apparent that PDA use in the PA community is on the rise and here to stay. There's a biological principle that energy flows toward greater organization. I assert that PDAs, with the appropriate applications, are a greater form of organization. Want more energy? Get a PDA!

References

1. Poll: PDAs in medicine. Online. Available at http://www.physicianassociate.om/ forums/ Aug. 21, 2001.
2. Personal e-mail communication with Kevin Marvelle at American Academy of Physicians' Assistants (AAPA) (Sept. 5, 2001), re: AAPA 2001 Market Research Survey.

Case Study: VNA Home Health Systems: By Jeneane A. Brian, RN, BSN, PHN, MBA

Who?

VNA Home Health Systems (VNAHHS) is a Medicare-certified home health agency and has been the industry pioneer in the use of PDAs for clinical documentation in the field. VNAHHS is located in a large metropolitan area and has been in business since 1947. The average age of the field nursing staff is 47 years. The agency was "paper based" before the implementation of a new enterprise-wide mobile documentation system in

January 2001. Mobile clinicians include nurses, therapists, social workers, chaplains, nurse aides, and physicians. VNAHHS self-developed its mobile solution and calls it the FreeForms System. VNAHHS believes its new system allows service delivery with more efficiency than the industry has seen to date.

Why a Handheld Solution?

One-hundred percent of the VNAHHS patient care workforce is mobile. Thus, they jumped on the PDA bandwagon as soon as devices became affordable and development software allowed for (relatively) easy software programming. Alternatives included only laptop solutions, which are expensive and unpopular with nurses and other field clinicians. Laptops are heavy, and home health laptop software is slow.

Here's what the agency was after:

- Improved quality of patient care
- Faster, more decentralized, decision making in the field
- Improved responsiveness to patients
- Reduced clinical documentation time
- Reduced information flow latency
- Increased staff morale and productivity
- Reduced travel costs
- Decreased facility costs

VNAHHS does business in busy Southern California counties, on a 24/7 schedule, and deals with patients from infancy to adult including hospice. They had high hopes for their system's impact, and they have not been disappointed.

What Do the Nurses Get?

VNAHHS issues PDAs equipped with proprietary documentation software and other third-party applications to all mobile clinicians (see Figs. 13-19a and 13-19b). Users are also equipped with portable keyboards to help with extended text entry. Patient data are organized in an electronic medical record format (see Fig. 13-19c). With each synchronization, clinicians receive their own list of active patient records (see Fig. 13-20). FreeForms clinical documentation software processes locally (on the handheld), stores locally, and data are synchronized via a land line-connected Internet-capable PC. The System supports bidirectional information flow, so all data in the patient's electronic medical record are updated on each data exchange.

Agency-provided third-party software includes drug reference applications such as Nursing Rx and Interact from Lexi Comp. Nurse specialists are welcome to download other reference software applications, most of which are available on PDAcortex.com. Hospice nurses prefer ePocrates drug software because the cost of the drugs is included in the program.

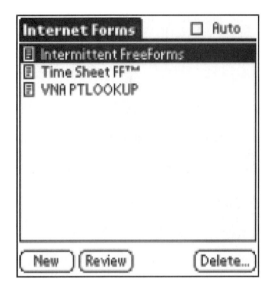

FIGURE 13.19a. This is the application screen for FreeForms. Clinical notes, time and attendance, and patient EMRs are synchronized back and forth. (Reprinted with permission from FreeForms.)

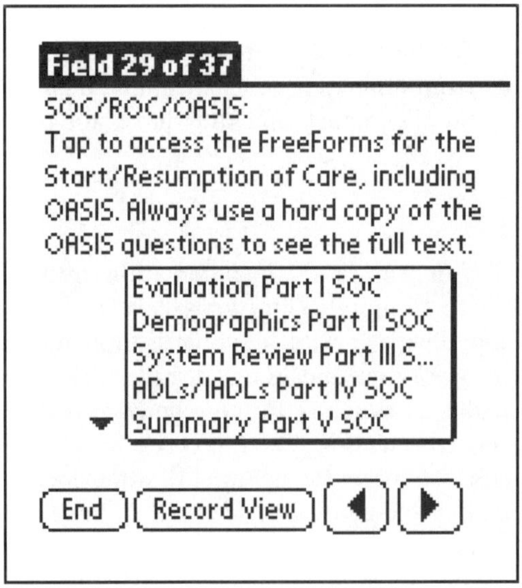

FIGURE 13.19b. All necessary forms for clinical documentation are available on the PDA. There are three text entry options: Graffiti, portable keyboard, or a secure Web site. (Reprinted with permission from FreeForms.)

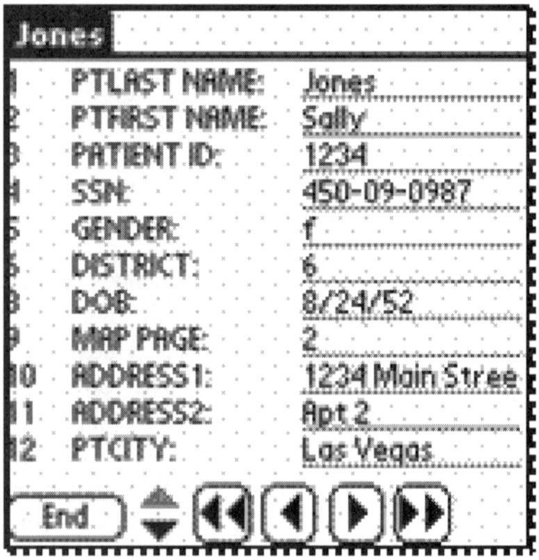

FIGURE 13.19c. Illustration of patient record. (Reprinted with permission from FreeForms.)

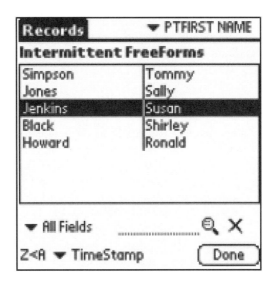

FIGURE 13.20. This is the list of homecare clinician's electronic medical records available on the PDA. All authorized members of the patient's care team can view the records. Read/write permissions apply. (Reprinted with permission from FreeForms.)

How's the System Used?

Of course, the main users of the mobile system are field clinicians. There are currently about 250 VNAHHS FreeForms users. Clinicians collect clinical data on PDAs and synchronize via the Internet to the agency's main office. Additionally, clinicians can edit or review synchronized data via a password-protected, secure VNAHHS Web site. This gives mobile workers a choice: they can enter data via the handheld, via the Internet, or both.

Clinical documentation editing permission is allowed up to 48 hours after a patient encounter. Once data have been synchronized to the server, it is pushed back out to the providers as part of the patient's electronic medical record and based upon the clinician's caseload. Data generated by one user cannot be viewed or edited by another.

Besides the field staff component, the FreeForms System includes a backend that has been written for use by in-house office staff. Both business and clinical managers use the backend system for time and attendance reporting, human resource forms input, and all kinds of statistical reporting for other business and clinical purposes. The backend system has been built in Microsoft Access using data stored on a Microsoft SQL server. In the office, data are sorted in a lot of different ways; records can be printed, and data are examined. Office user access is password and permission based. Patient information is printed only on demand. Clinical supervisors approve timecards, perform quality assurance audits on clinical documentation, and review the patient's digital chart via the backend mechanism. Data can be viewed in aggregate format, by individual clinician, or by patient.

What About Wireless?

The agency is already using wireless technology in those areas where it currently makes sense. The FreeForms synchronization platform supports wireless connections via the TCP/IP protocol ("the Internet protocol"). Clinicians have the ability to synchronize wirelessly; however, large amounts of electronic medical record data do not synchronize reliably with the slower speeds of 2G networks (typically, 14.4–19 kbps). As 2.5 and 3G networks begin to roll out, VNAHHS hopes to see a dramatic shift in the way field staff choose to synchronize. With the use of these high-speed wireless networks, they look forward to patient data available to clinicians in real time.

What Now?

Original goals to address the nursing shortage included improvements in clinician recruitment and retention. Since August of 2001, when the FreeForms System was implemented agency wide, VNAHHS has experienced a 37% increase in nurse recruitment, and nurse turnover has decreased from 27% during the first 90 days of employment to 4.5%. The recruitment cost per clinician has dropped 40%. The system has delivered.

In August 2002, VNAHHS is implementing always-on e-mail through the use of Palm i705 handheld devices. It is hoped that costs can be further reduced through elimination of pagers and cell phone expenses by the use of e-mail. The future is bright for PDA technology and the enterprise!

Summary

This chapter highlights some of the many innovative uses for handheld computers throughout our diverse healthcare system. Different types of providers can apply many of these uses, and the only limit is your imagination and the type of information that you need to practice.

In addition to the uses highlighted here, respiratory therapists, nurse practitioners, physical therapists, paramedics, and many other healthcare providers are using handheld computers.

Section III

Advanced Topics

14

Evidence-Based Medicine and Handhelds

SCOTT M. STRAYER AND MARK H. EBELL

Evidence-based medicine (EBM) is an important shift in the way we learn about and practice clinical medicine. It advocates basing patient care decisions on a careful survey of the best available evidence; the evidence more than the expert should determine what we do for our patients. Haven't we always done this, you might ask? Actually, no. There are many examples of common practices based on habit or tradition that on closer examination have been shown to be ineffective or even harmful, including the following:

- Not allowing infants to sleep on their backs
- Encanide or flecanide post myocardial infarction
- Antibiotics for bronchitis in otherwise healthy adults
- Patches for uncomplicated corneal abrasion
- Arthroscopic lavage and debridement for osteoarthritis
- Vitamin E and hormone replacement therapy to prevent heart disease

Many of these interventions made perfect sense based on physiologic principles or studies of intermediate outcomes, or observational studies, but did not stand up to the scrutiny of well-designed randomized controlled trials. As described in Chapter 10, "information mastery," proposed by Shaughnessy and Slawson,[1] takes EBM one step further by adding a focus on making sure information is relevant to your practice and by reducing the work needed to obtain it. They recommend, and we agree, that you emphasize patient-oriented evidence that matters (POEMs) in your reading. POEMs address a question about a common or important topic in your practice, measure patient-oriented outcomes (morbidity, mortality, symptom improvement, cost, quality of life), and have the potential to change practice if valid. Shaughnessy et al. also recommend that you let others do the work of scouring the literature for POEMs, critically appraising them, and summarizing them for you.

Although information mastery makes it easier to practice evidence-based medicine, it is still a bigger challenge than simply doing "the same old thing," doing something to a patient because "it's always worked for me" or "it's the Duke (insert your favorite school here) way to do things." Hand-held computers can make it easier to be a medical information master using some of the software that we discuss in this chapter.

For example, how about being able to look up that vaguely remembered POEM about who should be admitted for pneumonia and who shouldn't and using it before calling admissions? Would you find it useful to be able to calculate a patient's 10-year risk of a myocardial infarction using the Framingham data at the point of care, and be able to demonstrate to him the drastic reduction in risk by quitting smoking or controlling blood pressure? What about knowing the risk of an operative delivery in your patient who wants to be induced before her cervix is ripe? EBM software for hand-helds lets you do this and much more. Best of all, we believe that EBM at the point of care is a much more effective way for physicians to keep up to date and continue learning.

Why Is the Point of Care a Better Place to Answer Questions?

Experts who study adult learning have found that dark rooms with a slide projector, cold food, and bad coffee are not where adults learn best. Big surprise! These kinds of lectures can make us aware of our learning needs and holes in our knowledge base, so they aren't completely worthless. Plus, they can be an important source of free food and coffee. But actual learning doesn't take place for most adults until we have a problem, and solve it. For clinicians, that usually means a clinical question that arises during the care of a patient. Answering that question is how the clinician learns, and answering it with the best available evidence is what makes that clinician an "information master".

Of course, there are many barriers to answering questions with the best available evidence:

- Time
- Knowledge of resources
- Availability of resources, particularly evidence-based sources
- Skill at searching and using computers
- Ability to understand and/or critically appraise the search results
- Local practice culture, which may not support the process

Many of these barriers can be at least partially overcome by providing clinicians with a handheld information source for use at the point of care that quickly searches several evidence-based references at once and which provides "predigested" information that doesn't require further critical appraisal. In the next section, we'll discuss software for Palm and Pocket PC PDA's that has some or even all these characteristics.

Handheld Software for Information Masters

There are many excellent programs currently available that will help you take information mastery to the bedside. The basic types of software include medical calculators, information mastery references, database programs, programmable calculators, and Web-based content viewers. Many of these programs are presented in other chapters, but we wanted to consolidate them all here so you have ready access to an EBM list of handheld software that we use and recommend. One note of caution, however, is to always check the formulas and assumptions that are programmed into the software, and remember that the final decision for every patient should be based on a combination of the best available evidence, your clinical experience, and the patient's unique clinical situation.

The Programs

Medcalc | Palm OS | http://netxperience.org/medcalc | free download

Why memorize formulas, when you can easily access them and use them at the point of care with this free software program for the Palm OS? In addition to many clinically useful formulas, the program includes several important calculations for practicing evidence-based medicine, including likelihood ratios; numbers needed to treat; and posttest probabilities based on either sensitivity and specificity, or likelihood ratios. This is an excellent resource to help you critically analyze the literature (Figure 14.1).

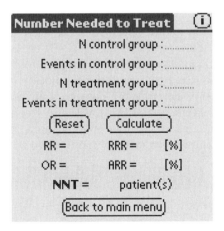

FIGURE 14.1. Number Needed to Treat in Medcalc. (Reprinted with permission from Mathias Schopp, MD.)

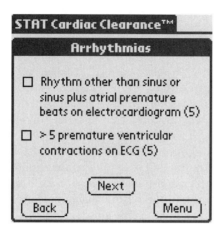

Figure 14.2. Risk factors in Cardiac Clearance. (Reprinted with permission from StatCoder.com.)

Stat Cardiac Clearance | Palm OS | www.statcoder.com | free download

Trying to remember the various risk factors for increased surgical risk can be difficult as you perform a preoperative physical for the local surgical group. How would you like to have both the American College of Cardiology/American Heart Association guidelines and those of the American College of Physicians available at your fingertips every time you need them? This handy little program lets you choose either guideline, walks you through the criteria, and based on your answers, stratifies your patient and makes recommendations for decreasing their surgical risk (Figure 14.2).

Stat Cholesterol | Palm OS | www.statcoder.com | free download

How many time have you tried to read the new National Cholesterol Education Program's ATP III cholesterol guidelines? Even if you've read them, do you really know how to apply this revised guideline at the point of care? Stat cholesterol guides you through the pertinent questions, and after entering the data on your patient, will produce your patient's risk factors, goal LDL level, and treatment recommendations based on the guideline. Lifestyle modifications are outlined, and the program lets you know when drug therapy should be initiated (Figures 14.3, 14.4).

MedRules | Palm OS | http://pbrain.hypermart.net | free download

How would you like to have 40 of the top evidence-based rules loaded onto your handheld computer for the price your last drug lunch? That's right, absolutely free. This program has clinical decision rules such as the Ottawa knee and ankle rules for predicting the need of an X-ray, a Bishop's rule

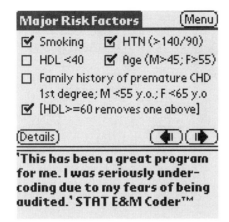

FIGURE 14.3. Major Risk Factors in Stat Cholesterol. (Reprinted with permission from StatCoder.com.)

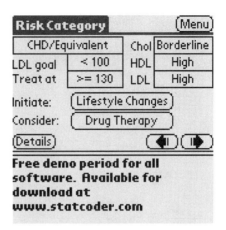

FIGURE 14.4. Treatment guidelines in Stat Cholesterol. (Reprinted with permission from StatCoder.com.)

calculator that lets you predict the outcome of labor induction, and many others that can be used at the point of care. The author updates the program regularly, and it expires periodically, prompting you to download the latest version. The program also includes the references from which the rules were derived, although it does not provide details about study design or tell us how well the rule has been validated (Figures 14.5–14.7).

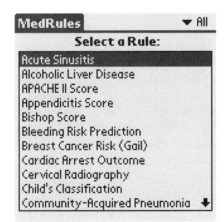

FIGURE 14.5. Rules screen in MedRules. (Reprinted with permission from Kent E. Wilyard, MD.)

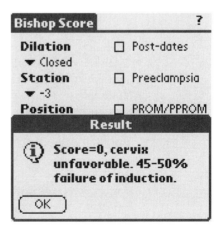

FIGURE 14.6. Bishop Score calculator in MedRules. (Reprinted with permission from Kent E. Wilyard, MD.)

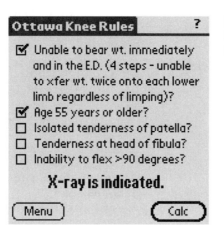

FIGURE 14.7. Ottawa knee rules in MedRules. (Reprinted with permission from Kent E. Wilyard, MD.)

InfoRetriever | Palm OS and Pocket PC | http://www.infopoems.com/ sample/sampledownload.cfm | see Web site for cost

This is the Cadillac of information mastery software for handheld computers. Maybe the BMW. Caveat emptor: Note that part of the reason we love this software is because one of the authors (Dr. Mark Ebell) created it! It is the only software designed explicitly with POEMs and information mastery in mind:

- It focuses on information that is relevant to primary care physicians—common and important problems, selected using the "POEMs" criteria
- Each item is evaluated for validity and tagged with a level of evidence, and most of the references are the highest quality evidence-based materials
- It reduces work by using a single search interface to search many references, putting diagnostic test information in a simple calculator, and incorporating more than 140 useful clinical decision rules

Table 14.1 shows the different references included in the Pocket PC and Palm versions of InfoRetriever.

InfoRetriever is available for the Pocket PC, Palm, desktop computer, and Web browser; subscribers also get a daily e-mail InfoPOEM update. Some sample screens from the Pocket PC version are shown in Figures 14.8 through 14.12. Tapping on the down arrow next to "Select a test" in Figure 14.12 shows a list of over 20 tests, sorted by likelihood ratio.

TABLE 14.1. References included in InfoRetriever.

Reference	Comment
Clinical decision rules	More than 140 useful rules as simple-to-use calculators, all evaluated for validity
Cochrane Database of Systematic Reviews	1700+ abstracts from the "gold standard" for evidence-based medicine (EBM)
InfoPOEMs synopses	2400+ brief, structured summaries of relevant research
Database of diagnostic tests and history and physical examination	Information on more than 2000 unique combinations of symptom, diagnosis, and test in a handy calculator
Drug database	Basic prescribing information for more than 1200 drugs
Photo atlas	More than 500 photos of common problems
Evidence-based guidelines	Summaries of key guidelines and pointers to evidence-based guidelines on the Web
5 Minute Clinical Consult	Comprehensive reference provides information to fill the gaps in evidence

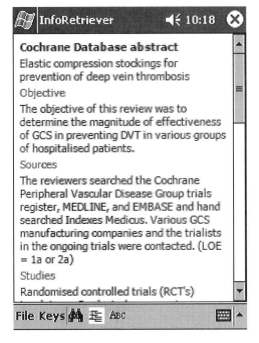

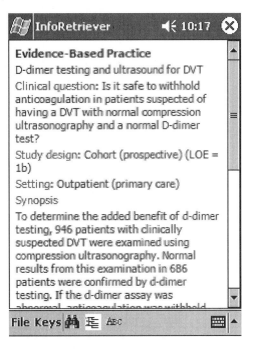

FIGURE 14.8. Abstract from the Cochrane Database of Systematic Reviews. (Reprinted with permission from InfoPOEM, Inc.)

FIGURE 14.9. POEM (patient-oriented evidence that matters) summary of a recent research article. (Reprinted with permission from InfoPOEM, Inc.)

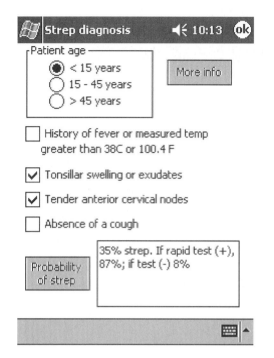

FIGURE 14.10. Clinical decision rule to assist in diagnosis of strep. (Reprinted with permission from InfoPOEM, Inc.)

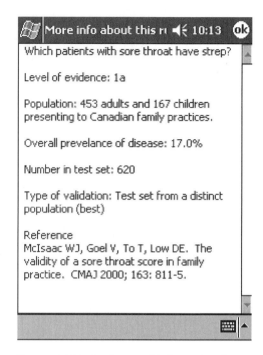

FIGURE 14.11. Background information for the strep score. (Reprinted with permission from InfoPOEM, Inc.)

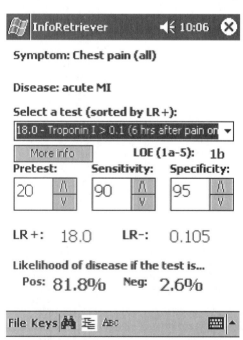

FIGURE 14.12. Diagnostic test information for acute myocardial infarction (MI) in patients with chest pain. (Reprinted with permission from InfoPOEM, Inc.)

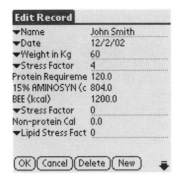

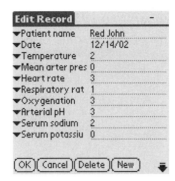

FIGURE 14.13. TPN (total parenteral nutrition) calculator for HanDBase. (Reprinted with permission from DDH Software.)

FIGURE 14.14. APACHE II calculator for HanDBase. (Reprinted with permission from DDH Software.)

InfoRetriever is updated every 4 months, and each item is indexed using both ICD-9 codes and the level of evidence. Subscribers also get a daily e-mail update with one or two recent POEMs.

HanDBase | Palm OS and Pocket PC | http://www.handbase.com | $24.95 HanDBase Applets | Palm OS and Pocket PC | http://www.ddhsoftware.com/gallery.html | free downloads

As described in Chapter 11, HanDBase is a nifty little database application that allows you to create simple databases or download databases created by others. The databases are known as "applets," and are available in a gallery at the HanDBase site. Many of these databases are evidence based such as the total parenteral nutrition (TPN) formula calculator (Figure 14.13) and an APACHE II score calculator for intensive care patients (Figure 14.14). If you're feeling brave, you could even program your own evidence-based calculators using the advice in our HanDBase programming chapter (Chapter 17).

Syncalc | Palm OS | http://www.installigent.com | $19.95

Syncalc is a robust scientific calculator program that also has the ability to be programmed by advanced end-users (see Chapter 16). The beauty of this program is that several savvy physicians have taken the work out of programming and have already completed downloadable "shortcuts" that allow you to conduct several calculations important to information mastery. The shortcuts are available on the Synergy Solutions, Inc., Web site.

DiagnosisPro | Pocket PC | http://www.medicalamazon.com/
diagforpocpc.html | $249.95

This program provides an extensive database of differential diagnoses. You select a combination of symptoms, and the program's expert system suggests a prioritized differential diagnosis. This program takes up quite a bit of room on your Pocket PC (17 MB with version 5.0), so make sure you have plenty of free memory.

Putting Web-Based Content in Your Hand

Another great way to master information using your handheld computer is to take Web pages and even entire websites with you using programs like iSilo or AvantGo. Perhaps you found a new guideline you would like to carry around with you, or you may want to put the current issue of American Family Physician in your hand. The Cochrane Web site (*www.cochrane.org*) has a great index to Cochrane abstracts that is perfect for either iSilo or AvantGo. We show you exactly how to use these two programs in Chapter 10.

Although more advanced users might urge you to wait until you can do this wirelessly from wherever you are located, there are limitations to this approach, including current wireless coverage, cost, and slow speed of wide-area wireless networks (taking up to a minute to load many Web pages). Local-area wireless networks are another option, but once again, you are constrained by availability, cost, security, and inconvenience. AvantGo and iSilo let you take Web content with you right now, wherever you go (so long as you remember your handheld computer!). As we already mentioned, they both work on Palm OS and Pocket PC handhelds as well.

You can use iSilo or AvantGo to convert Cochrane abstracts (Figures 14.15, 14.16), *Journal of Family Practice* POEMs (Figure 14.17), and guidelines such as the National Cholesterol Education Program's ATP III cholesterol guidelines. Almost any evidence-based Web site is fair game, and once it is on your handheld it becomes usable at the point of care.

Summary

For physicians who want to be medical information masters, a handheld computer is as vital as a stethoscope, and perhaps more so. Great software for EBM is available for both Palm and Pocket PC platforms; perhaps the most useful are the clinical decision rules and calculators that help turn an esoteric research paper into an eminently useful decision support tool for use at the point of care.

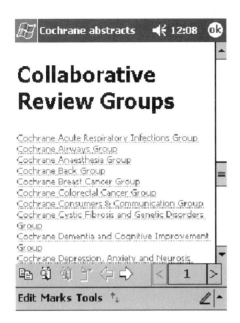

FIGURE 14.15. Cochrane abstracts Using iSilo. (Reprinted with permission from iSilo.)

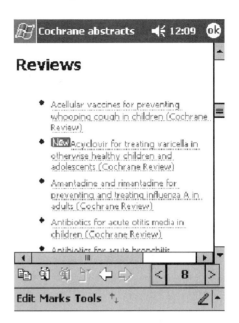

FIGURE 14.16. Detail of Cochrane acute respiratory infections group abstracts using iSilo. (Reprinted with permission from iSilo.)

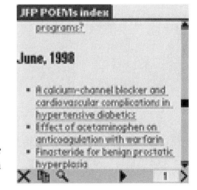

FIGURE 14.17. *Journal of Family Practice* POEMs Index using iSilo. (Reprinted with permission from iSilo.)

We have surveyed the current EBM software, but more is being developed all the time. As you evaluate new software that claims to be "evidence based," ask yourself these questions:

- Do the authors have clear, reasonable criteria for determining the relevance of the information?
- Do the authors explicitly evaluate the validity of the information?
- Do the authors tell you the level of associated evidence or strength of recommendation for every piece of information?

- Do the authors go out of their way to reduce work for you by doing calculations in the background, or is it just "shovelware" with lots of text shoveled on a handheld?
- How often is the information updated?

If the answer to one or more of these questions is "No," then consider looking further before spending your money.

Reference

1. Slawson DC, Shaughnessy AF, Bennett JH. Becoming a medical information master: feeling good about not knowing everything. J Fam Pract 1994;38:505–513.

15

Wireless 101

DAVID R. BLAIR

When you first get your PDA, the thought of a wireless connection probably won't even cross your mind. All the neat programs and other bells and whistles will keep you busy for some time. But sooner or later, any avid PDA user will end up yearning for more. The convenience of e-mail downloaded with each synchronization is really nice, but wouldn't it be even better to get the e-mail at the time it was sent rather than only at the time of synchronization? The programs on your PDA are helpful, but wouldn't it be nice to do a new search on the Internet, or interact with a database in real time? When you find that you are frustrated by the limits of a disconnected PDA, then you are ready to look at wireless.

When talking about wireless PDAs and networks to a bunch of physicians and healthcare providers, the obvious analogy from our medical experience is that of the fetal–maternal relationship. And why not? After all, handheld computing is in its infancy, particularly in the healthcare arena, and the umbilical cord–wire comparison is too rich to pass up. Handheld computers are currently at a stage where the technology has proven useful enough that many clinicians have made them a part of their clinical toolbox. Networking with the devices, particularly wirelessly, is more problematic. As of the fall of 2002, only the most skilled users can set such a system up and use it effectively and safely (in regard to network security). Even these users will encounter serious limitations and pitfalls due to the technology's relative immaturity. Robust applications are limited not only by the complexities of system integration, but also by the hardware. Developers and users need to be aware of these and work together patiently to create user-friendly, value-added products that benefit the clinician, the administrator, and most importantly the patient. Overzealous deployments on the one hand, and overregulation and bureaucratic constraints. On the other, limit the advancement of wireless technology in medicine. Meanwhile, other industries are blazing the way with innovations in wireless security, database creation and integration, and novel approaches to data entry. The challenge for the medical community is to integrate all these with a system of knowledge management so the best available evidence and the patient's medical information can be brought to the point of care anytime, anywhere.

In this chapter, I acquaint you with the general principles and terminology that surround wireless networks, the basic steps to get started wirelessly, and a few of the inherent weaknesses and strengths in the technology.

It's a . . . PDA!

So here we are in the delivery room, the proud parent of a 6-ounce bundle of joy. The cord has been clamped and cut. Our PDA is now wireless and ready to roam the world with us. Like all newborns, there are some things that our desktop computer's "little one" is able to do right now, and other things that must continue to develop. Being a proud new parent, full of excitement, fear, and uncertainty about your baby, you need a crash course in the basics of your wireless PDA. A quick view of the current landscape of wireless technologies is summarized in Table 15.1.

Before we discuss how to connect various handheld computers without wires to a network, we need to review a few basic concepts of how these connections are made. Like most "tech-speak," there are a series of acronyms and pet phrases that you must be able to throw around to look cool to other computer geeks. This lexicon is guaranteed to make even Bill Gates think you know what you are talking about at your next cocktail party.

- Wireless: without a wire (we'll start slow!).
- LAN: local area network. This is the group of computers and servers primarily that are connected together, usually at a single location or organization (Figure 15.1).
- WLAN: wireless local area network. Same as a LAN but, that's right, **WITHOUT WIRES** (Figure 15.2).
- WAN: wide area network. The best way to describe this is a network that extends over a broad area, typically a region–wide or nation-wide network of connections. The easiest example is a cellular network for wireless connections such as is used for cellular phones (Figure 15.3).
- PAN: personal area network. This is the opposite of a WAN in that this term refers to a short-range wireless network generally measured on the order of 10 to 15 feet from the user or device (Figure 15.4).

TABLE 15.1. Pros and cons of wireless PDAs.	
Pros	Cons
Cool	Relatively expensive
Anywhere, anytime Connection for e-mail and Internet	Slow
"Synchronization on the fly"	Security concerns
Remote connections and control for more robust computers	Electromagnetic interference concerns

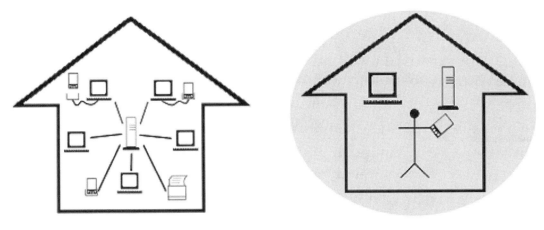

FIGURE 15.1. Traditional or wired local area network.

FIGURE 15.2. Wireless local area network (WLAN).

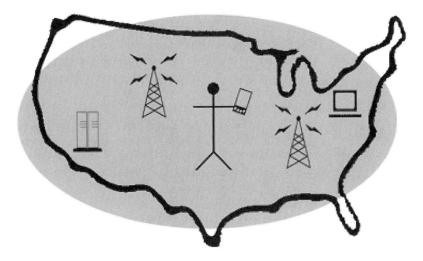

FIGURE 15.3. Wide area network (WAN).

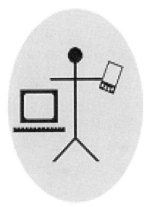

FIGURE 15.4. Personal area network (PAN).

Now that we have the frame of reference for the ranges and types of networks, we'll venture further into the alphabet soup of wireless computing.

Unplug and Play on the WANs, WLANs, and PANs

In a perfect world, all devices would communicate with one another automatically. Unfortunately, as with all new technologies, every company thinks that their own system should be the standard and everyone should choose their product to achieve a desired goal. Ah, the joys of capitalism!

When going wireless, knowing the type of network you will be connecting with is the first order of business. WAN connections can be done with a modem or data-capable cell phone connection. WLAN and PANs can be connected to with the built-in infrared (IR) port on the PDA or with a short-range radio card. A combination of the two is presently not available, although a few cards that have separate radios on the same card are beginning to pop up. This is not unlike the situation with phones: your cordless phone will not connect directly to your cellular system. And like cordless and cell phones, there are a number of different systems and standards on the market.

We'll first look at making connections to WANs. Choosing a wireless service can be confusing and frustrating. Just because you can connect in New York or Los Angeles, don't assume you will be able to in Peoria. Or if you can, you might pay through the nose for the connection. Also, although wireless is cool and convenient, it is rather slow, with maximum connection speeds on most networks of 19.2 kps. Ten years ago this would have been a blistering data transfer rate, but then again, a cool Web site at that time would have had text that blinked. Compare this with the typical home modem of 28.8 kps or 56 kps, or a cable modem that can achive 750 or more kps when downloading files. Consequently, connecting to the internet via a WAN connection today for viewing Web pages may prove painfully slow and costly, especially if graphics are involved. Never fear, however, as newer systems are in the works that promise to pass the speeds offered on dial-up and potentially approach the speeds of broadband. A number of the current standards will whither and die on the vine over the next few years and join the Betamax in the land of the dinosaurs. Table 15.2 shows you the current crop of standards.

Local Wireless

A WAN connection is neat for when you are jet-setting, but you might have to pawn the Learjet for a Yugo if you use the same connection while at home or in the clinic. WLAN and PAN connections are free once you

TABLE 15.2. Acronyms associated with digital wireless standards.[1,2]		
Standard	Typical speed (kps)	Definition
CDMA	9.6	Code Division Multiple Access: cellular phone technology that sends voice and data signals over a shared region of the spectrum. CDMA networks have been upgrades to many analog cellular systems in North America.
CDPD	19.2	Cellular Digital Packet Data: digital wireless transmission system that does not require a continuous connection. Data transmission at 19.2 kps. Availability primarily in urban regions of North America.
GPRS	171.2 (44.0 reported in actual use)	General Packet Radio Service: digital wireless transmission system that has direct compatibility with Internet transfer protocols. Offers data transfer rates approaching those available for desktop PCs. Protocol overlays GSM networks. As of fall 2002 widely available in Europe, almost nonexistent in North America, with only pockets of availability in metropolitan areas.
GSM	9.6	Groupe Speciale Mobile: (in English, Global Standard for Mobile) European digital cellular standard. Available essentially throughout Europe, independent of borders. Availability in North America very limited at this time.
Mobitex	8.0	Digital wireless transmission network that is similar to CDPD but has lower data transfer rate of 8 kbps. Widely available in United States with coverage for greater than 90% of population as of fall 2002.
TDMA	9.6	Time Division Multiple Access: digital wireless transmission system that is designed to allow a large number of users to access a single channel without interference. Available in North America but has fallen by the wayside to newer technologies.
EDGE	384	Enhanced Data Rates for Global Evolution (under development). Would operate over a GSM network and enhance data rate speed through phase-shift modulation.
3G/UMTS	384–2000	Third Generation/Universal Mobile Telephone System (under development). No one "standard" truly defined at the present.
PCS		Personal Communications Services: U.S. Federal Communications Commission terminology for digital wireless communication that allows devices and people to exchange voice and data signals. Not a standard for communications, but, more accurately, a system classification.

TABLE 15.3. Wireless standards for WLANs and PANs.

Standard	Speed (kps or Mbps)[a]	Range (feet)
IrDA (infrared)[3]	115.2 kps–4 Mbps (depending on encoding scheme)	6
802.11a[4]	54 Mbps	150
802.11b[5]	11 Mbps	1500
802.11g (Backward compatible with 802.11b)[6]	54 Mbps	1500
HomeRF[7]	10 Mbps	150
Bluetooth[8]	2 Mbps	30

[a] 1 Mbps = 1024 kps.
WLAN, wireless local area network; PAN, personal area network.

purchase the hardware, making them a much better option for daily use, not to mention the fact that the connection speeds are comparable to wired connections. However, the WLAN and PAN world is similarly confusing to the unacquainted, and again complicated by a number of "standards" for connecting. Darwin's favorite so far appears to be 802.11b, and 802.11g (also called "WiFi"); they are probably the only standards most folks need to think about for the next couple of years. But for those of you who are into being hip, you might want to take a look at the chart in Table 15.3. Bear in mind that these are the optimal figures for speed and range. Walls, people, radio interference, etc. will cut into this in practice, and the data rate will drop as you get further away from the base unit.

Got Wireless? Now What?

I would like to tell you that we were completely done with learning the wireless lingo, but alas, so far we have only discussed the basics of hardware and network radio standards. That and a buck fifty will get you a cup of coffee and a connection icon on your wireless PDA at a Starbucks Internet Café, but what are you going to do now? Making a connection is the first step, but now we need to get the software and the device configured to ride the wave of the future. Get your machete back out, hack through the next few terms, and then we will roll up our sleeves and get to the details of connecting the most popular PDAs to wireless systems. This lexicon will be a help for the newbies when we hit the nuts-and-bolts section on how to play with these new toys (Table 15.4).

TABLE 15.4. A glossary of wireless networking terms and acronyms.

Acronym/term	Meaning
ISP	Internet Service Provider—yes, the same one you use for connecting with a wired connection. They maintain your "on-ramp to the Information Superhighway."
Client	Any machine that connects to a network via a server. The term can also be used to describe the software that allows the machine to connect and exchange data with software on the server.
Thin client	A program that primarily serves as a way for a user on a client machine (a PDA) to interact directly with the software on the server. The server does the vast majority of the actual computing required by the program.
Thick client	A program that resides on the client machine (PDA) which interacts directly with software/data on the server, but the client program does the majority of the computational work.
Dumb terminal	A device that provides a "window" onto a server for running programs directly.
Telnet	Method for logging onto a computer/server as a terminal remotely from another computer/device.
TCP/IP	Transmission Control Protocol/Internet Protocol—the most widely used networking standard on the Internet.
WAP	Wireless Application Protocol—standard that allows for handheld devices, smartphones, pagers, and other wireless devices to access small chunks of information.
POP	Post Office Protocol—standard used for retrieving e-mail from a server.
SMTP	Simple Mail Transfer Protocol—standard used for transferring e-mail across a network.
VPN	Virtual Private Network—using the Internet as the vehicle for private network traffic in encrypted form (otherwise "private" is not likely to apply).
Browser	Client program that retrieves data from a server and displays them on the user's device. Typically considered a thin client.
HTML	HyperText Markup Language—the format for Web pages.

Getting Down to Business

Let's go out to the tool shed and set up a few wireless PDAs by the numbers. As in the rest of this book, we are going to concentrate on wireless PDAs running the Palm and Pocket PC operating systems. We also discuss the RIM Operating system in this section. Over the last year or so, making these WAN connections has become more straightforward, particularly for Palm and Pocket PC devices, as dual-function PDA/cellular phones have emerged. Regarding WLAN connections, devices with embedded 802.11b (WiFi) cards have begun to appear in increasing numbers, particularly in the Pocket PC arena. Given the ever-shifting landscape of devices on the market, the approaches here focus on the software side of making these connections, rather than the numerous hardware variations. The hardware requirements are summed up in Table 15.5. In the next sections, we show

TABLE 15.5. General hardware requirements by operating system to make wireless connections.

Operating system	Network type	Wireless "connector"	Additional hardware	Additional cost
RIM/ Blackberry	WAN	None additional (radio built into the device)	None	RIM service provider (may have limits on data downloads from Internet without incurring extra fees)
	WLAN	N/A	N/A	N/A
	PAN	N/A	N/A	N/A
Palm OS	WAN	Modem or data-capable cellular phone	Means to connect modem or cable to cellular phone	Wireless carrier or cellular phone provider and separate ISP
	WLAN	WLAN card access point (a pair of WLAN cards is the minimum requirement to connect one device to a network)	May need additional adapter for WLAN card to connect to PDA (also, WLAN card drivers are very limited for Palm OS at the present time, so even if you can physically connect the card, the device may not be able to use it; check with the card and PDA manufacturer before taking the plunge in a WLAN configuration)	ISP if Internet connection is desired
	PAN	IrDA, infrared port connection to LAN, PC, or printer depending on use; Bluetooth/ 802.11 series, minimum is card pair	IrDA, none; additional Bluetooth/802.11 series, means of connecting card to PDA (again, check with manufacturer for availability of drivers)	ISP if Internet connection is desired
Pocket PC	WAN	Modem/radio card or data-capable cellular phone	Means of connecting card to PDA or cable to cellular phone	Wireless carrier or cellular phone provider and separate ISP
	WLAN	WLAN card access point (a pair of WLAN	May need Additional adapter for WLAN card to connect to PDA	ISP if Internet connection is desired

TABLE 15.5. *Continued*				
Operating system	Network type	Wireless "connector"	Additional hardware	Additional cost
		cards is the minimum requirement to connect one device to a network)		
	PAN	IrDA, infrared port connection to LAN, PC, depending on use (printer connectivity not supported by operating system; however, some proprietary options are available); Bluetooth/802.11 series, minimum is card pair	IrDA, none; additional Bluetooth/802.11 series, means of connecting card to PDA.	ISP if Internet connection is desired

you how to get a connection from the device to either a WLAN or WAN with each of these operating systems, and then discuss what to do once we get them talking to each other.

The Palm OS: Can 24 Million (and Still Counting . . .) Users Be Wrong?

If you are in medicine and you have a PDA in your pocket, then odds are it has the Palm operating system on it. So now you want to expand to a connection on the fly, shed the cradle for syncing, and surf for the latest treatment recommendations at the bedside. Here is a more or less step-by-step guide to making wireless network connections that will get you going in that direction. To connect to a WAN connection is really no different than the steps for connecting your Palm device with a "wired" modem. The following hands-on exercise will walk you through it.

HANDS-ON EXERCISE 15.1. UNTETHERING YOUR PALM DEVICE: CONNECTING TO WIRELESS

Follow the steps in Figures 15.5 through 15.20.

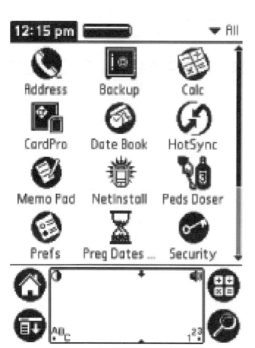

FIGURE 15.5. First, tap on the "Prefs" icon. (Reprinted with permission from palmOne, Inc.)

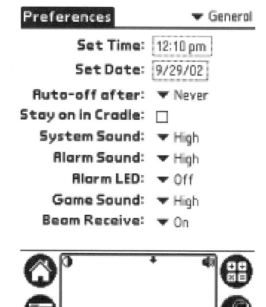

FIGURE 15.6. Second, tap on the upper-right-hand corner over "General." (Reprinted with permission from palmOne, Inc.)

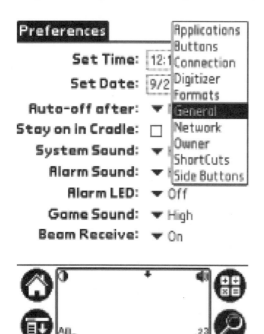

FIGURE 15.7. Third, select "Connection" from the drop-down menu. (Reprinted with permission from palmOne, Inc.)

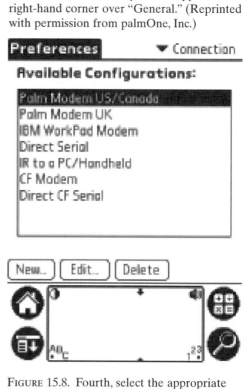

FIGURE 15.8. Fourth, select the appropriate type of modem. If you are connecting via a cellular phone, first try the "Palm Modem" for your region. Then tap on the button at the bottom labeled "Edit." (Reprinted with permission from palmOne, Inc.)

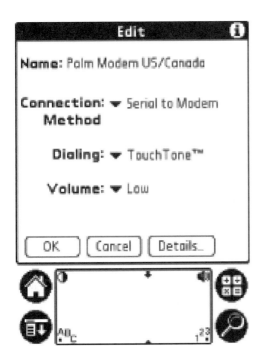

FIGURE 15.9. Tap over the options by "Connection Method." (Reprinted with permission from palmOne, Inc.)

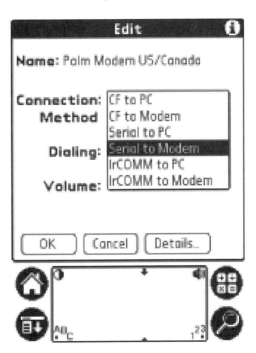

FIGURE 15.10. Select the means by which the modem or cellular phone is connected to the PDA from the drop-down menu. (Reprinted with permission from palmOne, Inc.)

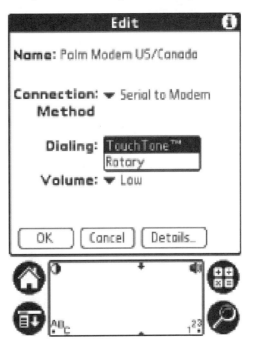

FIGURE 15.11. Next select "Dialing" options, but only if "Touch Tone" is not already selected. (Unless you have a rotary cellular phone—were those ever made?) Then tap "OK." You should be returned to the "Connection" page where you originally selected the modem. Now tap in the upper-right-hand corner to find "Network" in the drop-down menu and tap on it. (Reprinted with permission from palmOne, Inc.)

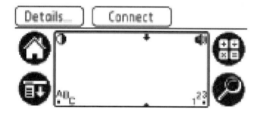

FIGURE 15.12. Click over "Service." (Reprinted with permission from palmOne, Inc.)

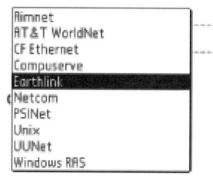

FIGURE 15.13. Select the Internet service provider (ISP) to which you will be connecting. If your ISP is not listed, then you should contact them to determine the settings necessary. Some, such as AOL, may have their own software and configuration. (Reprinted with permission from palmOne, Inc.)

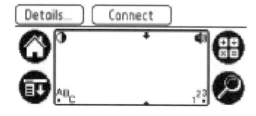

FIGURE 15.14. Fill in the appropriate username, and then tap on "Prompt." (Reprinted with permission from palmOne, Inc.)

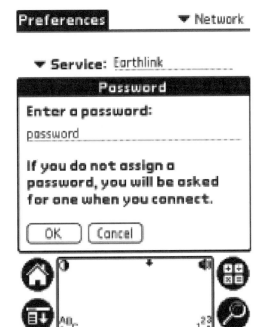

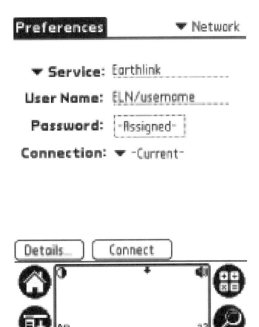

FIGURE 15.15. Enter password now or leave blank to be asked once connected. As you can see, the password appears in plain text, so you might not want to store it here. Then tap on "OK." (Reprinted with permission from palmOne, Inc.)

FIGURE 15.16. Now select the drop-down options next to "Connection." (Reprinted with permission from palmOne, Inc.)

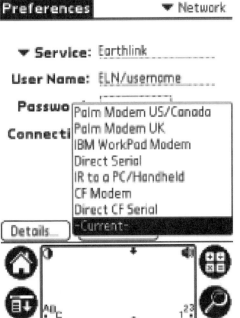

FIGURE 15.17. Find the means by which you will be connecting to your ISP. (Reprinted with permission from palmOne, Inc.)

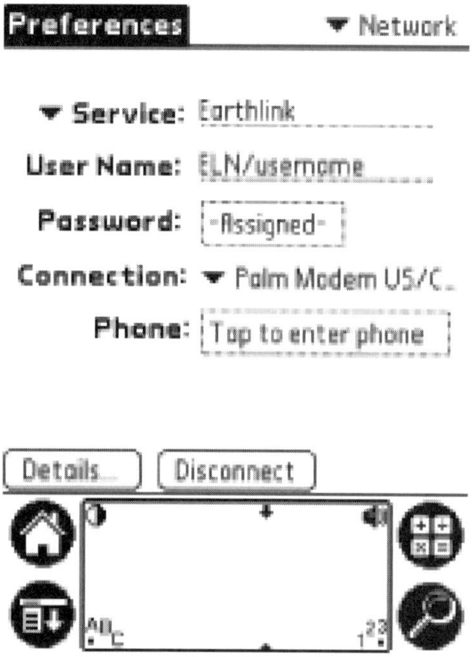

FIGURE 15.18. You will now tap over "Tap to enter phone #." If you selected "Current," this option will not appear. (Reprinted with permission from palmOne, Inc.)

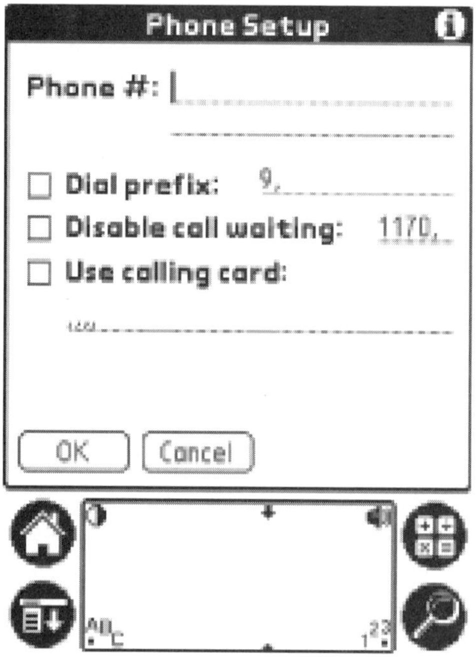

FIGURE 15.19. Enter phone number and select other options if desired. Again, for security reasons, you may wish to return to this page after hanging up if you are afraid that someone might swipe your calling card number. (Reprinted with permission from palmOne, Inc.)

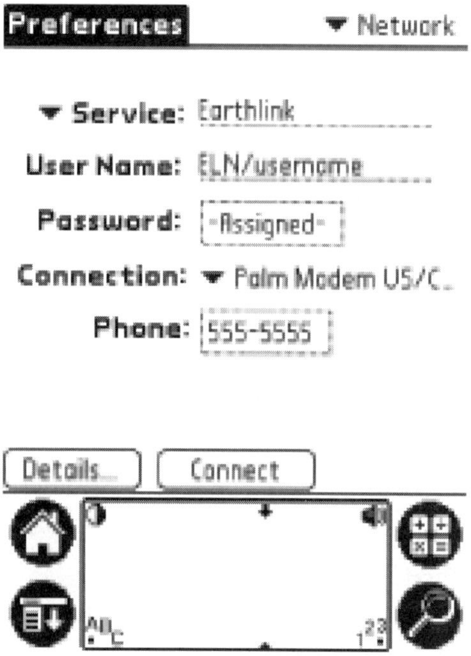

FIGURE 15.20. Tap "Connect" and you are rolling! (Reprinted with permission from palmOne, Inc.)

WLAN/PAN connections with Palm devices are probably most useful as a substitute for synchronizing with the cradle; this can be done most easily with infrared (IR), but is also possible with a radio device like a PCMCIA, Compact Flash (CF), or Secure Digital (SD) card plugged into a slot on the device, or with one of a variety of "sleds" that can attached to a Palm OS device. The software configuration for Palm OS devices is discussed in the next hands-on exercise.

HANDS-ON EXERCISE 15.2. USING YOUR PALM WIRELESSLY ON A WLAN/PAN CONNECTION

Infrared (Figures 15.21–15.23)
Modem (Figure 15.24)

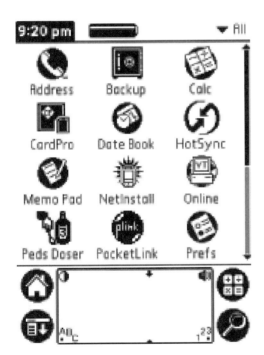

FIGURE 15.21. Select "HotSync" icon. (Reprinted with permission from palmOne, Inc.)

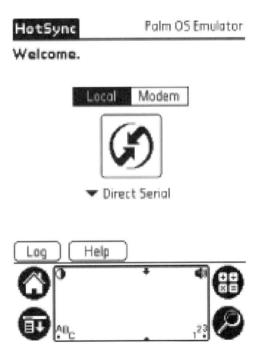

FIGURE 15.22. Next, select the drop-down menu next to "Direct Serial" for synchronization via infrared (IrDA). If you have a wireless LAN driver installed, it will appear here as well. (Reprinted with permission from palmOne, Inc.)

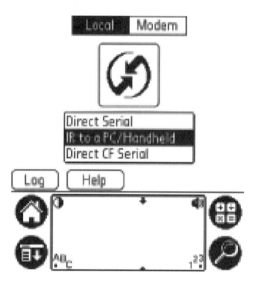

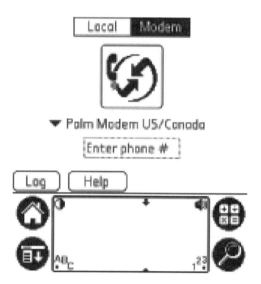

FIGURE 15.23. Select the IR option for IR syncing to PC, or the wireless LAN card driver if offered. (Reprinted with permission from palmOne, Inc.)

FIGURE 15.24. To connect to a LAN or PC via a modem or cellular phone, select "Modem" in the opening "HotSync" screen and the appropriate modem you will be using. Then tap on "Enter phone #" to plug in the number you will be calling. Now tap on the icon with the "HotSync" symbol in the center of the screen to start the synchronization. (Reprinted with permission from palmOne, Inc.)

Pocket PC: Up and Coming

Pocket PCs are becoming more and more popular, and who can blame folks? Cool screens, fast processors, easy expandability, familiar icons, multitasking, and easier enterprise management. Making the wireless leap is relatively easy with a Pocket PC 2002 device like the HP/Compaq Ipaq, Toshiba, Dell, or ViewSonic. To establish a WAN connection, follow our easy-to-use tutorial in the next hands-on exercise.

HANDS-ON EXERCISE 15.3. CONNECTING YOUR POCKET PC TO A WAN

See Figures 15.25 through 15.31.
WLAN is not much more difficult. In the next hands-on exercise we show you how to set up an 802.11b card for a WiFi network. Bluetooth and other protocols are done in a similar fashion.

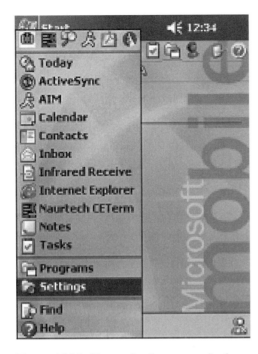

FIGURE 15.25. Tap on the Start menu in the upper-left-hand corner, then select "Settings." (Reprinted with permission from Microsoft Corporation.)

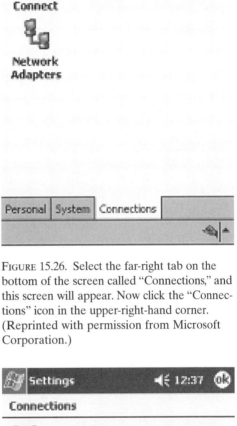

FIGURE 15.26. Select the far-right tab on the bottom of the screen called "Connections," and this screen will appear. Now click the "Connections" icon in the upper-right-hand corner. (Reprinted with permission from Microsoft Corporation.)

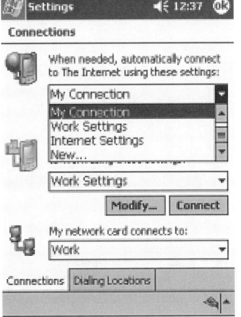

FIGURE 15.27. The screen will show three different options for how to connect to the Internet, at work, and via network card. Click on the drop-down options under "The Internet." Select "My Connection." (Reprinted with permission from Microsoft Corporation.)

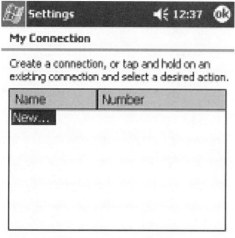

FIGURE 15.28. On first use of "My Connection," the following screen will appear. Tap on "New . . ." to configure your modem for this connection. (Reprinted with permission from Microsoft Corporation.)

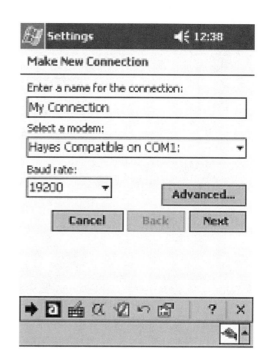

FIGURE 15.29. The modem options will appear, provided you have the appropriate drivers loaded. You should find your modem listed under "Select a modem." Check with the manufacturer of your modem for specific steps or alternate settings. Also, if connecting with a data-capable cellular phone, check with the phone manufacturer or the Microsoft website (www.microsoft.com/pocketpc) for additional details. (The ce.windows.net Web site is a rich source of technical information, with lots of "walk-throughs" and installation tips for Pocket PC users. Newsgroups are also a great source for tips on specific devices here.) When you're done, tap "Next." (Reprinted with permission from Microsoft Corporation.)

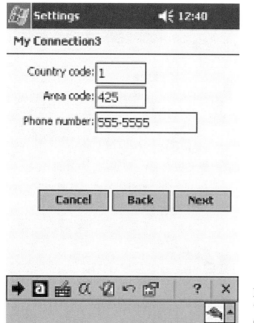

FIGURE 15.30. Enter dialing details and then tap on "Next." (Reprinted with permission from Microsoft Corporation.)

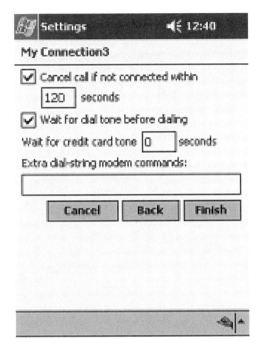

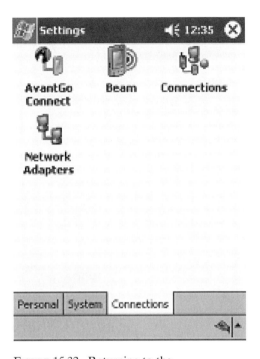

FIGURE 15.31. Answer specific questions on final screen, and then select "Finish." Now when you use your Pocket PC and open Internet Explorer, the modem will be triggered to dial up and connect. (Reprinted with permission from Microsoft Corporation.)

FIGURE 15.32. Returning to the "Connections" page, tap once on "Network Adapters." (Reprinted with permission from Microsoft Corporation.)

HANDS-ON EXERCISE 15.4. CONNECTING YOUR POCKET PC TO A WLAN

See Figures 15.32 through 15.36.

The Pocket PC 2003 Mobile operating system, being released at press time, promises ever easier wirless connections, automaticaly detecting and logging onto any available WiFi networks.

The Blackberry: Wireless Simplicity

The last wireless device we discuss is the RIM Blackberry (Research in Motion, Inc.). All wireless devices should be so simple to connect, but then again, without a wireless connection a RIM device is not much more useful than a pocket calculator, Rolodex, and memo pad. For those not familiar with the RIM device, it was originally designed as a wireless e-mail client and de facto two-way pager. And these are still its strong suits, but it has added wireless Internet browsing, and cellular phone capabilities that will

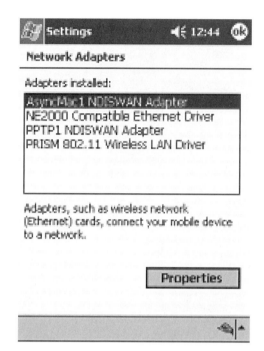

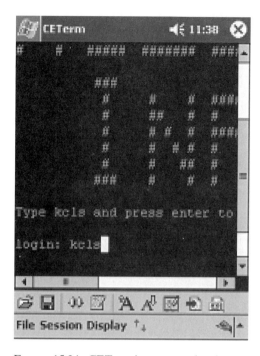

FIGURE 15.33. Find the Adapter that you will be using. Again, if you have the drivers installed correctly, it should appear in this window. Then tap on "Properties." The next screen will prompt you for specific information for configuring the card with information such as using a server-assigned IP address versus a specific IP address, and options for named servers as well. If connecting to a network, check with the administrator for these settings. If doing this at home, try the server-assigned default and keep your fingers crossed. The network settings can drive you nuts, and my experience has been that trial and error ends up being the best way to determine the best settings due to variations in computer and network settings. (Reprinted with permission from Microsoft Corporation.)

FIGURE 15.34. CETerm is an example of a shareware program available for connecting a Pocket PC to a mainframe computer. This is a "thin client" application that allows your PDA to function as a terminal on the network. The connection speed via modem/cell phone and WLAN cards is usually very adequate due to the text-based screens used on most mainframes. They're ugly, but they're fast, and the biggest drawback is the screen size. Most of these programs were written for a 640 × 480 pixel terminal, not a 320 × 240 Pocket PC. CETerm can be downloaded at http://www.naurtech.com/ceterm.htm. (Reprinted with permission from CETerm.)

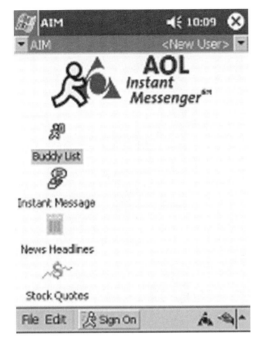
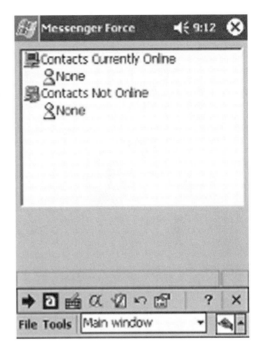

FIGURES 15.35, 15.36. Instant Messaging is becoming available for wireless PDAs, and AOL and MSN Messenger have versions available now. (Reprinted with permission from Microsoft Corporation and AOL.)

perhaps make it even more appealing in the future. Folks in medicine probably are the least familiar with these devices, but provided that they survive the telecom feeding frenzy, they will likely carve out their niche.

Corporate organizations love these things for many reasons, but mostly because of the inherent security they offer. In fact, they are the only wireless devices that have been granted a FIPS140-1 certification by the U.S. National Security Agency (NSA), and have announced plans to cooperate with the U.S. Department of Defense for secure e-mail communications.[9] If it is good enough for the NSA/DoD, it will be good enough for HIPAA! And if that isn't reason enough for medicine to look at these devices, you gotta love their simplicity for wireless connections.

HANDS-ON EXERCISE 15.5. USING A RIM BLACKBERRY DEVICE WIRELESSLY

Step one: find device (Figure 15.37)
Step two: push power button (Figure 15.38)
Step three: view e-mail; cruise Internet (Figure 15.39)

So, where do you get one, you ask? Before you run out and buy one and make a yearlong commitment for wireless service, compare it to the previ-

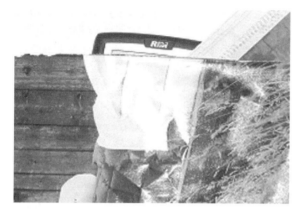

FIGURE 15.37. Find device. (Reprinted with permission from Blackberry.)

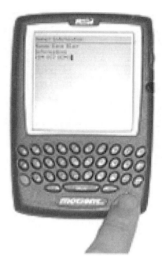

FIGURE 15.38. Push power button. (Reprinted with permission from Blackberry.)

ously discussed Palm and Pocket PC options. There are a number of downsides for use of the RIM by us medical types. The biggest shortcoming is the lack of readily available medical software compared with other devices. Right now, the only way to get the same information and tools that your colleagues with Palm and Pocket PC devices have is by using an Internet browser to connect to pages with this information posted on them in a

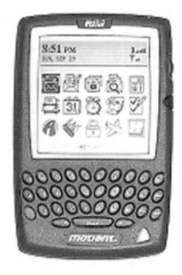

FIGURE 15.39. View e-mail; cruise Intrenet. (Reprinted with permission from Blackberry.)

format that the Blackberry Browser can understand. Doing this over a 19.2-kbps (or less) connection is painfully slow to say the least! Perhaps as Internet resources are better adapted to the smaller screens and slower connections (and as connection speeds increase as a lucky few already have in GPRS networks), this will improve, but progress remains slow in these areas, particularly since the "dot com burst" hit the technology sector in the United States. Also, if you hit one of the many "dead zones" inside a building, you are back to the calculator/Rolodex/memo pad mode. Costwise, a Blackberry will run you about $50 a month, depending on the contract and carrier. In short, if you are in medicine and plan to use your PDA to assist in patient care, consider your needs very carefully if you look at the Blackberry as of 2003.

Running in a Hospital with Scissors (or Why IT and Legal Departments Cringe at the Sight of an Intern with a Wireless PDA)

Wireless Lockbox

Wireless systems have been under considerable scrutiny recently, largely due to limitations of the Wireless Equivalent Protocol that ships with 802.11b networks.[10] In fact, the recently released NIST (National Institute of Standards and Technology) draft of Wireless Network security states in its Executive Summary:

Risks are inherent, however, in any wireless technology. Some of these risks are similar to those of wired networks; some are exacerbated by wireless connectivity; some are new. Perhaps the most significant difference from wired networks and the main source of these risks is that with wireless networks the organization's underlying communications medium, the airwave, is openly exposed to intruders, making it the logical equivalent of placing an Ethernet port in the parking lot.[11]

Interestingly, the same things were being said about wired networks only 5 years ago! Even infrared on handheld computers has been criticized for its inherent "insecurity" by many of the same agencies that have been known to tout its "security" given its directional nature (it can only be received over short distances, and only when pointed right at the other computer). Go figure. Anyway, like all new technologies, wireless connectivity will take its lumps until the kinks are ironed out. Medical information, although not needing the level of security required for top-secret information, should be reasonably secure. But what level of security is reasonable? The recently released HIPAA privacy guidelines are less than straightforward regarding a specific set of guidelines for privacy protection, especially as would apply to wireless transmission of such data. The "plain English" version of the regulation posted by the Department of Health and Human

Services states the following regarding incidental disclosure of patient-specific information:

Incidental Use and Disclosure: The final Rule acknowledges that uses or disclosures that are incidental to an otherwise permitted use or disclosure may occur. Such incidental uses or disclosures are not considered a violation of the Rule provided that the covered entity has met the reasonable safeguards and minimum necessary requirements. For example, if these requirements are met, doctors' offices may use waiting room sign-in sheets, hospitals may keep patient charts at bedside, doctors can talk to patients in semiprivate rooms, and doctors can confer at nurse's stations without fear of violating the rule if overheard by a passerby.[12]

Advocates of increasing technology use have seen this as a green light to move forward with Internet and wireless transmissions of patient identifiable data, so long as security measures are in place. At the other end of the spectrum are those who believe no truly secure measures exist and therefore these activities should not be undertaken, lest the U.S. federal government swoop down and slap them with a fine or jail time. The exact interpretation of the HIPAA rules remains to be seen, and not unlike a bunch of kids standing at the edge of a pool on a brisk late spring morning, no one wants to be the one to find out how cold the water is. No one will know for certain until someone jumps in and the degree of "reasonable measures" is tested in court.

Network administrators can configure the system so that it is relatively "airtight" in keeping unwanted folks outside of a WLAN. However, this requires constant vigilance on their part, and care on the part of end-users to keep their software up to date with the appropriate security patches installed. Another approach for insuring security of a WLAN is to have the transmission range limited to areas that can be monitored by the users and office staff. Like most things, though, you could never say that it is absolutely secure, as there are ways to enhance faint signals. Ultimately the old adage caveat emptor will apply in all cases, and this is true of any network, wired or wireless.

Someone Adjust the Antenna: I Can't Read the Tracing for All the Snow . . .

All wireless device users, but particularly medical personnel, need to be concerned about the potential for electromagnetic interference (EMI) of the devices in the environment where they are being used. Cellular phones were the first devices that brought this issue to light with stories of technical problems in electronic devices caused by cell phone transmissions.[13,14] An even greater concern is malfunctions of pacemakers and hearing aids in response to a variety of electromagnetic energy emitters.[15–17] The reality is that EMI has been an issue ever since the first electrical devices were introduced into medical practice. The simple fact is that devices that have or potentially could have interfered with each other have been in hospitals ever since the days of Edison, because electricity flowing through a wire is an electromagnetic transmitter. Conversely, any wire can function as a receiver of such electromagnetic energy. The difference with wireless devices is that they are new, and their signal strength is greater because they are intended to transmit and receive signals. So, should these devices be completely banned from a medical facility due to the infinitesimal chance that the device, if put close enough to another device, could interfere with its readings or behavior?

There is no easy answer, but there are a few important facts. One, EMI cannot be totally eliminated, so long as electrons are being driven through a wire somewhere. Two, the intensity of the interference will decrease as the distance between two devices increases. Three, shielding of sensitive devices or instruments will minimize the potential for interference. The term electromagnetic compatibility (EMC) is really what needs to be addressed in risk assessments, rather than EMI. EMC means that two devices (or a group of devices for that matter) can coexist without any significant unintended influence on one another.[18] Despite the press hype and the wringing of hands by hospital administrators, EMI is not a unique or new problem created by wireless devices. Awareness and thoughtful use are the weapons against ignorance and prohibition.

References for EMI/EMC in Health Care

- U.S. Food and Drug Administration's Center for Devices and Radiological Health: online home page: http://www.fda.gov/cdrh/emc/
- Center for the Study of Wireless Electromagnetic Compatibility: online home page: http://www.ou.edu/engineering/emc/
- IEEE EMC Society: online home page: http://www.ewh.ieee.org/soc/emcs/
- Medical Devices Agency, Department of Health, United Kingdom: online home page: http://medical-devices.gov.uk/

Packing Things Up and Heading for Home

For those of you who have hung on this long and are still reading, I have compiled a table of general considerations for comparing the three major operating systems and their wireless capabilities as of autumn 2002 (Table 15.6).

With the pace of technology, these characteristics will change, so research on your own part at that time will be the best advice. A number of good resources to look at are listed here.

Wireless medical applications:
- American Medical Informatics Association Mobile Computing Special Interest Group: http://mailman.amia.org/mailman/listinfo/mc-sig/

TABLE 15.6. Operating systems for wireless PDAs.

	Blackberry	Palm OS	Pocket PC 2002
WAN capable	Yes	Yes	Yes
WLAN capable	No	Yes	Yes
Wireless equipment needed To Cut the cord	None additional	Modem/WLAN card Adapter[a] Access point/ receiving card	Modem/WLAN card Adapter[a] Access point/ receiving card
Internet browsing	Yes[b]	Yes	Yes
Combination phones available (network type required)	Yes GSM	Yes CDMA GSM	Yes GSM
Telnet	Yes[c]	Yes	Yes
Transmission security	Triple DES, FIPS 140-1	WEP, WLAN Protocols vary	WEP, WLAN Protocols vary
Wireless printing directly from device via infrared	No	Yes (with optional software)	Yes (with optional software)
Wireless printing capable via radio connection	Yes (requires Internet-connected networked printer.)	Yes (via networked printer)	Yes (via network printer)

[a] Depends on the device as to whether an adapter is required, as now some devices are coming with slots that can accept SD/MMC, or Compactflash form factor radios. A few devices will even accept PCMCIA Cards.
[b] Internet browsing is available, but it usually requires an additional monthly charge or fee above that which is charged for e-mail access.
[c] Telnet is potentially available, but at present it is via an add-on software program that runs through a subscription based online service.

- FP Net Office Computerization Resources, PDAs and wireless: http://www.aafp.org/x433.xml
- PDA Cortex (*Journal of Mobile Informatics*): http://www.pdacortex.com/
- The U.S. Army's Telemedicine and Advanced Technology Research Center Wireless Medical Enterprise Working Group: http://www.tatrc.org/website_wme/
- Wireless Medical Applications Newsgroup: http://www.yahoogroups.com/group/wirelessmedicalapplications/

General wireless information:
- 802.11 Planet: http://www.80211-planet.com/
- Mobile Village: http://www.mobilevillage.com/
- Pocket PC wireless information: http://www.ppcw.net/

General PDA-related sites that have wireless information from time to time:

- PDABuzz: http://www.pdabuzz.com/
- Pocket PCThoughts: http://www.pocketpcthoughts.com
- DevBuzz: http://www.devbuzz.com
- CE Windows.net: http://www.cewindows.net
- PDAStreet: http://www.pdastreet.com/
- WiredGuy: http://www.wiredguy.com/
- PalmInfoCenter: http://www.palminfocenter.com/
- PDAGeek: http://www.pdageek.com/
- Pocket PC Tools: http://www.pocketpctools.com/

Wireless Present, Wireless Future

So let's return to the nursery again to look at our bundle of joy that we cut the cord on at the beginning of this chapter. You have survived the boot camp basics for wireless; some of you are thrilled with the possibilities, others are underwhelmed. To the skeptics in the group, don't forget that we are in the very early days of this technology. Despite the fact that the PDA may appear like its "mother," the PC, it will go through much more development and experience before it will rival the capabilities of an "adult" computer. Some of you will want to be active in aiding in this progress, others of you would rather wait to become more involved once the device matures a bit more. Either approach is fine; after all, not everyone enjoys changing diapers, even if it means missing a few moments of cute smiles and laughter. And there will be plenty of setbacks and disappointments in the next few years related to wireless medical applications. Such is life on the "bleeding edge" of technology. But the trials and tribulations of life with a new technology will ultimately be rewarded; otherwise, we would still be bloodletting and applying leeches to our patients. So I invite the most skeptical to look into my crystal ball in closing, to at least keep an eye open to a number of related advances that will make the untethered yet connected PDA as indispensable as a stethoscope in the years to come!

Ultimately, wireless will do for PDAs and handheld computers what the Internet did for personal computers. Trust me. But what form the devices take will be as varied as the users. Tablet devices have been toyed with over the last few years, but cost, weight, and fragility have kept them out of most clinics. This is changing with the arrival of the "Tablet PC devices coming to market in late 2002. They are projected to eventually cost under $500 by early reports; coupled with WLAN technology running at under $150 for access points and sub-$100 WLAN cards, this will compel more folks to look at making these a part of their tools of the trade. Not unrelated, the arrival of fuel cells should make the devices more user-friendly by dropping the weight and potentially eliminating the need for downtime while recharging a device.

On the security front, true wireless virtual private networking (VPN) technologies will answer the worries of IT departments everywhere. Hardware-based technologies like the recently released Air Fortress Gateway (http://www.fortresstech.com/) that the U.S. military is currently pursuing will likely fill the need for hospitals as well. Cool factor aside, it will take more than just being "hip" to convince many physicians, healthcare providers, and hospitals to shuck out ever more scarce resources for items that will be more prone to loss and breakage than desktop PCs. A number of trends will change this. Electronic medical records will become the norm, rather than the exception, in the not too distant future. Data entry at the point of care will be a key element that wireless devices will provide in an unobtrusive fashion, something that desktop PCs cannot offer. The efficiency and accuracy of this will be invaluable for the ever-evolving documentation expectations of both payers and the legal community.

These demands, coupled with ever-increasing pressures for compliance with clinical practice guidelines and evidence-based medicine, are changing the nature of medical practice for better or for worse. The physician's role is evolving from medical expert to knowledge manager. Many may take issue at this characterization; however, with the ever-accelerating pace of medical advances, the concept of a physician as a medical expert, memorizing all the facts and applying them, is a paradigm that is already on the wane.

Instead, the ability to rapidly acquire and review the most up-to-date medical studies and opinions in regard to a patient's condition and then select not only the most efficacious but also mutually acceptable course for physician and patient to pursue is becoming the keystone of our profession. This is a higher level of practice, which involves technology and thought, and is certainly not replaced by these technologies, but rather enhanced by them. Honestly, this is not really any different from the essence of what we have done for millennia; however, now the volume of information we must command at all times is humanly impossible to master, particularly in primary care specialties.

Point-of-care computing will soon become a necessity, not a nicety. This day is probably not as far off as many of us may think, but much will depend on factors far beyond advances in technology. Economic, cultural, and regulatory factors will dictate and shape the destiny of the fledgling wireless PDAs of today. The wheels were set in motion the moment the cord was cut. Where it will lead us, we can only dream and hope!

References

1. Mock D. Wireless industry primer: a guide to wireless for non-techies living and working in a techie world, April 2002. Available on the Web at http://www.wow-com.com/market_research/documents/WirelessPrimerL.pdf.
2. Mobile Streams, Ltd. Wireless clueless: your mobile reality check, data rate review. Available online at http://www.wirelessclueless.com/data.asp.

3. Infrared Data Association. Technical summary of "Ir DATA" and "IrDA Control." Available on the Web at http://irda.org/standards/standards.asp.

4. Geier J. 802.11a: An excellent long term Solution. 2002. 802.11Planet.Com. Available on the Web at http://www.80211-planet.com/tutorials/article/0,4000,10724_1436331,00.html.

5. Wi-Fi Alliance. Range and environment issues. Available on the Web at http://www.wi-fi.net/.

6. Vaughan-Nichols SJ. 802.11g: The next best thing or the next last thing. 2002. 802.11Planet.Com. Available on the Web at http://www.80211-planet.com/columns/.

7. HomeRF Working Group. HomeRF product profile, March 2001. Available on the Web at http://www.homerf.org/products/.

8. Bluetooth SIG, Bluetooth Specifications, Februrary 2001. Available on the Web at http://www.bluetooth.org/specifications.htm.

9. Dorobek CJ. Blackberry to carry DOD security. Federal Computer Week, Aug. 20, 2002. Available on the Web at http://www.fcw.com/fcw/articles/2002/.

10. Borisov N, Goldberg I, Wagner D. Intercepting mobile communications: the insecurity of 802.11. Proceedings of Mobicom 2001. 2001:180–189.

11. National Institute of Standards and Technology. Draft of NIST Special Publication 800–48. Wireless Network Security: 802.11, Bluetooth, and Handheld Devices. Washington, DC: NIST, 2002.

12. U.S. Department of Health and Human Services. Modifications to the standards for privacy of individually identifiable health information: final rule. Washington, DC: USDHHS, 2002.

13. Silberberg J. Electronic medical devices and EMI. Compliance Engineering 1996; Jan/Feb:77–78.

14. Lyznicki JM, Altman RD, Williams MA. Report of the American Medical Association (AMA) Council on Scientific Affairs and AMA recommendations to medical professional staff on the use of wireless radio-frequency in hospitals. Biomed Instrum Technol 2001;35(3):189–95.

15. Barbaro V, Bartolini P, Donato A. Electromagnetic interference of analog cellular telephones with pacemakers. PACE 1996;19:1410–1418.

16. Naegell B, Osswald S, Deola M. Intermittent pacemaker dysfunction caused by digital mobile telephones. J Am Coll Cardiol 1996;27(6):1471–1477.

17. Witters D. Medical devices and EMI: the FDA perspective. Available on the Web at http://www.fda.gov/cdrh/emc/persp.html.

18. Institute of Biomedical Engineering Technology. Electromagnetic interference: causes and concerns in the health care environment. Available on the Web at http://ibet.asttbc.org/emi.htm.

16
Programmable Calculators

PETER L. REYNOLDS AND MARK H. EBELL

What, Me Program? Are You Crazy?

It's safe to say that most people who read this book have either never written a computer program or, if they have long ago, never intend to do so again. The majority of off-the-shelf software these days consists of thousands of lines of code written by teams of programmers. So why even bother trying to write your own program—why not just jump ahead to the next chapter? My first answer is that programming is fun and you should give it a try before saying no. If you're not technically inclined, don't laugh quite yet—you might like reason number two. The second reason to try programming your own code is that if you want it programmed right, you have to do it yourself. Sound familiar? Well, it's really true when it comes to computer software, so keep reading.

If the thought of this much programming is too much to bear, then a custom software solution is another option, and might be your best bet. A list of potential freelance programmers for Palm OS devices is available at www.palm.com and other locations on the World Wide Web.

Programmable calculators meet the needs of specialized users by allowing them to further customize the software. There are two approaches to programmable calculators found in handheld calculator software. The first, sometimes called "plug-in" software, is difficult to implement but overall more powerful than other options. In this case, the user writes a software program using a desktop editor (such as Syncalc's Software Development Kit for Palm OS or Napier's VB Script editor for Pocket PC). The user may need to compile the program, and then installs the program onto a handheld device. The programmable calculator interface is used to access the software. Although the programmable calculator software itself provides a graphical user interface (GUI) and some programming logic, a good deal of technical expertise is needed. The time investment can be significant, too. The upside is that you can create complicated calculator functions without the hassles of programming a stand-alone application from scratch.

The "plug-in" approach is beyond the scope of this chapter and the interest of most everyday PDA users, but keep reading! The second approach is almost as powerful in most situations and much, much easier to master. Anyone who has used macro functions with word processing and other office software will pick it up right away. Just as with macros, these programmable calculators process a sequence of calculator functions provided by the user.

Programmable Calculators for the Palm and Pocket PC OS

SynCalc, one type of programmable calculator that accepts plug-in software, is found at http://www.installigent.com/software.php?productline_id=8. It runs on the Palm OS. There are also several Pocket PC programmable calculators. Napier is a very full-featured product and is the equivalent of SynCalc for the Palm in most ways (http://www.nca-corp.com/Napier/Napier%20Start.htm); best of all, it only costs $25 at this writing. A simpler program that is focused more on the health professions is MedFormulas, which is freeware (http://www.liesens.com/medformulas).

In the rest of the chapter, we'll go through a step-by-step example using SynCalc. It's really just a matter of translating the algorithm you wish to accomplish into a list of sequential calculator functions. Once you write a successful program, you can use it repeatedly. You can also modify it as needed over time. To download and use SynCalc, go to their site at http://www.installigent.com/software.php?productline_id=8 ($19.95). The general lessons that you learn in this chapter will also apply to Napier and MedFormulas for the Pocket PC.

Using SynCalc

As an example, let's imagine you're a physician or nurse practitioner seeing sick children in the wintertime. Many of the medications you prescribe are dosed based on the patient weight. To make you more efficient and less prone to errors, we'll write a program called "URI Meds" that calculates the dosage of several commonly used medications for upper respiratory infection. It's easier to begin programming if you start with some kind of template. We'll base our first program on an existing shortcut and write the code to calculate the dosage of Tylenol only. Then, once we've learned the basic syntax, we'll expand it to other medications.

Here's what this program will look like on your PDA when finished. Select "shortcuts" from the bottom right of the SynCalc Display (Figure 16.1).

Many of the shortcuts listed in Figure 16.2 can be downloaded free of charge from the SynCalc website. As a medical professional, be sure to check all programs for accuracy before using them in practice. Select the

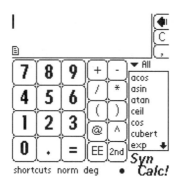

FIGURE 16.1. SynCalc for Palm OS. (Reprinted with permission from Installigent Team, a Zero-sixty Corp.)

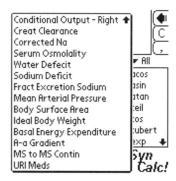

FIGURE 16.2. SynCalc pop-up with medical shortcuts. (Reprinted with permission from Installigent Team, a Zero-sixty Corp.)

URI Meds program, enter the patient's weight (Figure 16.3), and the correct dosage of medications is calculated (Figure 16.4).

IMPORTANT: Leave the "Auto-activate console?" checkbox checked as seen in Figure 16.4. Otherwise, the Shortcuts will not properly display results. If you accidentally uncheck this checkbox, you can display the Console again via the SynCalc main menu discussed later.

Here's the exact code as you'd enter it into the SynCalc editor:

```
C(in(Weight in pounds:)/2.2)@w=(w*15/160)@t=out(\n\nPatient weight
   %f kgs,w)= out(\nTylenol: %f tsp Q4,t)=out(\nIbuprofen: %f tsp Q6,t)
   =out(\nPen-Vee K: %f mg QID,(w*50/4))=out(\nAmoxicillin: %f mg
   TID, (w*40/3))=out(\nAugmentin: %f mg BID, (w*45/2))=
   out(\nAzithromycin: %f mg/dose, (w*5))=
```

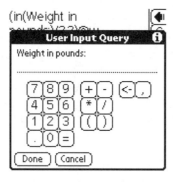

FIGURE 16.3. "URI Meds" Shortcut: Enter patient's weight. (Reprinted with permission from Installigent Team, a Zero-sixty Corp.)

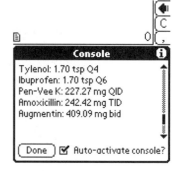

FIGURE 16.4. "URI Meds" Shortcut: Calculated dosage for common upper respiratory infection (URI) medications. (Reprinted with permission from Installigent Team, a Zero-sixty Corp.)

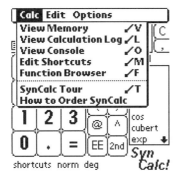

FIGURE 16.5. SynCalc program menu. (Reprinted with permission from Installigent Team, a Zero-sixty Corp.)

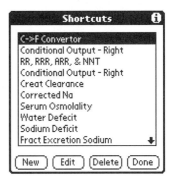

FIGURE 16.6. "Edit Shortcuts" menu option. (Reprinted with permission from Installigent Team, a Zero-sixty Corp.)

We'll go through the code line by line, but first let's get oriented to the SynCalc program editor. If you haven't already downloaded and installed SynCalc, you'll have to do so now. Choose SynCalc from the Application launcher and select the Menu function from the main SynCalc screen. Tap on "Edit Shortcuts" in the "Calc" menu (Figure 16.5). You should see a list of currently installed Shortcuts (Figure 16.6).

Some versions of SynCalc include a shortcut for temperature conversion from Celsius (C) to Fahrenheit (F). This short bit of code can serve as a template. If you see this choice, select it and tap "Edit" at the bottom of the screen. If not, you can tap "New" and copy the code from Figure 16.7 onto your screen. You can also skip using a template and begin entering your own code immediately.

The Edit Shortcut screen is divided into two parts. The name of each shortcut is entered in the top half entitled "Name." The algorithm used to calculate your solution is coded in the bottom half, entitled "Value."

IMPORTANT: If you edit the Name or Value of a shortcut, the original shortcut is completely overwritten and the starting information is lost.

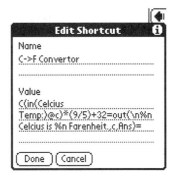

FIGURE 16.7. Shortcut code for temperature conversion. (Reprinted with permission from Installigent Team, a Zero-sixty Corp.)

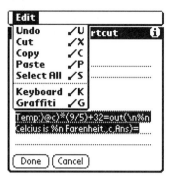

Figure 16.8. Editing with "Copy" and "Paste." (Reprinted with permission from Installigent Team, a Zero-sixty Corp.)

Another option is to copy code from an existing shortcut to a new shortcut using the Copy and Paste functions from the Edit menu (Figure 16.8). Try it!

We'll use this example to discuss the basic syntax of a SynCalc "plug-in" program. The temperature conversion code is as follows:

$$C(in(Celsius\ Temp:)@c)*(9/5)+32$$
$$= out(\backslash n\%n\ Celsius\ is\ \%n\ Farenheit., c, Ans) =$$

You will notice that the code is very compressed. The Palm OS environment is shorter on space than the typical office computer platform. The screen is small as well as the memory. In this case, formatting conventions that take up more space have been left out. The more compact code is hard for people to read, but the handheld computer can understand it just fine. Extra spaces and carriage return characters can lead to error messages, so be careful!

The principal commands used to write SynCalc shortcuts are summarized in Table 16.1. Note that the "C" command only clears the expression window on the main SynCalc calculator screen but not the Console pop-up window, where results are displayed by the "out" command.

TABLE 16.1. SynCalc command summary.

Command syntax	Explanation
C	At the beginning of a shortcut, tells computer to clear expression window
in(*Prompt Message Here*)	Request a value from the user via a pop-up window
@	Tells computer to assign the current value to a memory location
=	Tells computer to process all calculations up to that point in the program
out(*Response Message Here*)	Outputs text and values to the user via the SynCalc Console

TABLE 16.2. Formatting commands for SynCalc.		
Syntax	Output format	Example
%n	Normal number	"23"
%f	Fixed	"23.00"
%s	Scientific	"2.3000000e1"
%h	Hexadecimal	"00000049"

User-defined memory locations are identified with a single letter "a" to "z". There is an additional memory location used by SynCalc called "Ans". This system variable is extremely important as it contains the current numerical value being manipulated. It's the equivalent of the number you see on the display line of a pocket calculator or the expression window of the SynCalc main screen. Each time a new value is written to the location "Ans", the old value is lost. When a calculation is executed using the "=" command, the result is always stored in the "Ans" location.

You can output text as well as calculated numerical value. Although formatting is limited, values can be displayed in several different formats as listed in Table 16.2. "\n" and "\t" are special character strings indicating new line and tab, respectively.

The first command in our template code, "in(Celsius Temp:)", prompts the user to enter a value in response to the message "Celsius Temp:". The entered value is stored in "Ans". The next command, "@c", assigns this value to the memory location "c". Finally, the conversion calculation is completed and assigned to "Ans" by the "=" command. The original value of "Ans", the temperature in Celsius entered by the user, would have been lost except that it was also stored in the memory location "c" as a user-defined variable.

The results are output to the user by the command "out(\n%n Celsius is %n Fahrenheit.,c,Ans)", and the program is ended with a final "=". The formatting commands used in the output command are confusing but not complicated. The message to be displayed is followed by a comma-separated list of values stored in memory that will be included in the message. A place is reserved in the message for each of these variables using the syntax in Table 16.2. "\n" tells the program to move to a new line. The first "%n" reserves a place in the text message for the first of two comma-separated variables, "c", and the second "%n" reserves a place for the second variable listed, "Ans".

Now that we have an understanding of what the code means, let's edit the program to meet our needs. The original code, once again, is as follows:

$$C(in(\text{Celsius Temp:})@c) * (9/5) + 32 =$$
$$out(\backslash n\%n \text{ Celsius is } \%n \text{ Fahrenheit.}, c, Ans) =$$

We'll prompt the user to enter a weight rather than a temperature. It's a good idea to always specify the anticipated unit of measure in your prompt;

this will minimize errors later. As in the final code, I'll immediately change the weight in pounds to weight in kilograms by dividing by 2.2, and I'll store the resulting value in memory location "w".

$$C(\text{in}(\text{Weight in pounds:})/2.2)@w*(9/5)+32=$$
$$\text{out}(\backslash n\%n \text{ Celsius is } \%n \text{ Fahrenheit.}, c, \text{Ans})=$$

This code asks for weight and then returns a temperature, so we're not finished yet. The pediatric dosage of Tylenol is 15 mg/kg/dose, and liquid Tylenol contains 160 mg per teaspoon. Therefore, the dose calculation is "w*15/160". Note that as in most computer programming, multiplication is indicated with the "*". If we change the output text to match the new calculations, our code looks like the following:

$$C(\text{in}(\text{Weight in pounds:})/2.2)@w*15/160=$$
$$\text{out}(\backslash nA \%n \text{ kg patient receives } \%n \text{ teaspoon of Tylenol per}$$
$$\text{dose.}, w, \text{Ans})=$$

Try the program out and see how it works. If you enter a weight of 30 pounds, the output should look like that shown in Figure 16.9.

Because no one measures teaspoon medication dosages to the seventh decimal place, a different number format makes sense. Try changing the "%n" in the "out" command to "%f".

$$C(\text{in}(\text{Weight in pounds:})/2.2)@w*15/160=$$
$$\text{out}(\backslash nA \%f \text{ kg patient receives } \%f \text{ teaspoon of Tylenol per}$$
$$\text{dose.}, w, \text{Ans})=$$

Now the output makes more sense, as shown in Figure 16.10.

Your program may not run the first time because of errors. Don't forget to change the variable name in the "out" command from "c" to "w". A common source of errors is the use of parentheses. Parentheses tell SynCalc which calculation to complete first following the standard order of mathematical operations. Consider the following examples:

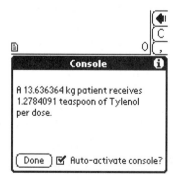

FIGURE 16.9. Drug calculation with "normal" formatting. (Reprinted with permission from Installigent Team, a Zero-sixty Corp.)

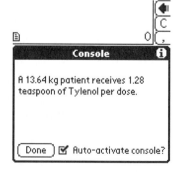

FIGURE 16.10. Drug calculation with "fixed" formatting. (Reprinted with permission from Installigent Team, a Zero-sixty Corp.)

$$(2+4)/2 = 3$$
$$2+4/2 = 4$$

Computer programs usually process multiplication and division operations before addition and subtraction. In the first line, the parentheses indicate that 2 and 4 are to be added together before dividing by 2. In the second line, the parentheses are left out, so 4 is divided by 2 and then added to 2. The subject of nested operations gives many nonmathematical, nonprogrammer types great heartburn. It suffices to say that an order of operations error is often to blame when your calculation produces an incorrect result. Always, double-check your program several times before depending on it in clinical situations.

As it turns out, the pediatric dosage of ibuprofen is the same as Tylenol. In the final "URI Meds" example, we store this value in the memory location "t" and use it for both.

    C(in(Weight in pounds:)/2.2)@w =
      (w * 15/160)@t = out(\n \nPatient weight %f kgs, w) =
      out(\nTylenol: %f tsp Q4, t) = out(\nIbuprofen: %f tsp Q6, t)

After each step in the algorithm, the "=" command tells SynCalc to complete the code up to that point. We've taken an existing SynCalc plug-in and modified it to calculate a new value. Once you become familiar with SynCalc plug-in programming, you'll be able to start from scratch. Just develop your algorithm, break it down into simple but very specific steps, and then translate these steps into language that SynCalc can understand. Table 16.3 shows one way you might proceed.

You can include calculations directly within the comma-separated list of values in an "out" command response message. For example, the command

    out(\nAmoxicillin: %f mg TID, (w * 40/3)) =

both calculates the three-times-per-day dosage of Amoxicillin based on weight in kilograms and displays the result. The drug dosages for Pen-Vee K, Amoxicillin, Augmentin, and azithromycin are calculated and displayed this way. Other medications can be added to the list by adding an additional "out" command following the same pattern. The final "URI Meds" program then looks like this:

    C(in(Weight in pounds)/2.2)@ w =
      (w * 15/160)@ t = out(\n \nPatient weight %f kgs, w) =
      out(\nTylenol: %f tsp Q4, t) =
      out(\nIbuprofen: %f tsp Q6, t) =
      out(\nPen - Vee K: % f mg QID, (w * 50/4)) =
      out(\nAmoxicillin : % f mg TID, w * 40/3) =
      out(\nAugmentin: % f mg BID, (w * 50/4)) =
      out(\nAzithromycin: %f mg/dose, (w * 5)) =

TABLE 16.3. Steps in a SynCalc program.

Algorithm	Simple steps	SynCalc code
1. Input weight in pounds	in(Weight in pounds:) → Ans	in(Weight in pounds:)/2.2)@w=
2. Change weight into kilograms and save value	Ans/2.2 → Ans Ans@w	
3. Calculate dosage of medications for Tylenol and ibuprofen	w*15/160 → Ans Ans@t	(w*15/160)@t=
4. Output weight in kilograms	out(\n\nPatient weight %f kgs,w)	out(\n\nPatient weight %f kgs,w)=
5. Output dosage of Tylenol	out(\n Tylenol: %f tsp Q4,t)	out(\n Tylenol: %f tsp Q4,t)=
6. Output dosage of ibuprofen	out(\nIbuprofen: %f tsp Q6,t)	out(\nIbuprofen: %f tsp Q6,t)=

That's it! You've completed the "URI Meds" plug-in. Be sure to test the program and double-check the values it outputs against a trusted source. Once you're sure you've got it right, it's ready for clinical practice. To learn more, download several Shortcuts from the SynCalc web page and read over the code. You'll be amazed how quickly you pick up new programming techniques.

Summary

Programming your handheld computer to perform complex, repetitive tasks is actually not as hard as most people think. Although preconfigured calculators are available for common tasks like calculating the body mass index and creatinine clearance, physicians who perform highly specialized calculations may find it best to 'roll their own' with the handy tools discussed in this chapter.

17

How to Make Your Own Database: Programming a Simple Procedure Log

JAMES M. THOMPSON AND SCOTT M. STRAYER

Don't Pay for a Handheld Database: Build Your Own!

Building a Procedure Tracking Log

Physicians often have to keep a record of all the clinical procedures they perform on patients. Most often they do it to get paid for their work—and then lose the bits of paper between hospital and office. Or maybe residents have to prove to their professors that they are actually learning skills—and then can't remember at the end of a busy rotation what they did, or when. Or a physician in practice might have to cough up a log every year to keep renewing hospital privileges, and not have any idea how to go back over 365 days to get the information together. Wouldn't it be much easier to tap that information into a handheld on the spot in a few seconds?

In Chapter 11 we reviewed database software products that you can use on a handheld computer for everything from your family's shoe sizes to tracking patients. Using the information we provided there, you should be able to pick an inexpensive software product suitable for building your own custom databases.

In this chapter we show you how to build and maintain your own databases using a clinical procedure log as an example. Forget about paying a software engineer: you can make databases like this yourself (for free) while in the dentist's chair, to keep your mind off the drill.

In this chapter we explain how to build a simple procedure log using HanDBase (www.handbase.com). Then we'll show you one way to convert this flat file design to a relational design and explain how to link the HanDBase database to more powerful desktop database software products. A great thing about HanDBase is that you can use its databases on either Palm OS or Pocket PC handhelds! Finally, we'll show you how to build a similar procedure log database within Microsoft Access using Pendragon Forms.

Most users will be content with this type of user-friendly database software. If you have a program like the ones described in Chapter 11 and run into a problem, talk to the company that made the product, because often they can provide programming expertise to find a solution with little-known features in their products. For very complex handheld database projects, you might want to consult a programmer who may use one of the heavyweight products mentioned in Chapter 11, or perhaps even hire a programmer to build your project in a low-level computer language like C++.

Key Points

1. You can build a simple procedure log database on your handheld in a few minutes.
2. You can share a HanDBase database with both Palm OS and Pocket PC users.
3. You can make the procedure log database more useful by modifying it with more complex features as you learn about them, like building in relationships between two or more tables.

Build Your Own

This is the "Do It Yourself" age, when everybody can roll their own—whatever. It is very easy to build your own database design. We'll show you the details later in this chapter, but here is a basic overview of the process.

The simplest database merely is a *table* comprising one or more *fields* that store data in *records*. To make a simple database you first make a table. To make a table you create and label fields, and then you define the type of data each field will hold, for example, date, text, time, or integer, depending on the feature set in the product you own. Then you enter data into the fields to create records. To make a simple relational database you build two or more tables, and then link certain fields in the tables together.

For Palm users, during the HotSync process a copy of the database structure moves from the handheld to the desktop, together with any data that might have been added to the table(s). At very least the desktop copy simply sits on the desktop's hard drive as a backup in case something goes wrong with the copy on the handheld. In the default setup, this backup copy typically resides in the C:\palm\yourpalm\backup folder, where "Yourpalm" is the folder name assigned to your handheld device.

For Pocket PC users, the ActiveSync process automatically backs up database programs, but "Files" needs to be set to "synchronize" in the ActiveSync settings (see the ActiveSync documentation for more details on this). HanDBase also creates a backup copy in the desktop files location on your hard drive if you have the synchronization software configured correctly.

All but the very simplest database products come with a companion desktop program that allows you to open the desktop copy of the database to add, delete, or edit records on the desktop, or even to modify the database structure. Products that support two-way synchronization load the changed data back onto the handheld the next time you synchronize the computer and handheld. HanDBase comes with a desktop companion that can do all this and more.

Key Points

1. The simplest database is a table composed of fields that store data in records.
2. To make a simple database you build a table, select the types of fields you want, and give them names.
3. To use the database, you simply enter data into the fields.
4. To make a database relational, you simply build two tables and link them together through a common field.
5. During HotSync, Palm databases are automatically backed up to your desktop computer.
6. During ActiveSync, Pocket PC databases are also backed up on your desktop computer.
7. Handheld database products come with a companion desktop utility that allows you to change the database design or edit database contents right on your desktop.

The Lazy Way to Get a Database: Download a Model from the Internet

Chances are that someone has already made a handheld database similar to your project. Do a search with an engine such as www.google.com to find the many Web sites that have database archives suitable for your product, or check out the product's home page. If you find a model that will run with your software, then download and modify it to suit your needs.

HANDS-ON EXERCISE 17.1. HOW TO BUILD A SIMPLE PROCEDURE LOG USING HANDBASE

How many times have you pulled your shirts out of the dryer to find an illegible scrap of paper that was supposed to remind you about the lumbar puncture you did in the hospital a few nights ago? In fact, this has happened to you so many times that your reapplication for privileges might not get approved this year because you don't have proof of your experience readily at hand. So instead of printing out a neat report in seconds, you have to take a day off from your clinic to plow through charts at the Medical Records Department. That's expensive.

Well, we've got a great solution for you. Here are directions for building a simple one-table, flat file database design for logging procedures performed by a physician, using HanDBase as an example. Most of the other middleweight database products work in a similar way. In these examples, we use Palm screenshots, but the procedures and screens are nearly identical for Pocket PC handhelds. Where there is a difference, it is noted.

Name the Database and Set up the Fields

Open HanDBase. Tap "New" to start building a new database. On Pocket PC's, you will tap on the "Create a new database" button.

Give the database a unique name, like "Procedure Log" (Figure 17.1).

When you tap "OK" on the screen in Figure 17.1, HanDBase creates the new database, then shows you a screen where you can start naming and configuring the fields (Figure 17.2).

Tap on "Field 1" (circled in Figure 17.2) to open a screen where you can define the first field for your procedure log database table (Figure 17.3).

Create a Date Field

Give Field 1 the new name "Date" by highlighting or erasing the words "Field 1" and writing "Date" (circled in Figure 17.4).

Tap on the "Field Type" drop-down list and select the field type "Date." When you do that, the screen changes to allow you to select more para-

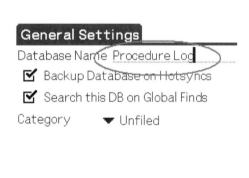

FIGURE 17.1. Name the Procedure Log database (Palm). (Reprinted with permission from DDH Software.)

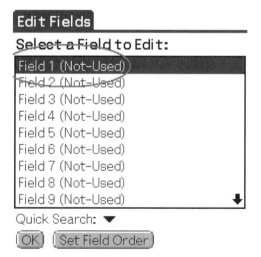

FIGURE 17.2. "Edit Fields" screen for a new database. (Reprinted with permission from DDH Software.)

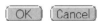

Edit Field 1
Field Name Field 1
Field Type: ▼ Not-Used

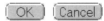

Edit Field 1
Field Name Date
Field Type: ▼ Not-Used

[OK] [Cancel]

[OK] [Cancel]

FIGURE 17.3. Create the first field for the database (Palm). (Reprinted with permission from DDH Software.)

FIGURE 17.4. Name the Date field (Palm). (Reprinted with permission from DDH Software.)

meters for a date field (Figure 17.5). Change the pixel width to 35 (circled). The default width of 58 pixels for this field's column will be too wide when you view the resulting screen to view record details. You might have to go back and adjust this setting later, to get the column widths right for each field. Trial and error works here. You can always go back and adjust the pixel width for any field later, if you don't like the way a screen comes out. You can also resize fields by just "dragging and dropping" them to the right width in the list view of HandBase.

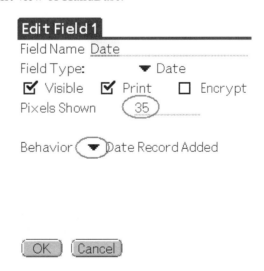

FIGURE 17.5. Setting the date field parameters (Palm). (Reprinted with permission from DDH Software.)

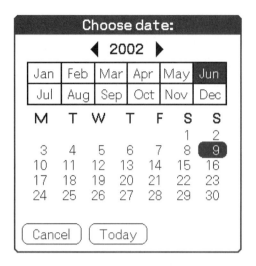

FIGURE 17.6a. The date picker screen (Palm). (Reprinted with permission from DDH Software.)

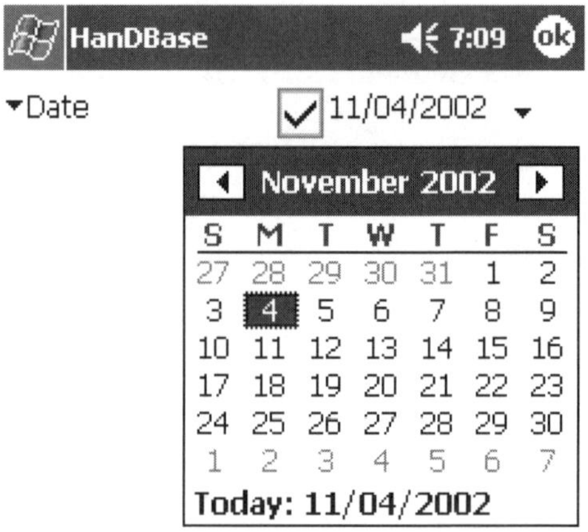

FIGURE 17.6b. The date picker screen (Pocket PC). (Reprinted with permission from DDH Software.)

Tap the drop-down list "Behavior" to pick the way you want the program to choose a date by default (circled in Figure 17.5). "Date Record Added" is convenient because it will automatically enter today's date. However, you will still be able to pick different dates from a handy calendar screen when you tap the down arrow beside the field name "Date" in the record view (Figure 17-6a,b). The date picker screen is a little different on the Pocket PC version of HanDBase. You can pick other default behaviors for the Date field too, depending on your personal preferences.

Key Point

1. The different ways you can set up a Date field to pick dates is a good example of how you can build handy features into your database with only a few screen taps, making it very fast and easy to use the database during a busy clinic day.

Create a "Pop-Up List" Procedure Field

Tap on Field 2 and create a second field called "Procedure." Make it a pop-up list for procedures. After you finish building the database structure, you can open the pop-up list to add all the procedures you can think of; here, I've added four (Figure 17.7). You can also add more on the fly while you use the database.

But, don't forget that pop-up lists only allow you to enter 60 choices, so if your list of procedures is longer, then you need to consider a different

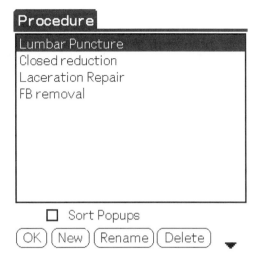

FIGURE 17.7. Pop-up list of procedures (Palm). (Reprinted with permission from DDH Software.)

solution. Later we'll explain how to build a second table for the procedures and link it to this one.

Key Points

1. Pop-up fields only allow you to list up to 60 different items.
2. For longer lists you can use other solutions, such as building a second table for procedures and linking it to the procedure log—these programmers think of everything!

Add Some More Fields, as Many as You Like

Carry on to build fields for data such as the following:

- Patient Name, text field
- Chart #, text field
- Price, floating field, two decimal places
- Multiplier, floating numeric field, one decimal place (modifies the base price for the procedure to account for increasing complexity)
- Extended price, calculated field (multiply price by multiplier)
- Physician, pop-up field
- Diagnosis, text field
- Notes, note field (for entering freehand descriptive information about the procedure)
- Age, integer field

- Gender, text field
- Location, pop-up (place where the procedure is carried out)

You might want to enter fields for anything else you might need, like perhaps these:

- A pop-up field for anatomic side (left, right, or bilateral)
- ICD (International Classification of Diseases) code
- American Medical Association's CPT (Current Procedural Terminology) code

HANDS-ON EXERCISE 17.2. TRY ENTERING A PROCEDURE TO THE LOG

Give yourself due credit—you've just become a programmer! Now, try out your brand-new procedure log by entering that LP from last night.

Add a New Record

Open it and tap "New" to enter a record. There are too many fields in this database for one screen, so you need to page down or tap the down arrow icon to see the rest of the record (Figure 17.8a,b). The "tabs" function available with the forms add-on available for HanDBase, and in other programs

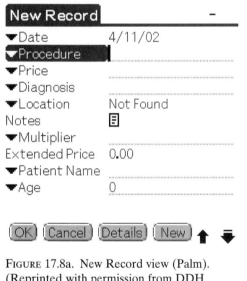

FIGURE 17.8a. New Record view (Palm). (Reprinted with permission from DDH Software.)

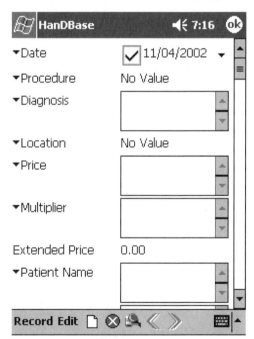

FIGURE 17.8b. New Record view (Pocket PC). (Reprinted with permission from DDH Software.)

like Smart List to Go, allows you to group similar fields in tabs that make it a bit easier to move around a record.

Now tap on the blank line alongside the Name field heading. Write in the patient's name. Carry on to fill in the data for the rest of the fields.

HANDS-ON EXERCISE 17.3. VIEWING SELECTED RECORD BY "FILTERING"

You finally get to sit down and eat lunch. Your pager goes off. It's the hospital administrator's secretary. She needs to know *right now* how many lumbar punctures you've done since January. "No problem," you say as you whip out your handheld and open your new procedure log database. A few screen taps later, you've filtered the database to show a list showing exactly what she wants. You simply count the number of records on the screen and tell her. Back at the clinic after lunch you can print out the filtered database to give her a hard copy with all the details, if she needs that too.

After entering a few records, try customizing the way you see the data by filtering the database. Filters are a very powerful way to customize views of the records in your database. Simply select the appropriate fields to filter on, and enter appropriate parameters for each field. Here is an example, using HanDBase.

Open the database, then tap "Filters" (Palm), or "Action," and then "Filters" (Pocket PC).

- Tap in the first checkbox to enable "Filter 1" (Figure 17.9).
- Select "Procedure" from the drop-down list of fields.
- Tap on "Must Contain," then "Lumbar" to filter the table for all the records containing the word lumbar.

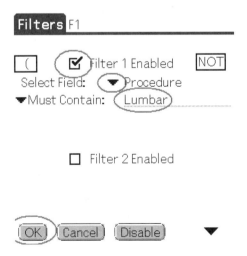

FIGURE 17.9. Setting up a filter (Palm). (Reprinted with permission from DDH Software.)

Tap "OK," and then you should see only the records with the word "lumbar" in the Procedure field.

To remove the filter and see all the records in the database again, tap "Filters" and uncheck the box for "Filter 1 Enabled."

You can enable up to six filters on the Palm or Pocket PC versions of HanDBase to exploit logical relationships between fields, setting up more refined filter views. For example, your first filter could be lumbar punctures, and the second filter could be for only those performed in the current year.

HANDS-ON EXERCISE 17.4. UPGRADE THE HANDBASE PROCEDURE LOG DATABASE FROM A FLAT FILE TO A RELATIONAL DESIGN

Although many users are very content with simple single-table, flat file databases, it is easy to build simple relational databases, with a little extra time on the learning curve. So get out your Nikes and start climbing—the view is excellent.

Remember we told you that a pop-up list could hold only 60 items? Perhaps the list of procedures you or your group performs is much longer. In this exercise, we show you how to build a second table for the procedures and then link it to the first. That's how you make a "relational" database.

A relational database basically consists of two or more tables linked by sharing one or more fields containing the same data. You might keep a list of patients in one table, then look up a patient's name from another table. Or you might want to put ICD and CPT codes in separate tables. Then you could look up the appropriate code by typing the diagnosis or procedure in plain English, and return the related alphanumeric code to the procedure log database.

Let's use the HanDBase procedure log as an example.

First, build a second table containing a list of procedures and prices relevant to your practice, then link that list to the procedure log table. That way you don't have to write in the procedure name each time you enter a new record, or remember the relevant fee. The linked field will bring up the procedure list table, then you can search for and tap on the appropriate record. HanDBase will import the appropriate information to the open record in your procedure log.

First: Build a Second Table Called "Procedure List"

Say you already have a defined list of procedures, complete with associated procedure code identifiers and fees. You wouldn't want to laboriously look up and type all that information into each record in your procedure log. Wouldn't it be much nicer if you could look up the related procedure from the log electronically? That's easy.

There are tables on the Internet that you can download which contain ICD and CPT codes. Some users have extracted the codes relevant to their practice, put them into HanDBase tables, and then linked to those for easy reference. A great example is the *Family Practice Management* journal's annual list of 600 commonly used codes in primary care. The list can be downloaded from www.aafp.org/fpm/icd9.html. It can then be used as a stand-alone reference, or incorporated into the procedures log as described next.

If the file was in csv (comma separated variable) format, or if you could put it into that format, then you could import that csv file using the HanDBase desktop companion. This would create a new table (call it "Procedures"), with three fields: "Procedure," "Code," and "Fee." HotSync, and that new table should appear on your handheld.

But if you can't import a prepared file, then simply build a new table called "Procedures" with those three text fields, then write in the data by hand. It shouldn't take long to type in a list of the procedures that you would typically use in your practice.

Link the Procedure List Table to the Procedure Log Table

Now link the Procedure Log table to the Procedures table. Select the database, then tap the "Details" icon (Figure 17.10a) to bring up the screen shown in Figure 17.11. For Pocket PC users, open the database first, select "File," and then "DB Properties" (Figure 17.10b). Then tap the "Fields" icon to bring up the list of fields (this screen is the same on both the Palm and Pocket PC).

Change the field type for the field "Procedure" in the database table "Procedure Log" to "DB Popup" (Figure 17.12). Point the field properties to the other database called "Procedures" by selecting the Other Field Name "Procedures" in that other database.

You also put the price for each procedure in the Procedures table. So change the properties for the price field to DB Popup too, and then point that field to Other Field #4 in the "Other DB" called Procedures. The screen should look like that shown on Figure 17.13.

Here is how the "DB Popup" field type works. Open the database, then open a new record. Tap on the little down arrow to the left of the field called Procedure. The Procedures table should pop up. Select the appropriate procedure by tapping on that record. The program should return you to your Procedure Log record and insert the name of the procedure. Then do the same for the Price field: select the procedure, and when the program returns you to the log, it will insert the correct price in the Price field automatically.

A word of warning: you can use the "popup appends" feature to add more procedures to each procedure field in a single record. You might be tempted to use that feature if you do two procedures on a single patient at one visit. However, it would make more sense to create a separate record for each

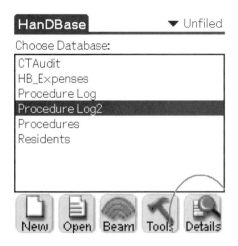

FIGURE 17.10a. Tap the "Details" icon to change the properties of a database (Palm). (Reprinted with permission from DDH Software.)

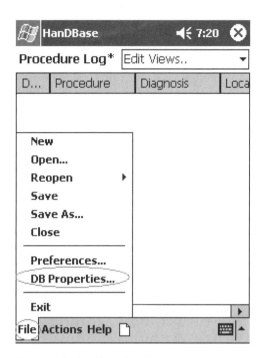

FIGURE 17.10b. Opening database properties on Pocket PC version. (Reprinted with permission from DDH Software.)

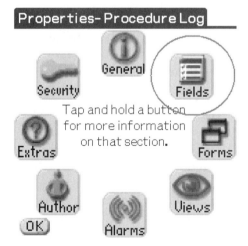

FIGURE 17.11. Tap the "Fields" icon to change the fields in the database (Palm). (Reprinted with permission from DDH Software.)

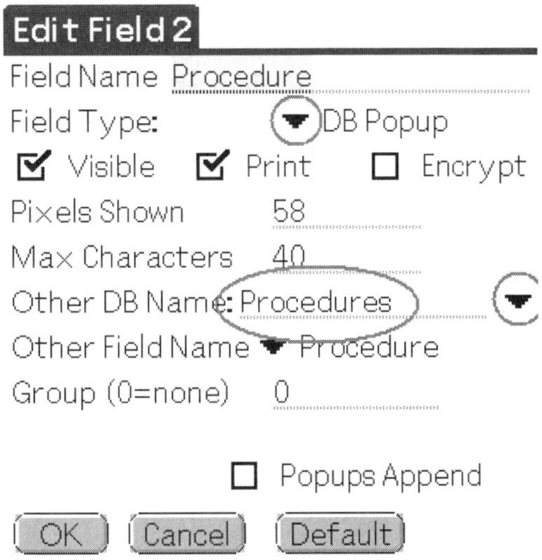

Edit Field 2

Field Name Procedure

Field Type: (▼)DB Popup

☑ Visible   ☑ Print   ☐ Encrypt

Pixels Shown   58

Max Characters   40

Other DB Name: Procedures   (▼)

Other Field Name ▼ Procedure

Group (0=none)   0

☐ Popups Append

[OK] [Cancel] [Default]

FIGURE 17.12. Linking the field called Procedure in the Procedure Log database to the field called Procedure in the Procedures database (Palm). (Reprinted with permission from DDH Software.)

procedure. You have to be careful with the popup appends feature, because it can make the database more complicated and harder to use.

HanDBase Relational Features Are Potent But Limited

There are limits to the degree of relational functionality that you can build into handheld databases, especially with the middleweight-type products. We decided not to go into all the technical details in this book, but be aware of two things. First: there are other relational features in the new version of HanDBase that we haven't told you about. Check the user's manual. Second: expert programmers can exploit relational database designs to

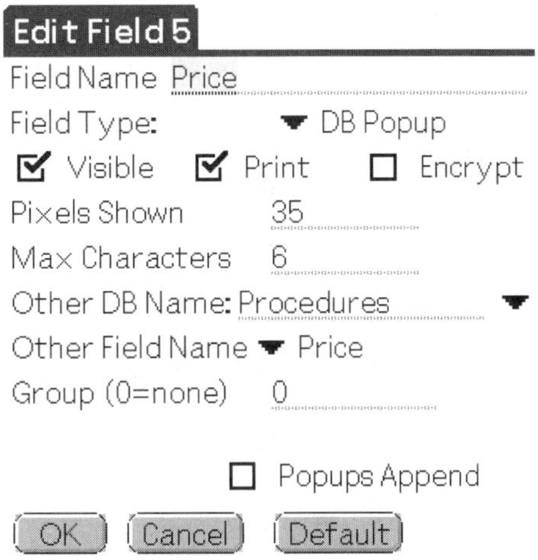

Edit Field 5

Field Name Price

Field Type: ▼ DB Popup

☑ Visible   ☑ Print   ☐ Encrypt

Pixels Shown   35

Max Characters   6

Other DB Name: Procedures   ▼

Other Field Name ▼ Price

Group (0=none)   0

☐ Popups Append

[OK] [Cancel] [Default]

FIGURE 17.13. Properties for the price field (Palm). (Reprinted with permission from DDH Software.)

huge advantage. If the standard features in your database software don't seem to do the job, then you might want to consult a database software engineer when you are thinking about building a database for multiple users, such as all the residents and staff physicians in your department or clinic.

HANDS-ON EXERCISE 17.5. TRACKING ALL THE PHYSICIANS IN YOUR GROUP WITH LINK AND LINKED FIELDS

To demonstrate how the link fields work in HanDBase, change your thinking about the way we have been using the Procedure Log. So far we assumed that the physicians doing the procedure would enter their own records of their procedures. They could filter the database by physician name to see all the procedures done by one physician. But say you already maintain a database of the residents in your program and would like the preceptors to log procedures done by residents that they are directly supervising. Or, in a clinic setting, your billing clerk in the business office might want to track all the procedures for all the physicians in your group. If you want to do that, then just substitute "physician" for "resident" in the following exercise.

The HanDBase "Link" and "Linked" fields in effect create a special relationship between two database tables so that several records in one database, called the "child," can be linked to one record in another, called the "parent." The parent database must have a Link field, and the child database must have a Linked field.

Create a parent database table called "Residents" and create a text field in that table called "Resident" (Figures 17.14–17.16). Create a "Link" field

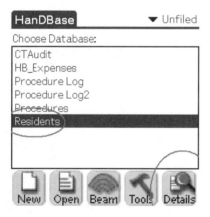

FIGURE 17.14. Select the Residents database and tap the "Details" icon to bring up the screen in Figure 17.15 (Palm). (Reprinted with permission from DDH Software.)

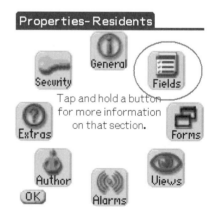

FIGURE 17.15. Tap the "Fields" icon to bring up the screen in FIGURE 17.16 (Palm). (Reprinted with permission from DDH Software.)

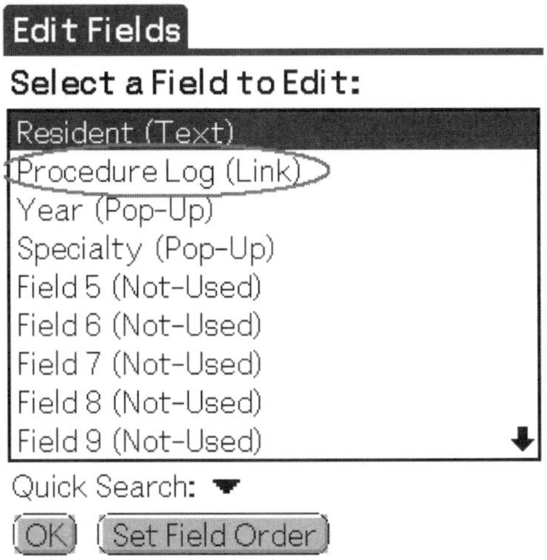

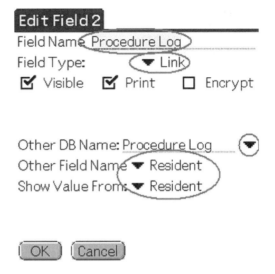

Edit Fields

Select a Field to Edit:

Resident (Text)
Procedure Log (Link)
Year (Pop-Up)
Specialty (Pop-Up)
Field 5 (Not-Used)
Field 6 (Not-Used)
Field 7 (Not-Used)
Field 8 (Not-Used)
Field 9 (Not-Used)

Quick Search: ▼

[OK] [Set Field Order]

Edit Field 2

Field Name: Procedure Log
Field Type: ▼ Link
☑ Visible   ☑ Print   ☐ Encrypt

Other DB Name: Procedure Log   ▼
Other Field Name ▼ Resident
Show Value From: ▼ Resident

[OK] [Cancel]

FIGURE 17.16. Select the field "Procedure Log" to change its properties (Palm). (Reprinted with permission from DDH Software.)

FIGURE 17.17. Settings to create the linked "Procedure Log" field in the "Residents" table (Palm). (Reprinted with permission from DDH Software.)

called "Procedure Log," and link it to a new field in the Procedure Log table called "Resident," as shown by the circles in Figure 17.17. This Link field will return the name of the Resident from the Residents table to the Procedure Log table when a record is viewed in the Procedure Log table. You can add other fields to the Residents table, such as "Year" and "Specialty."

Now modify the properties of the Procedure Log table to create the new "Resident" field. Specify Field Type "Linked," pick the "Residents" table for "Other DB Name," and point this field to Field #2 in the Residents table (Figure 17.18). This will link all the data in a record in the Procedure Log table to the "Procedure Log" link record field in the Residents table. Or, put another way, tapping on the Procedure Log field in the Residents table will bring up all the procedures logged for that resident.

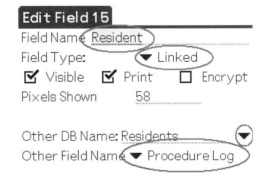

Edit Field 15

Field Name Resident
Field Type: ▼ Linked
☑ Visible   ☑ Print   ☐ Encrypt
Pixels Shown   58

Other DB Name: Residents   ▼
Other Field Name ▼ Procedure Log

FIGURE 17.18. Creating the linked "Resident" field in the Procedure Log table (Palm). (Reprinted with permission from DDH Software.)

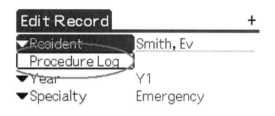

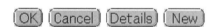

FIGURE 17.19b. Same screen on the Pocket PC version. (Reprinted with permission from DDH Software.)

FIGURE 17.19a. Record view in the Residents table. Tap on "Procedure Log" to see the list of the resident's procedures (Palm). (Reprinted with permission from DDH Software.)

What you have done is establish a true one-to-many link between the parent table (Residents) and the child table (Procedure Log). When you open the Residents table and select a resident's name, you will see a box called "Procedure Log" (Figure 17.19a,b), which represents the "Procedure Log" field in the Residents table. Tap on that box to bring up the Procedure Log table. You will see all the procedures logged so far for that resident, and be given an opportunity to log a new record for that resident.

Conversely, when you enter a new procedure record the resident's name is automatically entered into the Procedure Log table from the Residents table by the link feature (Figure 17.20a,b).

The "Relationships" field, new in HanDBase version 3.0, can also be used to make relationships between tables.

More sophisticated desktop database programs like Microsoft Access allow programmers to exploit relationships in much more rigorous and complex ways than are possible on handheld devices.

Key Points

1. A relational database made up of smaller databases is much more powerful and convenient than one big database table.
2. Relational databases are simply two or more tables linked together in some way.
3. Making a "relational" database sounds intimidating, but once you start up the shallow learning curve you'll find it isn't so bad after all.

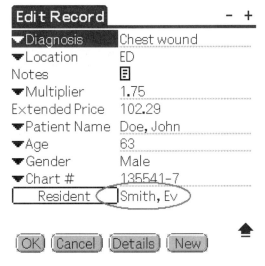

FIGURE 17.20a. Record View in the Procedure Log table, showing the resident's name from the Residents table (Palm). (Reprinted with permission from DDH Software.)

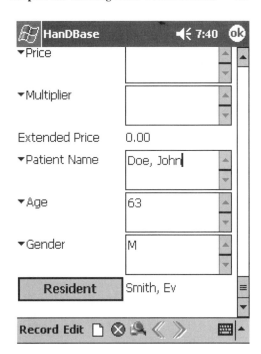

FIGURE 17.20b. Same screen on the Pocket PC version. (Reprinted with permission from DDH Software.)

HANDS-ON EXERCISE 17.6. WORKING WITH THE PROCEDURE LOG ON A DESKTOP COMPUTER

Option 1: The HanDBase Desktop Companion

A great feature of database products like HanDBase is that they come with a desktop program so you can open your handheld's databases on your desktop computer. HanDBase's desktop program even opens both Palm and Pocket PC HanDBase databases. Figure 17.21 shows what the procedure log looks like when I open it on my desktop computer with the HanDBase program.

The relationship between the Procedure Log table and the Procedures table is preserved on the desktop, allowing you to do your work on the desktop or your handheld. In Figure 17.22, notice how I was able to open the Procedures table simply by clicking on the Procedure field in the "Edit Record" window.

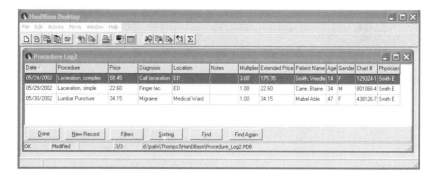

FIGURE 17.21. Procedure Log table on the desktop computer. (Reprinted with permission from DDH Software.)

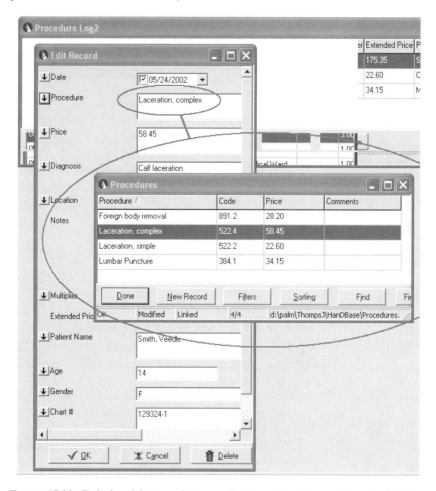

FIGURE 17.22. Relational features between the Procedure Log and Residents tables are preserved on the desktop computer. (Reprinted with permission from DDH Software.)

Option 2: Linking HanDBase to Microsoft Access and Other Desktop Programs

The HanDBase desktop program might suffice for most tasks, but you might want to link your handheld database to a more powerful program such as Microsoft Access so that you can do things such as print out fancier reports or do more complex analyses. That isn't too difficult. There are two ways to go: manually or automatically.

The manual way is to simply export the records from the Procedure Log table to a format that can be imported into a Microsoft Access database. This kind of procedure works in a similar way for many other desktop database software products like Excel, FileMaker, and others, although details vary between products. Use the following steps to link HanDBase data with a Microsoft Access table:

1. Build a table in Microsoft Access to receive the records (this assumes that you know how to use Microsoft Access).
2. Open the HanDBase table in the HanDBase desktop program. Click "File/Export" to see the window in Figure 17.23. Note that you can export to five different formats. Select "Comma Separated File" (.CSV).

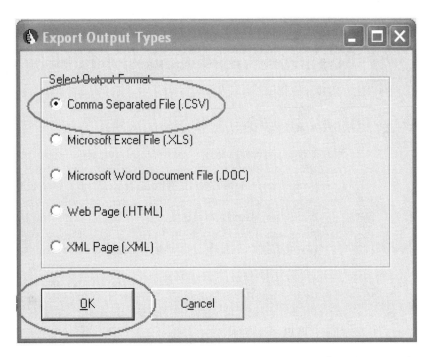

FIGURE 17.23. Data export options on the desktop computer (HanDBase version 3). (Reprinted with permission from DDH Software.)

Press "OK." Designate a file name in a folder on your computer to receive the data, and then click "Export Database."

3. Now open the Access table and import the .CSV file.

It is just as easy to export data from Access to HanDBase manually the other way. Export from Access in CSV format, and then import the CSV file into HanDBase on the desktop computer.

The automatic way is to use an optional utility called HanDBase Sync Exchange for Access. With this add-on tool available on the DDH Software Web site, you can synchronize your data directly with Access from Hand-Base. After each HotSync or ActiveSync, changes made in Access, the HanDBase Desktop, and the handheld will all be synchronized together, even for multiple users.

Key Points

1. You can work with your handheld database on your desktop computer too.
2. You can open the database with a desktop program designed specifically for your handheld software product, or you can link your handheld database to a more powerful software database system from another company, like Microsoft Access.

 HANDS-ON EXERCISE 17.7. BUILDING A PROCEDURE LOG WITH PEN-DRAGON FORMS FROM INSIDE MICROSOFT ACCESS

What Is Unique About Pendragon Forms?

So you're sold on the idea of building a database for your clinic group so that your clinic's business manager can track all the miscellaneous billings your docs generate on their rounds through the hospital and nursing homes. And your clinic staff are familiar with Microsoft Access. You could build it with HanDBase and then create links to Access, but there is another option: programs like Pendragon Forms (for Palm OS only) or Satellite Forms (available for Palm and Pocket PC). For the purposes of this hands-on exercise, we focus exclusively on Pendragon Forms.

Pendragon Forms is different from the middleweight database products like HanDBase, MobileDB, Smart List to Go, and JFile. In Pendragon Forms, you build the database from within Microsoft Access on a desktop computer. Pendragon Forms uses a special Microsoft Access database to build all the tables and forms within Access automatically; then, when you are finished creating your design, it freezes the database structure and uploads it to your handheld.

Once the design is loaded onto the handheld, you and your colleagues can collect and edit data on either their handheld or desktop computers. But, on the desktop you are always working inside Microsoft Access. This allows your business staff to use the full range on Access' powerful data-basing features to manage your billings.

Pendragon Forms' "build-freeze-deploy" model is similar to the way some other handheld database products are designed to work with other major desktop database systems, like Sybase (Palm) and Oracle (Palm and Pocket PC). Those products similarly create handheld databases that are tightly integrated with the associated desktop database system, and then freeze the design before uploading it to handhelds.

Compared to the middleweight handheld products, Pendragon Forms has more options for field types, and allows you to write scripts for advanced field functions. It is more expensive than the middleweights, but it is more like them because it is cheaper and simpler to use than the other heavy-weights.

If you plan to use this product, consider obtaining *The Official Pendragon Forms for Palm OS Starter Kit*, by Sancho and Phillips.[1]

Can I Use All of Access' Powerful Features on the Handheld?

When you build database forms for the handheld using Pendragon Forms, you cannot use the full range of Microsoft Access' powerful databasing features on the handheld. This is partly because the handheld does not have the computing power of a desktop computer. But it also partly due to prac-tical programming considerations. You pay for what you get. You could develop a very sophisticated handheld database with low-level computing language like C++ that would mimic most advanced database procedures, or use a heavyweight database product, but then you'd have to hire spe-cialized software engineers to help you.

Pendragon Form's developers found the right balance between advanced features and efficiency. You can learn quickly to develop quite advanced databases with Pendragon Forms, but you can also create quite simple, flat file databases in a few minutes. Here's how to build a simple procedure log.

First Open the Pendragon Forms Manager

First find the icon shortcut that opens the Pendragon Forms Manager and click on that. This opens two specialized Microsoft Access database windows: the Pendragon Access database (FORMS32K.mdb if you use Access 2000), and the Forms Manager window (Figure 17.24). The buttons on the Forms Manager window give you access to the tools you need to design the forms and tables for your procedure log, or any other database you care to create.

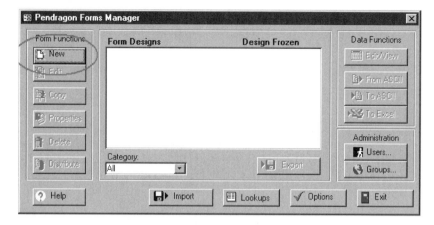

FIGURE 17.24. Pendragon Forms Manager window (Palm). (Reprinted with permission from Pendragon Software Corporation.)

Notice that the Forms Manager window does not show you all the standard Microsoft Access database design tools. That is because Pendragon Forms takes care of those details for you when it builds the table and associated form. Not only do you not have to know a low-level language like C++ to build your procedure log, you don't even need to know SQL or Microsoft's midlevel methods for building tables and forms!

You will need to know some of those things, however, if you want to get the most from the tables Pendragon Forms builds for you. We'll tell you more about that later.

Make the Procedure Log Form

Click on the "New" button under Form Functions to start building the form for your handheld. That opens a window Pendragon calls the "Form Designer." Give the form a name like "Procedure Log," make the first field a "Date Only" field type, and type the field name "Date" in the "Field" area, where the cursor is blinking (Figure 17.25).

Then Add More Fields to the Form

To add a second field to the form, click on the "+" button. Give that field a name and type. Continue on, perhaps adding these fields:

Patient Name, freeform text field
Chart #, freeform text field
Price, currency field
Physician, pop-up field
Diagnosis, text field

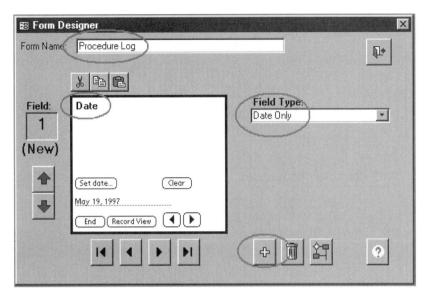

FIGURE 17.25. Pendragon form designer window, showing the date field and form name (Palm). (Reprinted with permission from Pendragon Software Corporation.)

Notes, text field
Age, numeric field
Gender, pop-up field
Location, pop-up (place where the procedure is carried out)

When you select the pop-up field type, the window changes to include a place where you can type in a list of physicians or locations (Figure 17.26). Pendragon Forms has a lot of neat tricks like that.

Save the Form

After getting all the fields set up the way you want, then click on the open door icon. That brings up the "Save Changes" dialog (Figure 17.27). Click "Yes."

Freeze the Form and Send It to Your Handheld

After saving the form, you will be returned to the Pendragon Forms Manager window. Notice that the form has not yet been frozen for distribution to your handheld. That's easy to do, but first make sure that you are happy with your form design. The kinds of changes you can make to a frozen form are limited.

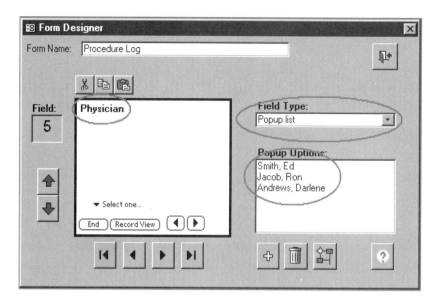

FIGURE 17.26. The Pendragon Forms pop-up field (Palm). (Reprinted with permission from Pendragon Software Corporation.)

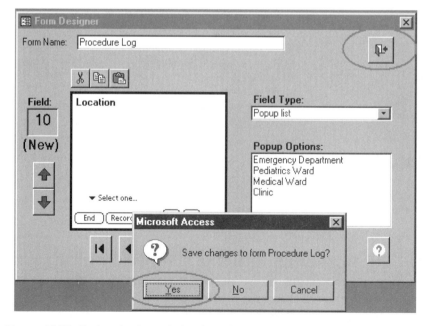

FIGURE 17.27. Saving the form design (Palm). (Reprinted with permission from Pendragon Software Corporation.)

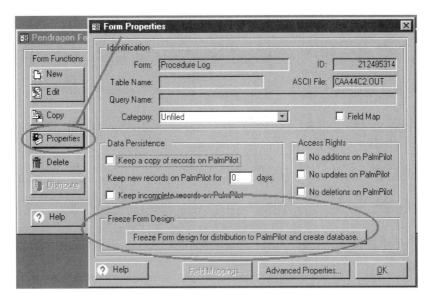

FIGURE 17.28. Freezing the form design (Palm). (Reprinted with permission from Pendragon Software Corporation.)

A number of things happen when you freeze the form. Pendragon tools work behind the scenes to build a version of the form that will work on your Palm OS handheld, and then queues it up for installing to your handheld at the next HotSync. And Pendragon's Access macros go to work to build a Microsoft Access table in the database, mapping the fields in the Access table to the fields in the handheld version. That way the Pendragon Forms conduit can move data between the handheld and the desktop at every HotSync.

To freeze a form, select the form from the list and click on the "Properties" button. That brings up the window shown in Figure 17.28. Click the button "Freeze Form design for distribution to PalmPilot and create database."

Creating Calculated Fields with Pendragon Forms

Notice that we left out the "multiplier" and "extended price" fields that we used in the HanDBase example above. This doesn't mean that Pendragon Forms does not allow calculated fields on the handheld: quite the opposite. The "Advanced Field" properties button (Figure 17.29) in the Form

FIGURE 17.29. Advanced Properties icon (Palm). (Reprinted with permission from Pendragon Software Corporation.)

Designer window allows users to write "Scripts" that enable very sophisticated calculations and can trigger other types of events. We won't go into that here. Sancho and Phillips describe all these procedures quite clearly in their book.[1]

Converting the Procedure Log to a Relational Design Using Pendragon Forms

The pop-up field lists cannot be modified after you freeze the design and distribute it to your handheld. This brings up an important limitation of Pendragon Forms. You cannot send your new form to your handheld until after you "freeze" the design. So if you want to add new physicians or locations to the pop-up lists in those fields, then you need to redesign and redistribute the form, overwriting existing data sets on the handhelds.

A more flexible method would be to use lookup field types. That gets into relational database design, but using Pendragon Forms that's no more difficult than pushing fairly obvious buttons.

The process for making your procedure log relational rather than flat file, using Pendragon Forms, is similar in principle to the way we did it for the HanDBase example above, but of course the procedures are different. Again we refer you to Sancho and Phillips,[1] although the program is so easy to use that it shouldn't be hard to figure it out. In fact the procedures are so simple that you probably won't even realize that you are building a relational database, because Pendragon Forms keeps the messy details hidden away under the hood.

Try Using the Pendragon Forms Procedure Log Database on Your Handheld

Once the Procedure Log form has been "distributed" (installed) on your handheld, you can use it pretty much like the HanDBase database above. In fact, the two look pretty similar on a handheld, although Pendragon Forms has some interesting and useful tricks for entering data to some of their fields that HanDBase doesn't have.

1. Tap on the "Forms" icon to open Pendragon Forms on the handheld.
2. Select the form called "Procedure Log" by tapping once on its name.

Figure 17.30 shows the first screen you see when you launch Forms on your handheld. There is only one form listed. I called it "Procedure Log2." Select that form.

Figure 17.31 shows the "record view," listing as many fields as will fit onto the handheld's screen. To see more, if there are more, page down. Tap on

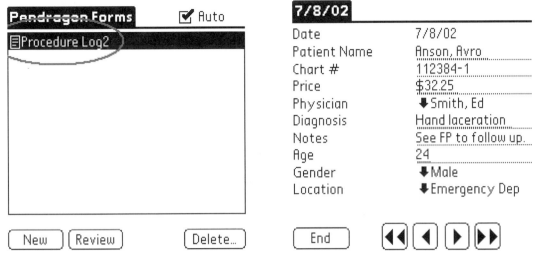

FIGURE 17.30. List of forms on the handheld (Palm). (Reprinted with permission from Pendragon Software Corporation.)

FIGURE 17.31. Record view (Palm). (Reprinted with permission from Pendragon Software Corporation.)

the field label in the left column to open the "field view," or just enter data in the right column in this view.

Figure 17.32 shows the "field view" for the price field, and Figure 17.33 shows the physician pop-up field. There are similar handy field views for all the other fields.

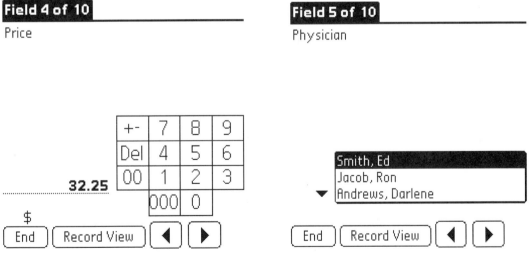

FIGURE 17.32. Field view for the price currency field (Palm). (Reprinted with permission from Pendragon Software Corporation.)

FIGURE 17.33. Field view for the physician pop-up field (Palm). (Reprinted with permission from Pendragon Software Corporation.)

Try Using the Pendragon Forms Procedure Log Database on Your Desktop Computer

After entering some records into the Procedure Log form on your hand-held, then HotSync your handheld to your desktop computer. The Pendragon Forms conduit will automatically move the data from the handheld to a table in the Pendragon Forms Microsoft Access database. Pendragon Forms automatically created that table when you froze the form design.

You can find out which table it is by checking the form's properties in the Pendragon Forms Manager window. Expect to find a code number with a bizarre identifier something like "FORM_ID_212512643" (that's what it was called on my computer). You can find that table in the list of tables in the window for the associated Pendragon Forms database. If you use Access 2000, then the database is called FORMS32K.mdb, and the associated window in Access is called "FORMS32K : Database."

If you understand how to use Microsoft Access, then once you've got the name of the table you can build queries, reports, and forms based on that table to manipulate the data it contains. Or you can set up a routine to export the data to an external table. The details for these procedures are beyond the scope of this book, but there are many good books on the market to help you understand how to use Access.

Pendragon Forms comes with powerful features for linking data tables, or linking to external programs using ODBC (the Open Database Connectivity standard).

Using the Data in Programs Such as Excel and Word

Pendragon Forms makes it very easy to use the data in all kinds of other programs. The Forms Manager window has buttons for exporting data from the form directly to Excel, or to the ASCII text file format for importing into a word processor. Once the data is in Excel, you can export it easily to even more file formats.

Sharing the Procedure Log in a Group of Pendragon Forms Users

You can set up a group of people to share the Procedure Log this way:

1. List each person's handheld user name in the list under the "Users" button on the Pendragon Forms main window on the desktop computer (Figure 17.34).
2. When each member HotSyncs to that computer, he or she will get a copy of the Procedure Log form on his or her handheld.
3. Each physician uses the form to log his or her procedures.
4. Each time the group's members HotSync again with that computer, their data flow into the related Microsoft Access table on the desktop com-

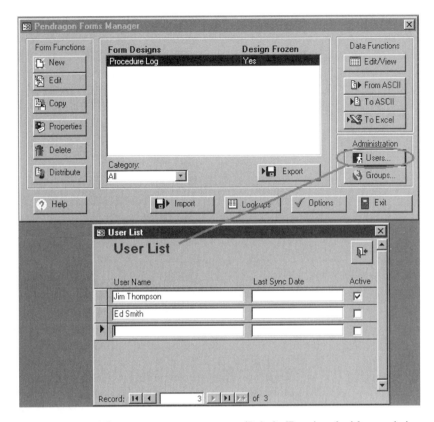

FIGURE 17.34. Adding more users to a group (Palm). (Reprinted with permission from Pendragon Software Corporation.)

puter, accumulating there with logged procedures from everyone else's handhelds. Special software tools are available from Pendragon Forms to allow users to synchronize with the main database from other computers over a network and the Internet.

More Users Cost You More Money

Pendragon Forms will interrupt you with a delightfully polite screen message when you attempt to add more users than your license allows. The message tactfully reminds you to contact Pendragon Forms about the cost of extending your license for larger groups. The message reminded me of an infinitely polite elderly grandmother, gently asking for another pillow in our hectic Emergency Department. Different database products handle this issue differently, and the industry's procedures for licensing their software to groups seems to be continually evolving. So heads up on that one.

Key Points

1. With Pendragon Forms (Palm) you build your database design on a desktop computer within Microsoft Access, not on your handheld.
2. Pendragon Forms (Palm) and Satellite Forms (for Palm and Pocket PC) help build databases integrated with Microsoft Access.
3. Pendragon Forms is an inexpensive example of a type of handheld database software where you build and freeze the database design within a desktop computer database system, then load the database onto handhelds to collect data.
4. Some database software companies require you to buy group licenses if you intend to use your database on more than one handheld computer.

Summary

In this chapter, we gave you an overview of how handheld databases are constructed. Then we showed you how to use HanDBase to build a simple, one-table, flat file procedure log database. After that we showed you how to use the simple relational features in HanDBase to convert the procedure log to a relational design, and demonstrated the advantages of doing so. We explained some of the ways you can use your HanDBase procedure log on your desktop computer, including ways to link it to other more powerful desktop database software products. We also described how to share the database among several users. Finally, we showed you how to build a similar procedure log from within Microsoft Access using Pendragon Forms.

Reference

1. Sancho D, Phillips I. The Official Pendragon Forms for PalmOS Starter Kit. New York: M & T Books, IDG Books Worldwide, 2000.

18

Creating Your Own Programs

MARK H. EBELL

So . . . you want to write your own programs for the Palm or Pocket PC. One of the thousands of programs written by professional programmers just won't do, eh? Your own custom database (Chapter 11) isn't powerful enough, hmmm? Well, aren't we special!

In this chapter, I'll survey some of the tools used to "roll your own" programs for the Palm and Pocket PC. No, you won't learn how to write software—my goal is to help you understand the strengths and weaknesses of each of your options. While there are dozens of minor languages, most are not well implemented or serve a particular niche. The programming environments discussed next are the most popular and useful.

What Is Programming?

Programming a computer is the process of creating a user interface (e.g., buttons, lists, and menus) and then writing a set of instructions that tell it in great detail what to do. For example, when a program starts, a set of instructions ("code") may tell the PDA where to find a database file and then load some initial data into a list for the user. When a button is pushed, another segment of code tells the program what to do.

Below is a very simple program for the Pocket PC that lets you choose a dose in mg/kg for amoxicillin, then calculates the proper dose for children of different weights. It is shown first in the programming environment, in this case embedded Visual Basic (Figure 18.1).

The developer chooses "controls" and draws them on a "form." Then, code is attached to the "Form_Load" event that adds doses to the drop-down box. Finally, a simple command figures out which dose was selected, calculates the appropriate dose for a child of this weight, and displays the answer. Some of this is pretty intuitive: the ".AddItem" method adds an item to a list. Some of it isn't: the "listIndex" tells me which item in the list was selected, and is 0 for 20 mg/kg, 1 for 40 mg/kg, and 2 for 10 mg/kg.

It's appearance on a Pocket PC is show in Figure 18.2.

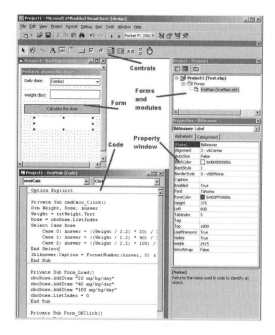

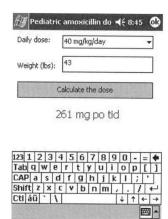

FIGURE 18.2. Sample program created with embedded Visual Basic. (Reprinted with permission from Microsoft Corporation.)

FIGURE 18.1. Embedded Visual Basic programming environment. (Reprinted with permission from Microsoft Corporation.)

Now that you are an expert programmer, let's consider some of the issues in choosing a programming environment.

What to Look for in a Programming Tool

There is a trade-off between power and ease of use in many products, just as there is between component stereos versus boomboxes and manual versus automatic transmissions. Programming tools are no exception. At one end of the spectrum are C++ compilers that require you to keep track of pointers and heaps and all sorts of arcane things. On the other hand, they create compact, very fast code that runs on a variety of devices. At the other end are programs like NSBasic and AppForge that provide a simpler interface but also create code that is slower and fatter.

Cost is another important issue—some tools are free, while some cost hundreds or even thousands of dollars. Ease of distribution is another. Although programs written in C++ can be distributed as a single file, those written with interpreted language require you to provide "run-time" files. These runtimes can conflict, leading to headaches for you and your users. Some runtimes even cost you money to distribute, a nonstarter for most developers. Table 18.1 summarizes the key characteristics of the programming tools that we discuss in this chapter.

TABLE 18.1. Comparison of programming tools for the Palm and Pocket PC.

Programming tool	Device	Cost	Core language	Compiled[a]	Runtime required
CodeWarrior www.metrowerks.com	Palm	$499	C/C++	Yes	No
embedded Visual C www.microsoft.com/windowsmobile/information/ deprograms/default.mspy	Pocket PC	Free	C	Yes	No
embedded Visual Basic www.microsoft.com/windowsmobile/information/ deprograms/default.mspy	Pocket PC	Free	Basic	No	Yes
NSBasic/Palm www.nsbasic.com	Palm	$149.95	Basic	No	Yes
NSBasic/PocketPC www.nsbasic.com	Pocket PC	$149.95	Basic	No	Yes
.Net Compact Framework msdn.microsoft.com/vstudio/device/compact.asp	Pocket PC	$1079[b]	C# or Basic		No
AppForge www.appforge.com	Palm, Pocket PC, Symbian/Nokia	$899 ($129 for Palm only)	Basic	No	Yes[c]

[a] Compiled languages are faster and more compact than interpreted.
[b] $579 for upgrade from any other Microsoft programming language.
[c] $10 fee for Pocket PC, free for Palm.

There are lots of options, as you can see, and quite a range in price. Let's look at each in a bit more detail.

CodeWarrior for Palm (Metrowerks)

CodeWarrior is an industrial-strength programming tool primarily aimed at professional developers that uses the C or C++ language. Like the .Net Framework (discussed below), it is not for the faint of heart and has a price to match. On the other hand, this is what they used to write the Palm operating system itself, if that gives you an idea of its power. For creating tight, fast, professional code for the Palm, CodeWarrior is the best choice. If you're a hobbyist or part-time developer, and especially if you don't know C, keep reading.

Embedded Visual C and Embedded Visual Basic (Microsoft)

These sister applications from Microsoft are a great deal—they're free! They don't require any other programming languages, and run in Windows 98, ME, 2000, NT, and XP. Note that the emulation features, which simulate a little Pocket PC on your screen for testing purposes, do not function in Windows 98 or ME.

Most professional software (i.e., the kind you have to pay for) has been created with one of these languages, the majority with embedded Visual C (eVC). eVC has all the strengths and weaknesses of any C compiler: terrific power, and a very steep learning curve. It is only recommended for those with 2 or 3 months to spare just getting up to speed.

Embedded Visual Basic (eVB), on the other hand, is easy to pick up for anyone who has done previous programming, even those simple Basic language programs in high school that made the computer say "hello world" when you pressed a certain key. This is especially true if you are familiar with its big brother Visual Basic for Windows. I showed you a very simple application created in eVB earlier in the chapter 3. It took all of 5 minutes to write and download to my Pocket PC. This is the strength of eVB: it's cheap, it's easy, and it's fast.

But (you knew this was coming) . . . it is also slow, a little buggy, and creates bloated installation packages. That simple program that I created would be about 3 kilobytes (KB) written in eVC, but would weigh in at well over 1000 KB written in eVB. Why? Its those pesky run-time files. While in theory they come preinstalled on every Pocket PC, you can't count on it, so you end up bundling a half dozen or more of these files with your tiny little program. This is less of an issue when your program is 3 or 4 MB (or 37 MB, as in our InfoRetriever software), but is a real disincentive for the hobby programmer who just wants to create a quick little program.

Programs written in eVB are slower than eVC programs, but comparable in speed to NSBasic and AppForge applications. There is a very active user community that has developed work-arounds for many of the language's shortcomings, and several dozen add-in programming controls from third-party vendors. Visit www.devbuzz.com or www.pocketpcdn. com for more information, as well as Microsoft's own developer site (http://www.microsoft.com/mobile/developer/default.asp). You can easily and quickly build links to the address book and calendar, wireless networks, databases, and the Internet. You can build in a Web browser, manipulate XML documents, and much more.

.Net Compact Framework (Microsoft)

This is the future of programming, according to Microsoft. The .Net Framework includes a half-dozen programming languages for desktop computers (e.g., C++, Visual Basic, C#) and what it calls the "Compact Framework" (CF) that lets you create programs for Pocket PCs and other mobile devices that run the Windows CE operating system. The Compact Framework has just been released in its final form in mid-2003. Because Microsoft does not plan any further support for the eVB and eVC programming tools, most serious programmers will probably migrate to .Net over the next few years.

.Net CF promises to allow reuse of code from programs originally written for the desktop computer. Of course, although code can be reused, the user interface would still have to be designed from the ground up for mobile devices. They also promise that the language will create software that is faster and less prone to "dll hell," the bugs created when conflicting run-time libraries exist on the same device.

Don't even try to run .Net CF unless you have 256 MB of RAM on your desktop computer and Windows 2000 or Windows XP, not to mention a very big hard drive. This is a serious programming environment for serious programmers, and is not well suited to the casual or hobbyist programmer. If you are reading this chapter, this probably isn't the programming tool for you.

NSBasic (NSBasic)

NSBasic comes in three flavors, one each for Palm, Windows CE (Pocket PC), and Newton. Newton? That was the grandpapa of handheld computers, and had a terrific operating system ... unfortunately, it was too bulky and arrived a bit before its time. The Palm and Windows CE versions of NSBasic are now in version 3.0 and 4.1, respectively, making it a mature language. NSBasic is a great language for clinicians who want to create programs for their own use or to share with colleagues, but has enough power that it can be considered for commercial applications as well.

As with other interpreted languages, the major drawbacks are that it requires a run-time file (although this can be built into the program) and is slower than compiled programs. Strengths of NSBasic include ease of use,

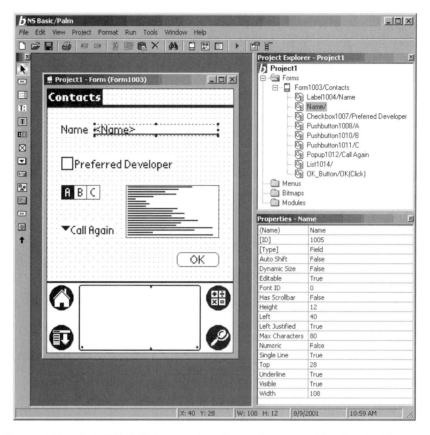

FIGURE 18.3. The NSBasic/Palm programming environment. (Reprinted with permission from NSBasic.)

low cost, and great technical support from the software's author (George Henne) and an enthusiastic community of users. Its chief competitor is App-Forge. While AppForge is a bit slicker and has a few more features, NSBasic has the advantage of being much less expensive and not requiring that you own Visual Basic 6.0. The disadvantage is that it takes more effort to move or "port" code from Visual Basic 6.0 to NSBasic than to AppForge.

A screenshot of NSBasic/Palm is shown in Figure 18.3.

AppForge/MobileVB (AppForge)

AppForge, which has recently changed its name to "MobileVB," has several unique features that make it worth considering. If you are already familiar with Visual Basic 6.0, perhaps the most widely used programming language for desktop computers, then it is an easy transition to learn AppForge. It is also the only programming tool that lets you use a single code base for

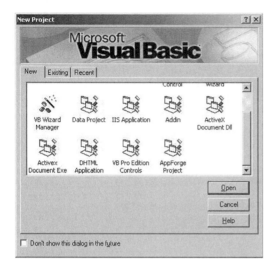

FIGURE 18.4. Selecting a type of project with AppForge in Visual Basic 6.0. (Reprinted with permission from Microsoft Corporation.)

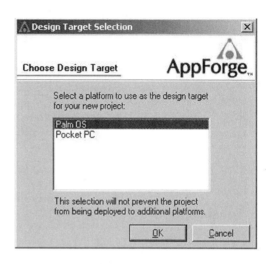

FIGURE 18.5. Selecting a device target within AppForge. (Reprinted with permission from AppForge.)

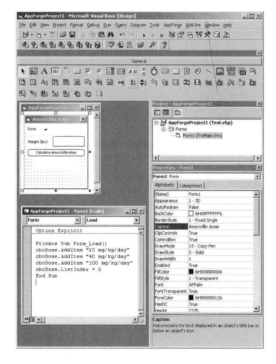

FIGURE 18.6. The AppForge/MobileVB programming environment, running within Visual Basic 6.0. (Reprinted with permission from AppForge and Microsoft Corporation.)

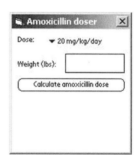

FIGURE 18.7. Example of a program created with AppForge, running in the "emulator" on the desktop computer. (Reprinted with permission from AppForge.)

TABLE 18.2. Resources for handheld device programmers.

Web sites
  Palm/CodeWarrior
    MetroWerks (http://www.metrowerks.com/MW/Develop/Desktop/PalmOS/Default.htm)
    Palm home page for developers (http://www.palm.com/developers/)
  eVB/eVC
    DevBuzz (www.devbuzz.com)
    Microsoft (http://www.microsoft.com/mobile/developer/default.asp)
  AppForge
    AppForge home page (www.appforge.com)
  General Pocket PC
    Pocket PC developer network (www.pocketpcdn.com)
  .Net Compact Framework
    GotDotNet community (http://www.gotdotnet.com/team/netcf/)
    Microsoft (http://msdn.microsoft.com/vstudio/device/compactfx.asp)
    DevBuzz (www.devbuzz.com)

Books
  Wigley A. Microsoft .NET Compact Framework (core reference). Redmond Washington Microsoft Press, 2002.
  rattan N. Pocket PC: Handheld PC Developer's Guide with Microsoft Embedded Visual Basic. Upper Saddle River, N.J.: Prentice Hall, 2002.
  Jamsa KA, Jamsa K. Instant Palm OS Applications. New York: McGraw-Hill Osborne Media, 2001.
  Foster LR. Palm OS Programming Bible, 2nd Ed. New York: Wiley, 2002

creating programs for the Palm, Pocket PC, and even Nokia mobile phones that use the Symbian operating system.

After installing AppForge/MobileVB, you now have a new kind of project when you first launch VB 6.0 (Figure 18.4).

Select an AppForge project, and you are prompted to choose Palm OS or Pocket PC as your target device (Figure 18.5).

If you select Palm OS, this is what your programming environment looks like. Note the new controls in the toolbar and a new menu (Figure 18.6).

Each of the new controls has a little "i" in the lower-right corner that stands for "ingot," which is what the AppForge calls their controls. You can't use the built-in VB controls, which remain in the toolbar but are not functional. In the screen above, I have quickly drawn a few controls. Pressing the right-hand arrow or selecting "Start" from the Run menu quickly compiles the program and runs it in a simulator windows, as shown in Figure 18.7.

AppForge/MobileVB is a comprehensive and easy-to-use tool for programming. Compared with NSBasic, its programs run at about the same speed, but it is more expensive, requires Visual Basic 6.0, and its run-time file is quite a bit larger (350 KB vs. 88 KB for NSBasic). On the other hand, I found that it was a more efficient programming tool, saving me time and allowing me to reuse code from Visual Basic projects. If your only interest is in Palm programming, check out the Palm-only version for $129.

Summary

Programming isn't just for teenagers, nerds, and bearded computer gurus. New tools like NSBasic and AppForge allow you to quickly and easily create programs for either Palms or Pocket PC's, and you can't beat the price of embedded Visual Basic and embedded Visual C for creating Pocket PC software. See Table 18.2 for a list of resources, then start cranking out the code!

19

Beyond the Beam: Server-Based Synchronization

Dale Patterson

Beyond the Beam

By now, you have become very comfortable using your handheld computer. You have ready access to all your information ranging from phone numbers to medical references, and now depend on the schedule program to get you to the right place at the right time. Maybe you even developed your own database program to keep track of procedures. It has truly become indispensable to your practice and your life.

If you are in a solo practice, the stand-alone handheld computer may be all you need. If you are in a group practice or a residency program, you have probably found yourself wishing others had access to the information you carry with you in your pocket. Beaming information back and forth with colleagues works well, but wouldn't it be nice to have an up-to-date, centralized database of phone numbers, pager numbers and addresses of all of your employees and partners that updates every time you synchronize? Or maybe you would like to be able to place meeting schedules on all your partners' handhelds so they are never late for a meeting again (OK, at least they will know they are late)? All these are possible with server-based synchronization.

Servers are also being used to track procedures in residency programs, place standardized references on the handheld computers of physicians, and synchronize billing information in large practices. Sure, some of these require additional software and even custom programming, but with a minimal investment in a server application, many of these functions are easily adapted to any group setting.

This chapter discusses the use of server synchronization and explains how to get started. We also cover some simple practical applications including address book synchronization, group scheduling, data or reference dispersion, and procedure tracking.

Server Basics: What Can It Do for Me?

A synchronization server is a software program that works like the synchronization program that came with your PDA. It may replace the built-in application or can be used in addition to it, depending on the intended use. Unlike the standard program, the server allows multiple handhelds to share information or link to the same data. It also allows the server administrator to choose what information is synchronized or pushed in either direction. When set up on a network system (see Chapter 15), it allows synchronization from multiple locations by numerous handhelds.

A real-life example of the capabilities of a synchronization server is its use at a residency program. Residents and faculty use their handhelds on a daily basis and synchronize with their own desktop computer to back up and update their personal information. However, they can also synchronize with the server, which is linked to the clinic's computer network. When they synchronize with the server, the call schedule is inserted and updated in the calendar application of their handheld computer. In addition, their handheld's address book has a "Work" category that is updated with the most recent pager numbers, phone numbers, and addresses of all clinic employees. An emergency recall roster is updated in their memo pad, and group-purchased medical applications are installed on the handheld. In addition to gaining all this information, the procedures recorded on a handheld database are extracted and automatically linked to a database on the network. Finally, all the old call schedules, former employees, and out-of-date programs are removed from the handheld. All this is accomplished without modifying or transferring personal information stored on an individual handheld. As you can see, a large amount of data can be transferred to and from the handheld, and with a little innovation, the uses of the server are unlimited.

Commercial Servers: What Is Out There Already?

Although Palm Inc. previously offered a server product, they stopped supporting this system in December 2001. Fortunately, several other products are commercially available that allow server synchronization. Because of the rapid progress in this technology, new products and updates are frequently available. The author of this chapter is most familiar with the software produced by Extended Systems, in Boise, Idaho (www.extendedsystems.com). The XTNDConnect Server supports both Palm OS and Pocket PC systems, in addition to several other less well known formats. Synchronization is compatible with Microsoft Exchange, Lotus Notes, ODBC (Open Database Connectivity)-compatible databases, and numerous other applications. In fact, the previous example of a residency programs application of server technology is currently being accomplished with XTNDConnect. Other server synchronization programs include Enterprise Intellisync (www.pumatech.com), Synchrologic Mobile Suite (www.synchrologic.com), and Mobile Net Connect Server (www.ibm.com).

XTNDConnect includes all the software needed to get started with server synchronization. In addition to the server software, a server administration program, client program, proxy program, and monitor program are included. While the server software allows the exchange of data and manages the synchronization, the administration program enables the server administrator to select the data that are shared or "exchanged." The client program is placed on each handheld to allow connection to the server and is available for Palm OS, Pocket PC, and other handhelds. The proxy program can be placed on desktop computers linked to a network to allow connection to the server from a desktop synchronization. This allows "remote synchronization": you don't have to go to the server to synchronize, the server comes to your desktop. The monitor program allows the administrator to see who has synced recently and to track any errors that occur when someone attempts to link to the server. Yes, errors do occur, especially early on in the process. But with the monitor program and a little trial and error, they can easily be fixed, and synchronization can become seamless and error-free.

The power of the XTNDConnect system lies in its simplicity; you don't have to be a computer programmer to set it up and run it. The "Setup Wizards" included in the software make installing the server a breeze. Anyone with experience in network administration or software programming is more than qualified to install and run the server. Someone with experience with Windows and a desire to run the server could probably have it up and running in a short time. The conduits that exist in the program itself save time and frustration by providing preprogrammed links to the standard applications already on the Palm OS or Pocket PC. To set up address book synchronization, for example, the administrator simply picks the data source (where to get information; e.g., Microsoft Access) and selects "Address Book" as the destination. XTNDConnect then gives you a list of fields (e.g., name, address, city, phone, e-mail address) that can be mapped between the handheld and the data source. When synchronized, the information in the data source will be synchronized to the designated fields in the handheld. Preprogrammed conduits also exist for program installation, backup features, memo pad synchronization, date book synchronization, e-mail synchronization, and a host of other applications.

The server synchronization software can replace the standard synchronization programs that come with each handheld or can be used in conjunction with them. Features are completely customizable and can be turned on and off easily by the server administrator. Filters and options

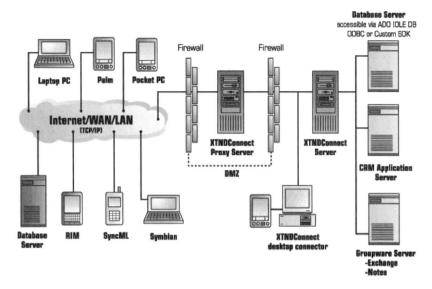

FIGURE 19.1. Schematic overview of XTNDconnect server. (Reprinted with permission from Extended Systems.)

enable the administrator to backup the entire handheld or specify which fields are uploaded. Data can be synchronized, pushed to the handheld only, or retrieved from the handheld only, similar to the synchronization with the standard desktop software. See Figure 19.1 for a schematic overview of the XTNDConnect server.

All the interfaces with XTNDConnect use the familiar Windows interface, and online documentation and support are readily available. The server is highly customizable and therefore requires that each handheld be given a username for synchronization. A profile is created for each user, including Lotus and Exchange server settings that allow personalized synchronization with these programs. Groups can also be established for multiple users who synchronize the same information including call schedules, address books, and programs. For example, you could create separate groups for first-year residents, second-year residents, and third-year residents, or for nurses and physicians in your practice. Server costs are based on the number of handhelds synchronized and are charged at startup and annually. A free trial is available at the Extended Systems Web site (www.extendedsystems.com).

In the next sections, we show you in more detail how to use server synchronization to share and synchronize addresses, schedules, and software with your colleagues.

Address Book: Keep Me in Touch!

As previously mentioned, the address book feature of your handheld is easily synchronized by a server program. This can be accomplished through the Exchange server linking to a company address book or by linking to a database source. In our example we will see how to link a Microsoft Access database to the standard address book feature of the handheld.

Although the development of databases is beyond the scope of this book, it is fairly likely that many readers are already familiar with databases and are probably using them on a daily basis. Microsoft Access is one commonly used database program. In our example, a database already existed for employees and was readily available in the Access format.

For simplicity, the headings in the database will be last name and pager number. Of course, in reality there are many more fields that need to be synchronized. For a server program to recognize a database, it must first be designated as an Open Database Connectivity (ODBC) data source. This is accomplished from the control panel of Windows. If you are unfamiliar with this process, detailed instructions are available through Windows help topics.

Once a data source is designated, the actual synchronization is programmed in the server administration program. For our example, we will focus on XTNDConnect and synchronize to our Microsoft Access database. The title of our database is "C:/Employees.mdb." It includes the fields "Name" and "Pager," which represent the last name and pager number of each employee. It also includes the "Category" field. This field is identical for all our entries, and we will call it "Work." It is important to keep this different than any existing category names on the handheld (Figure 19.2).

The first step to mapping this synchronization is to establish an "action set." An action set tells the server what to do. In this case we choose a "Data-

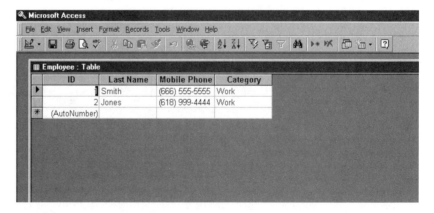

FIGURE 19.2. Screenshot of Microsoft Access employees database. (Reprinted with permission from Microsoft Corporation.)

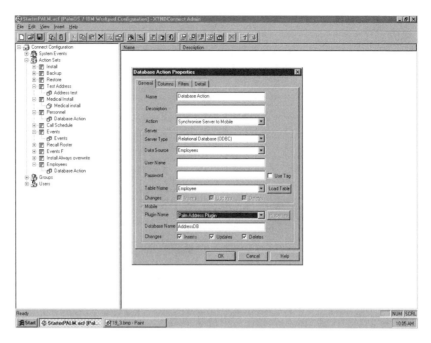

FIGURE 19.3. Screenshot of XTNDconnect demonstrating action sets. (Reprinted with permission from Extended Systems.)

base Action" (Figure 19.3). We then select the database from a list of available databases and choose an "address book" link. When we enter this information, the available fields are displayed for both the database and the handheld. By linking "Name" to "Last Name" and "Pager" to "Pager," the transfer of database information will be permitted. By linking the "category" fields to each other, all the information transferred to the handheld will be placed in a "work" category in the address book (Figure 19.4.).

Other options to consider include one-way or two-way synchronization. For our purposes, one-way sync allows the database to be updated by one individual and overwrites the new information to each user's handheld at each synchronization. Users should be cautioned to only view the information in the "Work" category and not to make changes, as they will be lost at synchronization. In some instances, it may be more appropriate to allow the handheld to update the data source. If this is the case, any changes on any handheld will change the data on the original database. With this simple customization of the server program and maintenance of an accurate database, each user will have up-to-date information for all contacts, including whatever information the administrator chooses to link for synchronization.

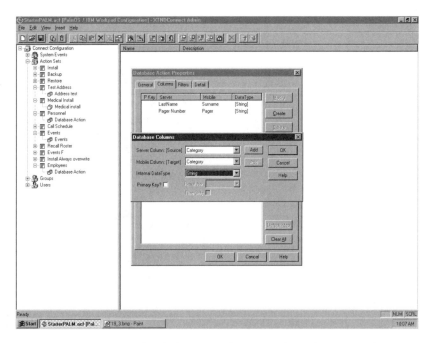

FIGURE 19.4. Screenshot of XTNDconnect demonstrating column mapping. (Reprinted with permission from Extended Systems.)

Schedules: Get Me Where I Need to Be

Scheduling can also be accomplished using a server application. The process is very similar to that employed for the address book application previously discussed. For this example, we will use a group call schedule with two physicians on call each day.

It is necessary to create another ODBC data source; this can be done with Access or even Excel if you already have a schedule in this program. The essential elements (fields) for a schedule are "date," "title," and "call." The date field is self-explanatory. The "title" field is what will show up in the one line on the handheld when the day is viewed, for example, "Call schedule." The "call" field is the information about who is on call that will be placed in the note portion of the schedule entry. Once the source is established the steps are as follows:

- Choose a database action
- Select a schedule or calendar action
- Choose one-way synchronization (unless you want others to change the call schedule)
- Link the fields (date to date, title to title, call to note)
- Keep the schedule updated at the data source

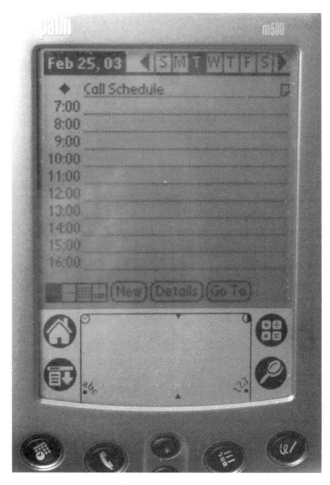

FIGURE 19.5. Image of Palm Handheld demonstrating call schedule insertion. (Reprinted with permission from palmOne, Inc.)

When these steps are followed, each user will have the most up-to-date call schedule in an untimed item in each day's schedule called "Call Schedule." When they tap the note, a list of the people "on call" that day is displayed (Figure 19.5).

Programs: Can I Have That Calculator Everyone Else Has?

A server can also install applications on individual handheld devices. The easiest way to do this is to establish a folder on a drive accessible to the server and place applications needing installation in that folder. Using

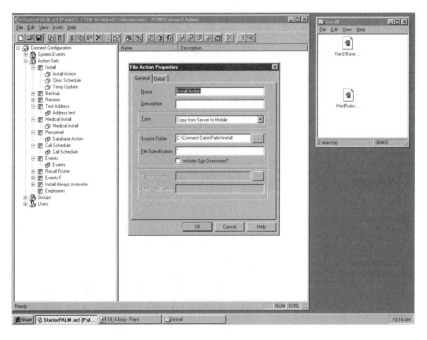

FIGURE 19.6. Screenshot of XTNDconnect demonstrating installation of programs. (Reprinted with permission from Extended Systems.)

the "Install" tool on the server, specify the folder location, and the next time the user synchronizes, the applications in the folder will be installed (Figure 19.6).

Although this may be the easiest use of the server, several areas of caution are advised. Copyright infringement is a serious concern when installing applications to multiple handhelds. The installation of "freeware" programs is acceptable, but the installation of proprietary material necessitates the procurement of appropriate licensure. Once a license for a particular program is purchased for the appropriate number of users, it can be installed via the server.

Another caution is programs using multiple files or requiring other programs to run. Programs like HanDBase that look for other files are usually not problematic, but programs such as Epocrates that require a desktop interface and installation tool are difficult to install from a server. Furthermore, these programs are usually large and consume much of the allotted memory of a handheld device. When installed from a server, they may overload an individual's handheld and produce uncertain results. It is best to limit server-installed applications and data to 25% to 50% of the available memory of a handheld and make this well known to the users. Finally, current server applications do not support installation to a memory card on

Palm OS devices. These cards greatly increase available memory, but they do not add to the memory accessible to the server.

In summary, it is simple to install programs and files via the server. However, to prevent synchronization problems and copyright infringement, limit installation to small programs that are "freeware" or have appropriate licensing.

Procedures Tracking: How Many Deliveries Have I Done?

If you are affiliated with a training program or perform procedures in your practice, you have probably encountered a need to track the number of procedures that are performed by a given physician. Residency graduation requirements, residency review committees, and hospital credentials committees may request these data. In the past, we have relied on 3×5 cards, logbooks, and other handwritten forms of documentation. Some have chosen not to document at all, and have had to do the tedious work of "reviewing" charts and operative logs to estimate a reasonable number of procedures performed. Your handheld can make procedural tracking almost effortless.

Using a program like HanDBase, write a simple database for the handheld. Procedures can be recorded with minimal entry of text by the use of pull-down menus and default entries. More information about database creation is available in an earlier chapter. With minimal programming, a customized procedure tracker can be devised that will fulfill the requirements of any credentialing or review committee. Advanced features can also be added that allow for tracking of biopsy results and recording of relevant statistical information.

For the physician in private practice, this type of procedural tracking will provide numerous benefits and may be all that is needed. For those in the residency setting or a large group practice, the desire to collect these data from multiple physicians on a continuing basis is probably a continuing need. By combining the server technology in this chapter with simple database programming, it is possible to collect data from numerous physicians and compile it in a traditional database format with the use of handheld computers.

There are several hardware requirements to establish this type of system. Each user must have a handheld device. The network synchronization hardware must be in place, including suitable desktop computers and cradles. Finally, a central computer capable of running an acceptable database program such as Microsoft Access must be available. One possible solution to the lack of a commercial server in a small group setting would be synchronization at one desktop computer to allow the compilation of procedural information. The benefits of both these types of system are seen in Table 19.1.

TABLE 19.1. The type of synchronization needed for common tasks.			
	One handheld, one desktop	Multiple handhelds, one desktop	Multiple handhelds, network server
Record procedures	Yes	Yes	Yes
Track statistics/biopsies of one physician	Yes	Yes	Yes
Merge data of several physicians	No	Yes	Yes
Select files to be extracted from handheld	N/A	No	Yes
Update date book and address book simultaneously	N/A	No	Yes
Sync from a cradle anywhere on the network	No	No	Yes

There are also significant software requirements. The software needed for the server has already been discussed. In addition, a handheld database program must be installed on each unit and a desktop-based database program must be available. In the example here, we will use HanDBase as the handheld database and Microsoft Access as the desktop-based database program. The server is XTNDConnect, as previously described.

A simplified description of the process involves three steps. First, the data are collected at the point of service by the individual physician on the handheld device using HanDBase. Next, the handheld is synchronized on the server and the database file is extracted to a designated folder. Finally, using Microsoft Access, the files collected on the server are integrated into the main database of all physicians using the system (Figure 19.7).

Using HanDBase to collect data at the time of service saves time and improves accuracy of reporting. Procedures are not "forgotten." Cards are not lost. Using pulldowns and defaults minimizes data entry. Once a procedure is synchronized, it is part of the permanent data set.

Synchronization can be done in three ways. For the individual user, to sync at the desktop is sufficient. HanDBase has a desktop application that allows you to review data on the desktop, and the data can be exported to more sophisticated database programs. For multiple users without a server, it is possible to have all of them synchronize to a single desktop computer and manually compile the data into Microsoft Access by "exporting" the files backed up into an Access database. The new version 3.0 of HanDBase also offers an optional multiuser synchronization module and conduits to Access that may streamline this process.

This type of system also eliminates other uses of the server, and also has the drawback of "backing up" all the files on an individual handheld to the desktop. The settings of the Palm synchronization software do not allow backup of specified files. The built-in applications and some add-on soft-

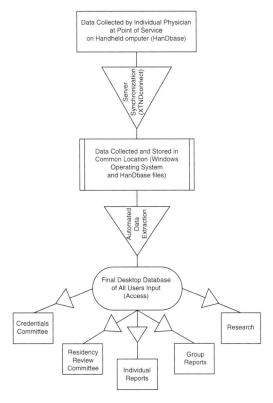

FIGURE 19.7. Schematic overview of procedure database and synchronization.

ware allow synchronization to be set to "do nothing," but there is no pro-
vision to extract some files and not others. This limitation, unfortunately,
means that personal information may be backed up to the one desktop
computer with which all users must synchronize.

The use of a server and a network is definitely the most versatile and customizable way to gather data from numerous users. Specific files can be designated for uploading to the server while personal files are not uploaded.
Users can synchronize from anywhere on the network, including the
desktop computer in their office or cradles placed strategically in the clinic.
In addition, they enjoy the numerous other benefits of the server, as discussed elsewhere in this chapter.

Compiling data is the final step of the group synchronization of procedural information. Database design can get complicated, and it is helpful
to have the assistance of a trained programmer when creating the initial
database. Furthermore, an experienced programmer can automate the
extraction of data and build in useful functions, such as the removal of

duplicate procedures. If a customized database is not practical or affordable, a ready-to-run procedures database is available free of charge at www.mdpr.org/CHHAMP/Downloads/Forms/AllItems.htm. Although not ideally customized to the users' location and needs, it can serve well when used "as is" or serve as an example to help develop custom applications.

While automated integration of procedural data is the "holy grail" of procedural tracking, with a little programming and minimal cost it is possible to track an individual's or small group's procedures.

Summary: Servers Can "Serve" Information to a Group

As you can see, a server is a powerful tool that can be used with a variety of handheld devices. The customized uses of the server are limited only by your imagination and resourcefulness. The server allows the users to choose what data are shared among the group and which are kept private on their individual handheld. It allows for shared phone books, schedules, and memos. It streamlines the integration of multiple databases and permits the pooling of large amounts of data. Once implemented, the exchange of data by the server is limited only by the available memory of the handhelds with which it synchronizes.

Although it may seem that this function is only applicable to advanced users, the use of a server can be beneficial to anyone who wishes to share information among multiple users. Because the cost of the server usually depends on the number of users, it is as readily available to small groups as it is to large. Although it may be helpful to have a dedicated administrator trained in networking, it is certainly possible to install and run a handheld server with little or no formal training.

20

Teaching People to Use Handheld Computers

PETER L. REYNOLDS, SCOTT M. STRAYER, AND MARK H. EBELL

Yes, handheld computers can simplify and improve healthcare delivery. No, not everyone agrees. On the individual level, some people naturally gravitate toward technologic solutions like handhelds. Others, however, just don't get the appeal. They're simply not interested. A third group of people, maybe the largest group overall, likes the idea of handheld computers but hesitates to invest time in anything new. If you've got a good thing going ("My inpatient-billing 3-by-5 index cards work just fine, thank you very much!"), why take chances with the unknown.

Our experience as teachers shows that these three group—early adopters, nonadopters, and slow adopters—must be recognized and approached differently. Implementation of handhelds within a large organization, such as a training program or hospital staff, succeeds best when each type of adopter receives training specific to their needs.

So, you may ask, what else is new? Target training to the needs of the learner—everyone knows that. Well, in practice, targeted training rarely happens. Take, for example, the first group, the early adopters. If you give an early adopter a current-generation handheld computer, in no time at all, they have mastered the basics and are telling everyone how wonderful life has become. No joke—something about these devices lights the techno fire within a nerd. Often, however, organizations drag their feet with new technology and make Huge Mistake #1.

Huge Mistake #1

Store all newly purchased handhelds under lock and key, and only release them to users once they've completed their mandatory 2-hour "Handhelds and Me" training.

Amazing, isn't it, that you'll trust a nurse to calculate dopamine drips or a resident to deliver a baby, but you won't trust them to take a $200 handheld computer out of the box by themselves. Instead of Huge Mistake #1, consider Wonderful Training Tip #1.

Wonderful Training Tip #1

> When deploying handheld computers in your organization, buy them and hand them out when they arrive.

Early adopters will love you and train themselves. With great books like this one available, they'll find and implement useful medical applications quickly. Most slow adopters, on the other hand, will play Tetris and that's about it (because they've got that good 3-by-5 card thing going). Some, believe it or not, will be won over by the early adopters and become fanatics themselves. Nonadopters, unfortunately, will probably take their handheld home in the unopened box and go out for sushi. You win some—you lose some. Regardless, you've already got a significant number of users training themselves without drafting a single lesson plan.

More importantly, you haven't wasted time training an uninterested, unreceptive audience. It takes time to move an organization to the point where they can embrace handheld computing as a group. Handheld applications like schedule dissemination and charge capture save time and money. They only work, however, if a majority of people come on board. Likewise, handheld applications are easy to sabotage. If you force nonadopters to use a handheld without gradually warming up to the idea, their resistance will likely grow, not diminish. That's Huge Mistake #2. Don't do it. Resistance tends to rear its head in the form of dead batteries, lost styluses, synchronization trouble, and all sorts of other handheld maladies, all of which hurt your cause.

Huge Mistake #2

> Deploy handhelds and, from day one, force all providers to submit billing charges using charge capture software only.

Instead, encourage experimentation and gradually introduce new applications as per Wonderful Training Tip #2. Ideally, you want an 80% to 90% adoption rate for a given application before you make its use mandatory. In the example of charge capture, if 9 of 10 providers use billing software, by our experience, 9 of 10 providers will be billing for more money with lower administrative overhead. At some point, the nonadopter holdout has no choice but to switch over or take a pay cut. Also, don't worry too much about folks playing games, showing family photos, and beaming jokes back and forth. Early on, Tetris and Solitaire are just as good for acclimating users to their handheld as more intimidating medical applications. Eventually, if handheld computers really are all we say they're cracked up to be, they will win over your slow adopters and nonadopters.

Wonderful Training Tip #2

> Let users play games on their handhelds. Encourage slow and nonadopters to use medical applications but wean them from their 3-by-5 cards slowly.

By the way, all these tips and examples are based on real people and circumstances. One physician all but left her Palm OS handheld in the box for 2 years. It took about a year more for her to master her appointment calendar, and now she's using ePocrates and loving it. It's a happy tale of a nonadopter turned enthusiast; admittedly, a particularly long tale, but a happy one. There is reason for hope—most people come around. Thus we come to Huge Mistake #3 and Wonderful Training Tip #3.

Huge Mistake #3

> Give up your handheld training program if you meet resistance.

Wonderful Training Tip #3 (paraphrased from Abraham Lincoln's original treatise on handheld computing)

> You can please all the slow adopters some of the time,
> And you can please some of the early adopters all of the time,
> But you can't please most of the nonadopters most of the time,
> Unless you wait a long time.

TABLE 20.1. Approaches to teaching handheld computing.

Type of handheld user	Teaching tips
Early adopter	Hands-on, self-directed training
	Formal training courses to introduce a wide range of medical applications early and speed progress
	Get them devices early; let them help direct further training for slow and nonadopters
Slow adopter	Encourage hands-on experimentation
	Encourage discussion with early adopters to pique interest and increase confidence (small group discussions)
	Offer incentives to use medical applications; measure rates of utilization and relative outcomes (charge capture, etc.)
Nonadopter	One-on-one training
	Require users to bring handheld devices to certain events (small group discussions, training courses, etc.)
	Be patient; recurrent one-on-one training

Formal training definitely has its place in the world of handheld computers. Just don't forget the importance of hands-on and peer-to-peer training, and consciously incorporate these aspects into your training plan. Busy health care providers, particularly physicians, respond best to training that they believe will directly improve their quality of care. For many, especially those wary of technology, this belief is best gained by peer-to-peer demonstration over time.

Table 20.1 summarizes teaching approaches for different types of handheld adopters. As for training content, we believe this book serves as an excellent outline. Begin with the basics. Go on to specific medical applications. And give people time before fully incorporating handheld-only solutions into your organization.

What follows are several tutorials on using alternative training tools, emulators and others, that allow you to project an image of a functioning handheld device onto a large screen. This ability becomes important for teaching larger groups for two reasons. First, as it turns out, the average handheld screen is too small to effectively train more than two or three people at a time. Second, when you demonstrate using a projected handheld image, students can easily follow along using their own handheld device simultaneously. You get to "see one" and "do one" at the same time—it's perfect!

Installing and Using the Palm OS Emulator for Presentations

Have you ever wanted to show your colleagues a great program for the Palm, but were limited by its small screen? Well, there is a way to project all your "killer apps" onto a screen so that everyone can share in your wealth of knowledge, but it takes a little bit of effort to install the program and run it. The effort will be well worth it, however, as your colleagues "ooh" and "aah" at all the incredible programs you show them for their handheld computers.

The program is called an emulator, and can be downloaded from the Palm Web site and installed on your computer. To project it, you also need to install a "ROM Image," a process that I will describe in laymen's terms (it took me several months to figure this one out using the tech manuals for the emulator). Then, you need to install your Palm programs onto the emulator, which is a little simpler. Finally, a good LCD projector will be needed to show these images to your eager colleagues. Please note that you cannot change the emulator from computer to computer without installing the ROM image on that computer as well (unless you save it as a self-executable file). The easiest way to avoid any trouble is to install the emulator and the ROM image on your laptop and use that computer for the presentation.

So Where Do You Get This Emulator?

HANDS-ON EXERCISE 20.1. DOWNLOADING THE EMULATOR

The emulator can be downloaded from the Palm website at http://www.palmos.com/dev/tools/emulator. Download the most current emulator and skins (graphical images of Palm handheld computers) from the section entitled "Download the Emulator."

What Do I Do with This Emulator Once It Is Downloaded?

HANDS-ON EXERCISE 20.2. INSTALLING THE EMULATOR

After you have downloaded the emulator, you can disconnect from the Internet and begin the installation process. The file needs to be "unzipped" using a decompression utility like Winzip (available at www.winzip.com; select the "download evaluation version" for a free trial). If you need more help with decompression and using Winzip, please see Chapter 3, where we have a great hands-on exercise that describes this process. Make sure you pay attention to where the file is decompressed. In my case, it sets up a default location called "c:\unzipped\emulator." When you open up Winzip and click "Unzip now," it will tell you which directory is the target for the decompressed file. You will also need to unzip the "skins" file and locate it in the same folder as the emulator. All the skins need to be placed in a folder called "skins," which you will have to rename using Windows (Figure 20.1a).

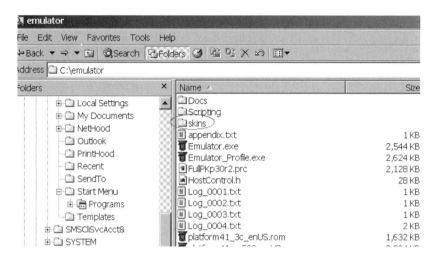

FIGURE 20.1a. Emulator folder with skins renamed. (Reprinted with permission from Microsoft Corporation.)

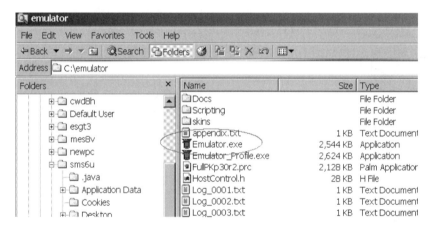

FIGURE 20.1b. Icon for Palm emulator. (Reprinted with permission from Microsoft Corporation.)

After you have unzipped the file, a window will open up with the files contained in the zip file. Alternatively, if you have to open it up later, just remember where it was unzipped. If you begin working on it right away, you will double-click on the file called "emulator.exe," which will have an icon of a Palm with a pilot's cap on it (Figure 20.1b). You will be asked if you want to add the emulator to the Start menu configuration, to which you can reply either "Yes" or "No."

Next, you will be brought to a box entitled "Palm OS Emulator." It will have the choices of "New," "Open," "Download," or "Exit" (Figure 20.2). To start a new session, just tap on "New." You can select which device you

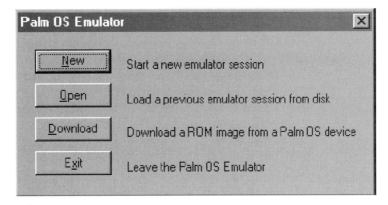

FIGURE 20.2. Starting an emulator session. (Reprinted with permission from palmOne, Inc.)

want from the "Device select" drop-down menu (choices include all the various Palm and Palm OS models). You can also select the "skin" or look of the Palm Pilot for your presentation (I would recommend the "generic" setting). Finally, you can select the RAM size. It is to your advantage to select the largest amount of RAM (i.e., 16384 K), as this will allow you to install more Palm programs later (Figure 20.3).

But wait, you aren't ready to run the emulator yet! The next step involves transferring the ROM image, and then you will be ready to project your emulator on any conference screen you choose.

HANDS-ON EXERCISE 20.3. INSTALLING THE ROM IMAGE

The first step of this process is to find the file "ROM transfer.prc" that came with your original emulator. It should be in the unzipped file that you stored earlier when you decompressed the entire "emulator.zip" file. When you

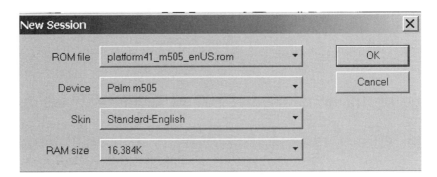

FIGURE 20.3. Selecting the attributes of the emulator. (Reprinted with permission from palmOne, Inc.)

open the unzipped file, you should find this Palm program that is installed in the usual manner (see Chapter 3 for details on Palm program installation). Just double-click on the program and it should automatically go into your Palm Install tool.

The computer you are using must have the Palm Desktop software installed and configured correctly and needs to synchronize via a cradle with your handheld. After you have installed the "ROM transfer" file to your Palm Pilot, open up the emulator and click the "Download" button (see Figure 20.2). You need to have the handheld hooked up and in the cradle. You will also need to disable the HotSync program by "right-clicking" on the icon of the blue and red arrows in the lower-right-hand corner of your computer's start bar, and hitting "Exit." A box will appear that asks you if you are sure you want to exit this program, and you should hit the "Yes" button. Now, hit "Download" and "Begin."

You will need to place your handheld in the cradle, turn it on, and open the "ROM transfer" program located under utilities. Press "Begin transfer" on the handheld, and then you will have to hit the "Begin" button on the computer to which you are transferring the ROM image. This process should take a few minutes, but a "progress bar" should come up immediately if you have followed the steps correctly so far.

You will be prompted to save the ROM files. Give them a meaningful name and remember where they are saved.

Now you can begin your first emulator session by tapping on the emulator and selecting "New" (see Figure 20.2). You can select the device, skin, and RAM size and when you will need to hit the "Browse" button and identify where you just saved the ROM files (see Figure 20.3).

HANDS-ON EXERCISE 20.4. AN ALTERNATIVE METHOD TO INSTALL THE ROM IMAGE

Another way to install the ROM image is to download it from the Palm site. You will need to register as a developer at http://www.palmos.com/dev/programs/pdp/join.html. This site can be accessed from the main Web site we told you about earlier. After registering, access the page for downloading ROM images to get your file. It will need to be decompressed, and after you have done this, you will just hit "Browse" to show where the ROM image is when you go to start your first emulator session.

HANDS-ON EXERCISE 20.5. INSTALLING PROGRAMS ONCE THE EMULATOR IS RUNNING

When you get the emulator to work, a large Palm clone will appear on your main computer that is about half the size of the screen (Figure 20.4). All the preinstalled programs on the Palm will be there. To show your colleagues a medical application, right-click on the screen, and select "Install Application/Database." Select "Other" from the menu that comes up to the

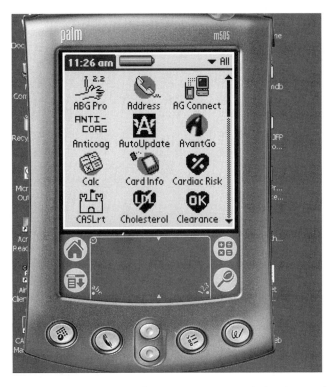

FIGURE 20.4. Emulator Palm clone. (Reprinted with permission from palmOne, Inc.)

right of that selection, and you will be taken to a file selection box. You can then grab any application on your hard drive (for example, in your Palm backup file located at C:\Palm\your user name\Backup) and install it on the emulator (Figures 20.5, 20.6).

Once you have saved all the programs you want on your emulator, you can right-click on the emulator screen and save the emulator under a certain name for that demonstration or particular lecture. Remember that you will only be able to install 16 MB of programs, so you may need multiple emulators if you have a lot of programs to show off.

Pocket PC Emulators

There is only one way to get a true Pocket PC emulator, and that is to install embedded Visual Basic, embedded Visual C, or the .Net Compact Framework on a Windows 2000 or Windows NT desktop computer. Unfortunately, older versions of Windows do not support the emulator. On the bright side, the eVB programming environment is free (www.microsoft.com/pocketpc),

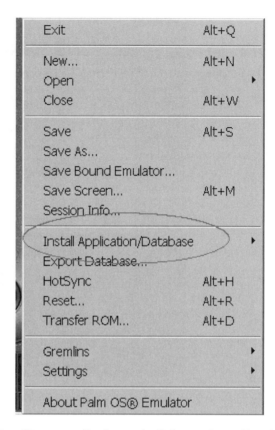

FIGURE 20.5. Installing an application to the Palm emulator. (Reprinted with permission from palmOne, Inc.)

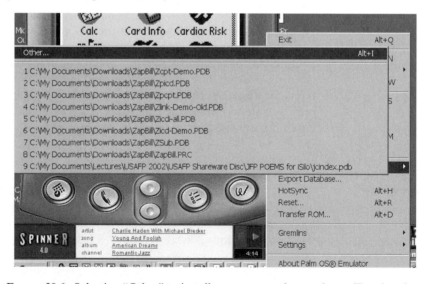

FIGURE 20.6. Selecting "Other" to install programs to the emulator. (Reprinted with permission from palmOne, Inc.)

but on the not-so-bright side it is a bit of a waste to install 40 MB of files just to get an emulator! Also, the emulator is very clumsy to work with, and is really only a tool for programmers to test their software, rather than a way to demonstrate Pocket PCs in a presentation.

So what should you do if you want to demonstrate how to use a Pocket PC to a roomful of eager learners (all your learners are eager, aren't they?) Not to worry—several free or inexpensive utilities are available that let you connect your Pocket PC to a laptop, connect the laptop to a projector, and then project the Pocket PC's screen through your laptop onto the screen. Then, anything you do on the Pocket PC is visible to your learners on the screen.

It's easy to set this up. Just go to http://www.microsoft.com/pocketpc, and click on the "Downloads" link. Then download the "Remote Display Adapter," one of the PowerToys that Microsoft has kindly made available at no charge. Make sure your device is in its cradle and synchronized, and then run the setup program (the icon is shown in Figure 20.7, the initial setup program screen is shown in Figure 20.8). The setup program will install a small program to your desktop or laptop computer and another to your Pocket PC.

When you are done installing, go to the Start menu under Windows and select "Remote Display Control" from the Programs menu.

Next, go to your Pocket PC, select Programs from the Start menu, and then select the cryptically named "cerdisp" from that folder (Figure 20.9). You will see the screen shown in Figure 20.10. Select "Connect" and you will see the screen shown in Figure 20.11.

Just agree—that tells it to use the "Peer to Peer Protocol" as a transport. There are other options, but I've never known anyone who had to use them.

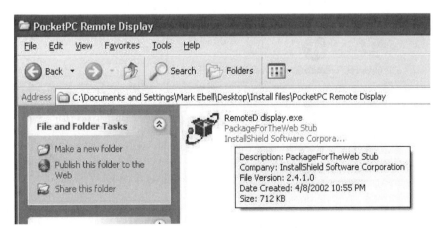

FIGURE 20.7. Icon for Remote Display. (Reprinted with permission from Microsoft Corporation.)

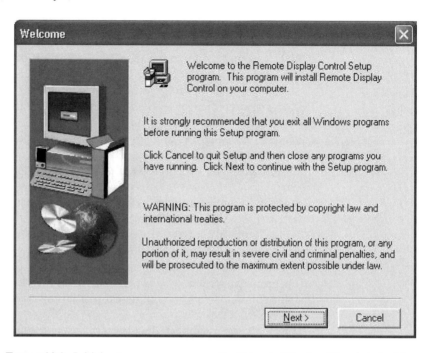

FIGURE 20.8. Initial setup program screen for Remote Display. (Reprinted with permission from Microsoft Corporation.)

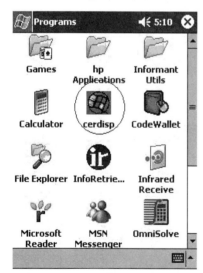

FIGURE 20.9. Locating the Remote Display program on your Pocket PC. (Reprinted with permission from Microsoft Corporation.)

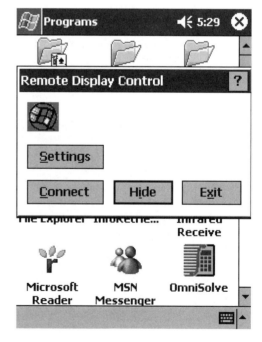

FIGURE 20.10. Opening Remote Display on your Pocket PC. (Reprinted with permission from Microsoft Corporation.)

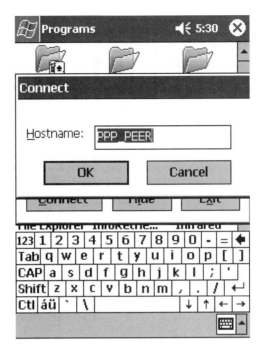

FIGURE 20.11. Connection type in Remote Diplay program. (Reprinted with permission from Microsoft Corporation.)

After you select "OK," wait a few seconds, and you should see the Pocket PC's screen appear on your desktop or laptop computer (Figure 20.12a).

One nice option is the ability to "Zoom" the screen. You can increase to two or even three times normal size. This is great when you have a laptop with a high-resolution screen and want the Pocket PC to take up most of it when you project it on a screen.

That's it. This free and easy-to-use software means that you can demonstrate anything on your Pocket PC for any size audience. The only downside is a slight "lag time" between when you enter your command on the Pocket PC and when you see the response on screen. You can also set the Remote Display program to send mouse moves from your laptop screen to the Pocket PC, but this just slows it down even further and isn't recommended. Another program that is commercially available (Pocket Controller, www.soti.net, $24.99) displays the actual device that you choose in addition to the Pocket PC screen (Figure 20.12b).

Now You're Ready

After all this hard work, the fun is about to begin. All you have to do is locate an LCD projector to plug into your laptop or computer, and run the emulator program to show your collection of Palm or Pocket PC applica-

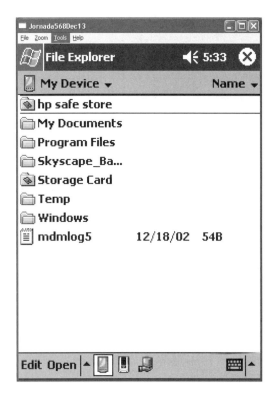

FIGURE 20.12a. Remote Display screen on your desktop or laptop computer. (Reprinted with permission from Microsoft Corporation.)

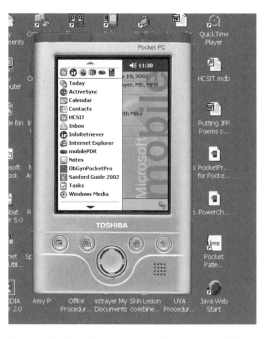

FIGURE 20.12b. Pocket controller with Toshiba e740 device. (Reprinted with permission from SOTI, Inc.)

tions. Be prepared for some astonished faces as you show fellow physicians how to conquer everyday tasks such as inpatient billing, looking up drug doses, checking your schedule, and oh yes, playing a game when you have a minute to take a breather!

Another Way to Present: An ELMO Unit

As you can probably gather, the emulator is a cheap way to demonstrate Palm programs, but maybe not the easiest. It works fine for many people, but if you have access to an ELMO unit, otherwise known as a video presenter (Figure 20.13), it provides a great alternative (ELMO was one of the first manufacturers of this type of technology, although others are now available). The ELMO unit has the advantage of presenting whatever you currently have installed on your Palm, Pocket PC, or whatever you are trying to show (including finger animals). The disadvantage is that it merely

FIGURE 20.13. Video presenter.

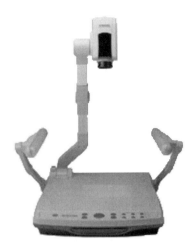

projects the images, but cannot be used to capture screenshots as we did in this book. All the screenshots shown were captured using either the Palm emulator or its Pocket PC brother that cones with eVB.

ELMO units come in various shapes and sizes, and also have varying price tags. Many academic centers and conference rooms already have them installed, or can get them set up through audio-visual support. Just check before your presentation. One disadvantage I have noticed when using one is that you usually have to sit down to use this type of technology.

Appendix

TABLE A.1. Palm® OS Devices.

Model	Cost	Batteries	Memory	Screen resolution	Color	Comments
Palm Zire	$	Rechargeable	+	+	No	Beginner model
Palm Zire 21	$	Rechargeable	++	+	No	Basic Model
Palm Zire 71	$$	Rechargeable	+++E	+++	Yes	Color, SD card, built-in camera
Palm Tungsten E	$$	Rechargeable	++++E	+++	Yes	Color, SD card
Palm Tungsten T2	$$$	Rechargeable	++++E	+++	Yes	Color, SD card, Bluetooth, compact design
Palm Tungsten T3	$$$	Rechargeable	+++++E	++++	Yes	Color, SD card, Bluetooth, stretch display, compact design
Palm Tungsten C	$$$	Rechargeable	+++++E	+++	Yes	Color, SD card, Wireless
Sony Clie PEG-SJ33	$$	Rechargeable	+++E	+++	Yes	Color, memory stick, basic model
Sony Clie PEG-TJ35	$$	Rechargeable	++++E	+++	Yes	Color, memory stick
Sony Clie PEG-TG50	$$	Rechargeable	+++E	+++	Yes	Color, memory stick, Bluetooth
Sony Clie PEG NX80V	$$$$	Rechargeable	++++E	++++	Yes	Built-in digital camera, memory stick and CF card, add-on 802.11b slot
Sony Clie PEG NZ90	$$$$	Rechargeable	+++E	++++	Yes	Built-in digital camera, memory stick and CF card, add-on 802.11b slot
Integrated PDA/Phones						
Palm Tungsten W	$$$	Rechargeable	+++	+++	Yes	GSM/GPRS standard
Kyocera 7135	$$$	Rechargeable	+++E	Resolution not available	Yes	SD/MMC slot, Integrated PDA and phone, dial from address book
Samsung SPH i330	$$$	Rechargeable	+++	160 × 240	Yes	Virtual key pad, CDMA standard

454

Model	Cost	Batteries	Memory	Screen resolution	Color	Comments
Handspring Treo 270/300	$ to $$$	Rechargeable	+++	Resolution not available	Yes	Compact, GSM/GPRS or CDMA standard depending on model, prices vary depending on mobile plan
Handspring Treo 600	$$$ to $$$$	Rechargeable	++++E	Resolution not available	Yes	Compact, SD/MMC slot, GSM/GPRS or CDMA, prices vary depending on mobile plan

Prices obtained from manufacturer's websites, March 2004.

Key

Cost	**Memory**	**Screen Resolution**
$ $0–$100	+ 2MB	+ 160 × 160 (lowest)
$$ $100–$300	++ 8MB	++ 240 × 320
$$$ $300–$500	+++ 16MB	+++ 320 × 320
$$$$ $500+	++++32MB	++++ >320 × 320 (highest)
	+++++64MB	

E-expandable

TABLE A.2. Microsoft™ Pocket PC Models.

Model	Cost	Batteries	Memory	Screen resolution	Color	Comments
Dell Axim X5 (300 Mhz)	$	Rechargeable	++	+	Yes	Internal SD/MMC and CF expansion slots, budget
Dell Axim X3 (400 Mhz)	$$	Rechargeable	+++	+	Yes	Internal SD/MMC slot, optional integrated wircless (X3i model)
HP iPAQ h1935	$	Rechargeable	+++	+	Yes	SD/MMC expansion
HP iPAQ 1945	$	Rechargeable	+++	+	Yes	SD/MMC expansion, integrated Bluetooth
HP iPAQ 2215	$$	Rechargeable	+++	+	Yes	SD/MMC and CF card slots, integrated Bluetooth
HP iPAQ h4155	$$	Rechargeable	+++	+	Yes	Built-in wireless, SD slot, Bluetooth
HP iPAQ 5555	$$$	Rechargeable	+++	+	Yes	SD expansion, Built-in wireless and Bluetooth, biometric security
Casio Cassiopeia E-125	$	Rechargeable	++	+	Yes	CF
Casio Cassiopeia E-200	$$	Rechargeable	+++	+	Yes	CF, SD
Toshiba e350	$$	Rechargeable	+++	+	Yes	SD
Toshiba e750	$$	Rechargeable	+++	+	Yes	Built-in wireless, CF, SD
Audiovox Maestro PDA-1032C	$	Rechargeable	++	+	Yes	CF, SD

Prices obtained from manufacturer's websites, March 2004.

Key

Cost	**Memory**	**Screen Resolution**
$ $200–$300	+ 16MB	+ 240 × 320 (lowest)
$$ $300–$500	++ 32MB	++ 320 × 320
$$$ >$500	+++ 64MB	+++ >320 × 320 (highest)

MMC = multimedia card; CF = compact flash card; SD = secure digital card.

Index